D0910157

RY

Eve's Herbs

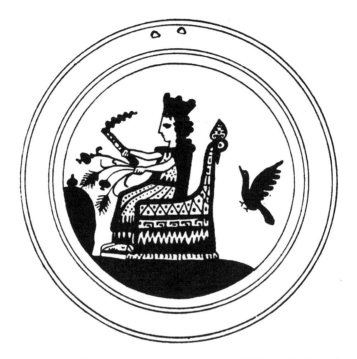

Demeter with pomegranates and grain (Athens National Museum 484). From Jane Harrison, *Prolegomena to the Study of Greek Religion* (Cambridge: Cambridge University Press, 1908), p. 274.

Eve's Herbs

A History of Contraception and
Abortion in the West

JOHN M. RIDDLE

HARVARD UNIVERSITY PRESS
Cambridge, Massachusetts
London, England
1997

CARL A. RUDISILL LIBRARY
LENOIR-RHYNE UNIVERSITY

RG
137.45
,R53
1997

Copyright © 1997 by the President and Fellows of Harvard College
All rights reserved
Printed in the United States of America

Library of Congress Cataloging-in-Publication Data
Riddle, John M.
    Eve's herbs : a history of contraception and abortion in the West
/ John M. Riddle.
      p. cm.
    Includes bibliographical references and index.
    ISBN 0-674-27024-X (alk. paper)
    1. Herbal contraceptives—History. 2. Herbal abortifacients
—History. 3. Birth control—Public opinion. 4. Abortion—Public
opinion. I. Title.
RG137.45.R53   1997
613.9'4—dc21   96-40383

Contents

Acknowledgments

The following colleagues read portions of or the full manuscript or reacted to specific problems by giving generously of their time and expertise: James Banker, Holly Brewer, Larry Champion, James Cooper, David Cowen, Alexander De Grand, Megan Fauls, Gerald Elkan, Monica Green, Paul Haagen, Gunnar Heinsohn, Kaye Hughes, Alison Klairmont-Lingo, Samuel Kottek, Samuel Levin, Cynthia Levin, Herbert N. Nigg, Everette Noland, John Orth, Ronald Sack, Kate Schmit, Otto Steiger, Samuel Tove, Maxim Weintraub, Steven Vincent, and the four anonymous readers of Harvard University Press. Also, I thank the librarians at the following institutions, who assisted me beyond the call of duty: the medical libraries at Duke University, University of North Carolina at Chapel Hill, North Carolina State University School of Veterinary Medicine, the Wellcome Medical Library, and the National Library of Medicine; the law libraries at the University of North Carolina at Chapel Hill, Duke University, and Supreme Court of North Carolina; and the main libraries at University of North Carolina at Chapel Hill, Duke University, and, above all, North Carolina State University, my home.

Eve's Herbs

Introduction: Roe v. Wade

"The right to privacy encompasses a woman's decision
whether or not to terminate her pregnancy [but] a
woman's right to terminate her pregnancy is not
absolute."

Roe v. Wade, 410 U.S. 113, p. 154

"Jane Roe" was a single woman by the name of Norma McCorvey.
She lived in Dallas County, Texas, and was pregnant early in 1970,
not for the first time. By chance, she met some lawyers and told them
of her desire for an abortion and lamented that Texas did not permit
her to receive a "legal" abortion. She could not afford to travel to those
states where, although abortion was restricted, a woman could receive
one without being exposed to the dangers of an illegal surgery performed clandestinely by an irregular practitioner. The lawyers, who
had been hoping to find a test case, suggested that she sue, claiming
her constitutional rights were abridged.[1] Long after her pregnancy was
over (sometime after May 1970), her lawyers were arguing through the
appellate process "on behalf of herself and all other women" in similar situations.[2] Her case was argued before the Supreme Court on December 13, 1971, and argued again on October 11, 1972. Henry Wade,
the district attorney, was destined to have his name linked to the case.

Jane Roe asserted that the constitutional rights that provided for her
privacy—those protected by the First, Fourth, Fifth, Ninth, and Fourteenth Amendments—were abridged. The State of Texas affirmed that
it had "compelling [reasons] to protect fetal life."[3] Parties to the suit
also were Mr. and Mrs. John and Mary Doe (also pseudonyms, the use
of which is a common law custom). They argued a similar constitutional deprivation because John and Mary Doe suffered mental anguish

1

over the possibility that failed contraceptive measures would lead to a pregnancy that could not be terminated. The Supreme Court threw John and Mary Doe's case out of court because they had no standing. Mary was not pregnant. That left Jane Roe in court. Her case altered the course of recent history in the United States.

Altering history's direction was, surprisingly, just the principal point of law that the majority on the Supreme Court considered an important issue. They thought modern legislatures had reversed women's rights as exercised historically until the nineteenth century. Justice Blackmun wrote for the majority: "We feel it desirable briefly to survey, in several aspects, the history of abortion, for such insight as that history may afford us . . . We have inquired into, and in this opinion place some emphasis upon, medical and medical-legal history and what that history reveals about man's attitudes toward the abortion procedure over the centuries."[4] In being guided by history, the Court was aware of philosophy but it would not necessarily be its guide: "the raw edges of human existence, one's religious training, one's attitudes toward life and family and their values, and the moral standards . . . [that] influence and . . . color one's thinking and conclusions about abortion."[5] In this case, the justices deliberately chose not philosophy but history as their guide in establishing law. Employing a standard textbook (Arturo Castiglioni's *History of Medicine*, 1947 ed.), the justices noted that the practice of abortion went back to ancient times ("at the time of the Persian Empire"[6]) and was available to women unless a father's right to offspring was being violated.

The Court was concerned about whether a physician had a moral duty not to perform abortions because of the Hippocratic Oath. The Court recognized Hippocrates as the "wisest and the greatest practitioner of his art" but was aware of differences in translation in respect to abortion. From Castiglioni's text, the Court read about a physician's prohibition to "give to a woman a pessary to produce abortion." It was aware of the alternative wording by Ludwig Edelstein, a distinguished medical historian at the Johns Hopkins University, whose translation read "give to a woman an abortive remedy."[7] Many medical schools employed translations according to Edelstein's interpretation.[8]

Indeed, other scholars made a similar translation.[9] The great French scholar of Hippocrates, Emile Littré, was aware of the word *pessary*, but he also considered the compassion for life expressed by Hippocrates in so many ways.[10] Littré recognized that the ancients believed there were circumstances in which an abortion was necessary.[11] The classical scholars of the late nineteenth and early twentieth centuries did not know that the ancients had effective birth control medicines. They believed that, given Hippocrates' reverence for life (as understood by their age), when specifying a pessary he was noting the means available for abortion in his own time. These scholars felt justified in translating the oath as prohibiting all abortions.

The Court's scholarship was better than that of some classical scholars on the matter of birth control. In 1943 Edelstein stated that some features of the oath were at variance with what we know to have been the attitudes of Hippocratic physicians and the prevailing culture. The ancients accepted not only abortion but suicide as well. Incontrovertibly, the author of the oath did not condone suicide. Because of its unusual ethics and its religious overtones, Professor Edelstein proposed that the oath's author was a member of a Pythagorean cult, as his views reflected those of only a small community among the ancients.[12] The Supreme Court found Edelstein's thesis "satisfactory and acceptable," thereby enabling them to dismiss the oath as an incorrect application of historical precedent.[13]

Common law on abortion directed the Court to recognize that women in England had for more than a thousand years been free to abort an unformed or "pre-quick" fetus (that is, before fetal movement). That was longer than there had been an England! Lengthy scholarly discussions developed in footnotes on how the common law principle arose. Whether abortion of a *quick fetus* was a felony at common law or even a lesser crime was disputed; but Edward Coke's opinion in the early seventeenth century that it was "a great misprision [misdemeanor], and no murder" was an important historical guide to many jurists in the early modern period. The Court noted "the paucity of common-law prosecutions."[14] Engaging in revisionist history (not necessarily to say incorrectly), the Court reviewed common law on abortion, notably through Coke, and cited an article by Cyril Means in the *New York Law Forum* (propitiously published in 1971, a year after Roe's pregnancy and just before the decision). Means believed that Coke may have been involved in a 1601 abortion case (cited in Chapter 5, below) and he "may have intentionally misstated the law."[15] In an astounding conclusion, the Court asserted that "it now appear doubtful that abortion was ever firmly established as a common-law crime even with respect to the destruction of a quick fetus."[16]

The Court reviewed British statutory laws restricting abortion, beginning with Lord Ellenborough's Act in 1803 and including the 1929 modification that emphasized "the life of a child capable of being born alive."[17] American law on abortion was reviewed from the received common law first restricted by Connecticut in 1821, by New York in 1828, and by Texas in 1840. The Court traced the breakdown in the distinction between the quick and the not-yet-quickened fetus sparked by medical advances and technologies that defined more certainly embryological development. It noted that by the 1950s most jurisdictions either banned abortions altogether or permitted them only to save the life of the mother. Two exceptions were Alabama and the District of Columbia, each of which permitted abortion to preserve the mother's health (not the more restrictive term, life). The Court concluded that even in the nineteenth century "a woman enjoyed a substantially broader right to terminate a pregnancy than she does in most States today."[18]

A principle in jurisprudence holds that the judges may be cognizant of that which is common knowledge. The Court knew what was happening. The birth control movement in the United States had been renewed in the 1960s after a relatively quiet period following World War II. The Court was aware that abortions were being administered in many states, in some with relative impunity, while others adhered strictly to the law.

The *New York Times* (31 January 1942) estimated between 100,000 and 250,000 criminal abortions within the city annually. By the 1960s the numbers increased, there and elsewhere. The Court took notice that fourteen states recently had liberalized abortion laws, and by the end of 1970 four more had joined them. In these states abortion was legal when performed in early pregnancy by a licensed physician, provided proper health and medical procedures were used.[19] In nonpermitting states, those women with resources could obtain an early-term abortion legally by traveling to permitting states, but the poor could not.

Neither the contraceptive nor the abortion drugs used earlier in the nineteenth century reappeared in the twentieth-century liberalization. After the Comstock Act was relaxed in 1930, Margaret Sanger and various women's groups opposed a move by the makers of patent medicines to supply oral contraceptive medicines.[20] These drugs were distrusted ("inferior," "unreliable," "definitely harmful") and, instead, contraceptive foams, jellies, and pessaries were preferred.[21] In the 1950s the researches of Gregory Pincus and John Rock resulted in the contraceptive pill, a combination of estrogen and progesterone hormones, which, when taken correctly, was a safe contraceptive.[22]

On the other hand, abortions were delivered by regular physicians operating on the edge of the law and by irregular physicians beyond the law. Abortion procedures were largely surgical, the quality varying from safe to dangerous. Most abortions were performed illegally prior to the 1960s, so stated a committee of U.S. historians in an *amicus curae* filed in 1988.[23] The committee concluded:

> Our experience from the 1890s until 1973 amply demonstrates that if women are denied access to legal abortions, many will turn in desperation to self-abortion, folk remedies, or illegal practitioners. Many will die. Others will suffer permanent damage to their reproductive capacity. Still others will bear children for whom they cannot provide adequate care.[24]

The majority and minority on the Supreme Court in *Roe v. Wade* were concerned by what was happening. The Court majority, in acting as it did, was guided by the past, the present, and its judgment about the future. The history of abortion must be matched with what was happening in the various states in the 1970s, "with the demands of the profound problems of the present day."[25] In a reference to "Mr. Justice [Oliver W.] Holmes," the Court signaled that it was guided by the felt necessities of the times.[26]

The various positions of the American Medical Association, the American Public Health Association, and the American Bar Association were read into the Court's opinion.[27] Even on the question about when life begins, the Court took a historical perspective. The ancient views of the Stoics and the Jews were reviewed, as were various Protestant and Catholic opinions.[28] Interestingly, the Court did not assume that the answer to the question would be determined by science or, by inference, that the most recent position would be the correct one.[29] The Catholic Church's current position was represented as being that ensoulment begins at "the moment of conception," based on the citation of Daniel Callahan's book published in 1970, two years before the decision.[30]

In 1964 Pope Paul VI reaffirmed the words of Pope Pius XII in 1951 that "innocent human life" ought to be protected from "the first moment of its existence."[31] The argument was made that the fetus was a person and, therefore, protected by the Fourteenth Amendment. The Supreme Court specifically rejected the claim. Justice Rehnquist raised the possibility in his dissenting opinion when he observed that, when the Fourteenth Amendment was enacted in 1868, thirty-six states had anti-abortion laws and that therefore the intent was not to withdraw a state's right to legislate this matter.[32] In the Fourteenth Amendment the justices in the majority found grounds to strike the Texas statute because that state was prohibited from abridging a citizen's privilege or immunity without due process of law. By being denied an abortion when her life was at risk, a woman was denied due process, said the seven-justice majority.[33]

Numerous criticisms followed, with many critics averring that the majority found a woman's right to privacy greater than a "person's" right to life.[34] Critics challenged the Court's interpretation of history. Arguments were developed that claimed that the ancients recognized life in the womb. For example, the Egyptian prayer to Aton (fourteenth century B.C.E.) spoke of "giving life to the son in the body of his mother."[35] (The Aton prayer, however, was misunderstood by the Court's critics because, relying on an English translation, they mistook the Egyptian to mean recognition of human life in a fetus.) Edelstein's article was misapplied, these same critics charged, because, despite the fact that the oath was originally taken only by a small sect, it came to be regarded as a functional, practical ethic for all physicians.[36]

Critics notwithstanding, the Supreme Court was persuaded in part by the historical argument that women traditionally had exercised a choice about pregnancy in the early term before a fetus was, in the Court's word, "viable."[37] What the justices did not know—because no one did at the time—was just how viable in earlier years women's knowledge concerning contraception and abortion was. Neither did they know how that knowledge was nearly lost. Eve's herbs, the secrets of women, were almost forgotten.

In 1992 I wrote *Contraception and Abortion from the Ancient World to the Renaissance*, in which I revealed the secrets of women that I had uncovered after years of research. My thesis was that ancient women took certain substances, mostly herbs, in order to control their reproduction. These herbs were named primarily in the medical records of the day, but in literary, religious, philosophical, and legal documents as well. I researched modern scientific and anthropological studies of the ancients to learn if they told us whether ancient people had effective agents for influencing reproduction. Little was found about male contraceptives, but there was considerable evidence in the records that women had both contraceptive and abortifacient pharmaceutical agents. Women thought that what they took worked successfully, and I found that modern scientific reports tend to confirm their practices as probably being effective.

The reaction to the book was gratifying because a thesis that would have appeared extravagantly speculative decades earlier was accepted by readers and critics. Only in recent decades did scientific studies reveal that plants have chemicals that induce reproductive hormonal reactions in mammals, including humans. What I did was to relate modern studies in science and anthropology to the historical data. When it ruled on *Roe v. Wade* the Supreme Court did not know about the scientific studies of the knowledge women had in the remote past. Experts in science, history, and medicine received favorably the thesis presented in the book, but a few historians and demographers were skeptical.[38]

Some demographers are unpersuaded that, even if effective birth control agents existed, evidence could be found that indicated family limitation.[39] Demographers have constructed mathematical models that indicate when societies go through transitions from no family planning to the use of methods to limit family size.[40] The data for the models are, however, based on the experience of the nineteenth and twentieth centuries, for which evidence is considerably more abundant than for previous periods. When investigators turn to the premodern era, their mathematical models, and their imaginations, twirl. Like demographers, historians also were skeptical for a reason. If once women had effective means of birth control, why were these methods unknown in modern times? Historians are not accustomed to attributing to ancient science accurate observations that are not confirmed by modern science. Generally we regard science as cumulative knowledge about the physical universe. In the first book I took note of the question about lost knowledge and postulated some possible explanations. The explanations were not complete and the problem of how the information was lost nagged. I determined to focus on the modern period until I found some better answers to the concerns of both the demographers and the historians. This book is the product of that inquiry.

Besides wanting to understand how the information was lost, I wanted to have a better idea of just *what* was lost. I went to China in 1994 to learn how women use natural birth control drugs. A number of modern scientific studies about the actions of herbs have been published in Chinese and Indian journals, many of which are cited in this book. In those countries scientific and medical experts, especially medicinal chemists, employ laboratory and clinical studies to examine traditional antifertility medicines. Many of the herbs employed in modern Chinese and Indian medicine are the same as those once used by ancient and medieval peoples. In Shenyang at Liaoning University, the College of Pharmacy, and in two local hospitals, I found physicians and pharmacists, men and women, who helped me to understand the practical matters that would be of concern to a person taking drugs made from natural products. The subject is sensitive, and I am very grateful to a number of people, none of whom I shall name, who helped me.

At first I wanted to write the history of abortion and contraception from both Western and Eastern perspectives. In the end I decided to limit the discussion to the Western world (including some Islamic culture) and merely to express my gratitude to the Chinese for their assistance. Documentary evidence from a woman's perspective is difficult to find in the classical and medieval periods, and leaving a written record was perilously fraught with danger during the early modern period, when witches were burned. The closer the story comes to the twentieth century, the more I have concentrated on events in the United States and England.

The clues I found to the disappearance of women's knowledge surprised me, even though I felt well grounded in the subject after writing the first book. From the medieval Inquisition I traced back the knowledge given in testimony by two alleged heretics before the church tribunal in the early fourteenth century. In Chapters 2 and 3 I discuss some of the herbs that were available to ancient and medieval people and review the attitudes, practices, and laws about reproductive control. Although this subject was partially covered in the first book, these chapters strive to place the drugs more in the context of ancient culture and to bring new information to light. Here I mention only the most important herbs, not all the herbs described in the first book.

Chapter 4 begins with the early modern period, when the craft of women was tragically misunderstood as witchcraft. The succeeding chapters unfold chronologically from early modern times to the twentieth century. In these chapters I tell how ancient craft information about herbs still lingered in modern times. That is one of the surprises I discovered. The herbal lore moved from the fourteenth through the seventeenth centuries of persecution to the nineteenth and twentieth centuries of prosecution. Another surprise was that although there were many victims, I found few villains. Changing attitudes toward human life both influenced and were influenced by the complexities of human society. At times I found both fault and folly, but those times are few. This book is my attempt to tell the story of Eve's herbs with as little judgment as possible.

Word Usage

A fews words about terminology are necessary. Demographers use the word *fertility* to connote the number of children a woman has and *fecundity* to designate the ability to have children. Popular usage of these words reverses the meanings. The Romance languages add to the problem. For example, fertility is *fécondité* in French and fecund becomes *fertilé*.[41] To the confusion is added medical references to "fertility" and "antifertility drugs" to signify what the demographers say is promoting and diminishing "fecundity." Also, in medicine *fecundity* coincides with the usage demographers give to it.[42] Because this book is written for a lay reader and employs medical and demographic studies, I use the term *fertility* to embrace both meanings: the ability to bear children *and* the number of those born.

1

A Woman's Secret

"What shall I do if I am pregnant by you?"
Woman to a would-be suitor, around 1301

She stood before the Inquisition on that twenty-second day of August, 1320. Although accused of heresy, Béatrice was neither defiant nor humble. She lived life with emotion, devotion, and flair. Mother of four loving and loved daughters, wife to first one and then another member of the lesser gentry, Béatrice lived life, in the words of the a poet of the thirteenth century, as one of the "fair and courteous ladies, who have friends—two or three—besides their wedded lord."[1] She stood before the Inquisition because she was accused of being an Albigensian heretic. This form of heresy is traced back to tenth-century Bulgaria where a group calling themselves the Cathari ("the Pure") stressed their convictions about a dualistic competition between the god of light and the god or devil of evil. We do not know whether Béatrice was a true "purist" or heretic, or even whether she was found innocent or guilty. The last part of the record is lost, but the first part of the unique Inquisition survives to tell us intimate secrets about Béatrice's life, her lovers, and her use of birth control drugs.

The bishop from the nearby town of Pamiers was in Béatrice's village of Montaillou in the Pyrenees mountains near the ridge that sloped downward and southward into Spain. Presiding over the Inquisition that examined Béatrice on suspicion of heresy, Bishop Jacques Fournier was particularly interested in a love affair Béatrice had had with a rogue priest, Pierre Clergue, that had begun about nineteen years earlier. Béatrice had come to the mountain village as a widow after the untimely death of her first husband, Bérenger de Roquefort. Pierre, a priest in the village, had heard that his bastard cousin, Raymond Clergue, known as Pathau, had raped Béatrice while she was married. Undoubtedly he was told that she did not appear resentful, not that it would matter too much, because Pierre considered women as opportunities for conquest. Among those whom he seduced were Alazais Fauré and her sister, Raymonde, Grazide Lizier, and Mengarde Buscailh, just a few of those known to us, and those known probably were in a minority. Many women gave in to his seductive, priestly—albeit heretical—charms. In the eyes of the Church, Pierre Clergue was an Albigensian heretic.

Should a priest seduce women? Yes and no, according to Pierre's convictions. Sexual activity outside marriage was, he conceded, a sin. But since all other good things in life were as well, it was equal to other activities, therefore acceptable. His distinctly nontheological words were: "One woman's just like another. The sin is the same, whether she is married or not. Which is as much as to say that there is no sin about it at all."[2] A male's answer, to be sure.

Bishop Jacques Fournier was interested in the details of how Béatrice was lured into Pierre's web and entangled in heresy and sin. Those things were defined by the Church, not by the inhabitants of the mountain village. What knowledge of birth control Béatrice brought into this first of her many love affairs is not known, either because she concealed the information or because the Inquisitors failed to probe the depths of her experiences. We possess, however, the testimony of both Béatrice and Pierre before the judicial panel over which Fournier presided. The record of their testimony gives us the rare opportunity to hear from ordinary people (if we may assume Béatrice and Pierre were ordinary).

Without formality or hesitation, Pierre proposed lovemaking when he first met Béatrice as a new widow who came to his church. "What shall I do if I am pregnant by you?" she reacted with neither outrage nor indignity. He responded that he had "a certain herb (*quamdam herbam*)" that would prevent a woman from conceiving. "What is this herb?" Béatrice queried in apparent or feigned ignorance. She had heard of such herbs; she guessed it was the same one that cowherders put over a pot to keep milk with rennet from curdling. Do not worry about what herb it is, Pierre returned. The important thing was that it worked and he had it in his possession.[3] For his own reasons, he did not wish to tell her the herb's name.

Béatrice gave the Inquisition some details about how the herb was used to prevent pregnancy. This information is preserved in a rare, chance survival of ecclesiastical proceedings in the village of Montaillou. The details are very important, because we learn from the people's own words what the common folk did. From numerous medical and legal documents we know that people long ago employed contraceptives and early-term abortifacients in order to have control over reproduction. Historians and demographers have assumed that these drugs (for that is what they were) did not work. Before modern times birth control drugs could, at best, be regarded as magical delusions along with exorcism, the evil eye, and other examples of acceptable magic and condemned witchcraft. Much information about these antifertility agents was lost, making the record that Béatrice gave all the more important.

The information she gave to Bishop Fournier and his minions— including a number of scribes who logged the sessions—is unprecedented in recorded history. Among the surprises is that birth control was practiced among common folk, or the nearly common folk. Béatrice was lesser nobility, but she lived her life among the peasants of this and nearby villages. Béatrice's later lovers, among them a young man when she was much older, were members of the peasant class.

In our age prominent historians (among them Norman Himes, Emmanuel Le Roy Ladurie, Angus McLaren, John Knodel, Etienne van de Walle, A. J. Coale) contend that what practical knowledge there was of effective birth control measures in Béatrice's time was confined to the beds of the elite, the smart, and the educated.[4] Historians have long believed that the upper classes were the first to discover withdrawal before male climax in vaginal intercourse. People in other classes were not sufficiently intelligent to understand it all, so historians believed. Peasants and workers, bakers and candlestick makers, all reproduced like rats in hay until the advent of the modern era, assumed to have begun around 1780. It is widely agreed that the modern era of birth control began about the time of the French Revolution, scarcely more than two hundred years ago.

What was it that Béatrice told the clerical court? Not much, unfortunately for us. But what she did say cautiously is revealing and consequential. Her words are the first direct evidence from *hoi polloi* that the masses employed birth control devices. It is not that we do not have many sources in medical writings recording prescriptions for both contraceptives and abortifacients. It is not that we do not have demographic evidence that indicates that the people in the many generations before Béatrice were doing something to limit reproduction. Despite the records of birth control drugs and the evidence that people practiced family limitation in meaningful ways, historians have been reluctant to accept the testimony of the historical records.

The appearance of birth control recipes in ancient and medieval Western medical tracts, as well as in Vedic and Chinese works, indicates only that they were known. The texts tell us little about the actual usage of such drugs. The fact that few recipes provide much detail suggests that most of them were orally transmitted. On the other hand, modern scientific and anthropological studies confirm that many of the herbs that appear in the written documents and that were used for birth control were effective.[5] If that is so, we must admit that people have long employed chemical means to check fertility. But how many people? Enough to account for modern estimates of earlier population sizes? Enough to explain why, for long periods, some regions (such as Campania and North Africa) had apparent population decline together with economic prosperity, while populations in other regions declined where economic conditions were less vigorous? Why, in other regions, did not economic prosperity and population increase correspond?

Historical demographic studies indicate that premodern peoples may have regulated family size purposely. Population figures for the long period of the Middle Ages are difficult to ascertain. Even so, we know, as did people during the Roman Empire and early Middle Ages, that for long periods the size of families was static or shrinking. Around 200 A.C.E. the population of the Roman Empire (including its Asian and African portions) was around 46 million, 28 million in Europe, and non-Roman Europe had a population of approximately 8 million.[6] Another estimate: in the first five centuries A.C.E., the population of Europe is estimated to have declined from 32.8 million to 27.5 million. During this time, it was the population within the bounds of the Roman Empire that declined most, while that of the rest of Europe increased slightly. According to Josiah Russell, a medievalist whose population studies are celebrated, by the year 1000 the population of the same region was 38.5 million, or less than 6 million more than what it had been a millennium before.[7]

Russell's projections are compared with those of other scholars in Figure 1. The fundamental point is the basic agreement among scholars about the pattern of population change: decline until the seventh century, a slow recovery followed by a greater advance after or during the tenth century, and, finally, a downturn in the thirteenth with a recovery beginning around 1440.[8]

Interestingly, much the same pattern of population growth, stagnation, and decrease is estimated to have been played out on a global scale (see Table 1). Historians and demographers have long sought either to explain how premodern peoples engaged in population control or to deny purposeful control at all. Demographers distinguish between birth control and family limitation, the latter being the desire of married couples to have a sufficent number of children. Wars, famine, climate, pestilence, and exposure of children always explained some results, but those calculations were not sufficient to explain the few children born, especially in times of seeming health and prosperity. One example of such a time, when food seldom was a problem and there was relative peace and prosperity, was during the early Roman Empire. In Chapter 6 there is more discussion of demographic data for the modern period; let us look at some specific ancient and medieval data.

In discussing the policy to regulate the size of the ideal city-state, Plato said that there were "many devices available; if too many children are being born, there are measures to check propagation."[9] Through Plato, Socrates identified those devices when he said that "midwives, by means of drugs and incantations, . . . cause abortions at an early state if they think them desirable."[10] In the second century B.C.E., Polybius complained about the economic viability of Greek cities because, he said, families were limiting their size to one or two children.[11] Lawgivers, Aristotle said, should encourage people to reproduce more abundantly if the city is too small or to employ birth control measures if it is too large.[12] A Roman writer, Musonius Rufus (ca. 30–101 A.C.E.), was much more specific when he wrote that lawmakers who wanted to increase population size forbade "women to abort . . . and to use contraceptives."[13] Thus, the combined testimonies of Plato, Aristotle, Polybius, and Musonius indicate that people were employing early-term abortifacients and, just as Pierre presented to Béatrice, contraceptives.

Europe, Including European Russia:
Population Estimates, A.D. 0–1650

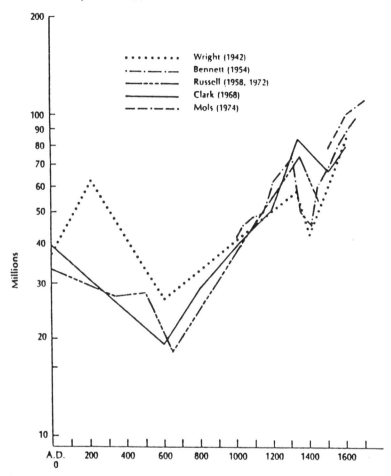

Figure 1. Estimations of Europe's population (including European Russia), 0 A.C.E.–1650. Citations are to the following references:

Wright, Quincy. 1942. *A Study of War,* 2 vols. Chicago: University of Chicago Press.

Bennett, M. K. 1954. *The World's Food.* New York: Harper and Bros.

Russell, Josiah C. 1958. *Late Ancient and Medieval Population.* Philadelphia: American Philosophical Society.

———— 1972. "Population in Europe, 500–1500." In *the Fontana Economic History of Europe,* ed. Carolo M. Cipolla, 1: 25–70. Glasgow: Collins.

Clark, Colin. 1968. *Population Growth and Land Use.* New York: St. Martin's.

Mols, Roger. 1974. "Population in Europe, 1500–1700." In *The Fontana Economic History of Europe,* ed. Carolo M. Cipolla, 2: 15–82. Glasgow: Collins.

Source: Graph prepared by John D. Durant, "Historical Estimates of World Population: An Evaluation," *Population and Development Review,* 3 [1977]: 253–296 at 270.)

Table 1. World population estimates

Year	Population (in millions)	Year	Population (in millions)
400 B.C.E.	153	1200	400
0 A.C.E.	252	1250	417
200	257	1300	431
400	206	1340	442
500	207	1400	375
600	208	1500	461
700	206	1600	578
900	222	1700	680
1000	253	1800	954
1100	299		

When David Herlihy studied family size in Florence and Verona in the late Middle Ages, he discovered very low birth rates in these cities even though the women there typically married at sixteen to eighteen years of age. The question is, how many years of pregnancy opportunity would an average woman have for the years of her married life? Life-span statistics are difficult to ascertain, but the average age of women in Florence in 1427 was 27.3 years, and their median age was 22.[14] By comparison, Veronese women in 1425 averaged 31.9 years of age with a median of 29. In fact, 24.5 percent of the women at Verona that year were fifty years old or more.[15] By contrast, aggregated data from medieval English graves show that only about 10 percent of the English population were sixty years or older.[16]

Because some women in the 15–44 age group would die before the age of 44, while some widows of comparable age would not remarry, it is reasonable to estimate twenty years of potential childbearing in a woman's life. Assuming a period of fifteen months for contraceptive protection from lactation, medieval women would be expected to have an average of from 4.2 to 5 children,[17] depending on the criteria used for mortality during the child-bearing years.

The most prominent scholar on the subject of early demographics, Josiah C. Russell, has postulated that a fertility rate of about 3.5 children per married woman was necessary to maintain a population—and the figure takes into account a high mortality rate during childhood.[18] Russell's figure is much lower than those of R. S. Bagnall and B. W. Frier, who studied Egyptian census data in the first three centuries of our era. Believing that Egypt's population remained relatively stable during the census periods, Bagnall and Frier calculated that the fertility rate for replacement (stable size) was about 5.7 children (or 2.9 daughters), and they assumed a much higher infant mortality rate than Russell's.[19] An estimated 85 percent of births in Egypt were to married couples; therefore, the data indicate that family limitation specifically, not aggregate fertility, was an important factor in the population levels of the Roman Empire (assuming Egypt reflects Empire-wide behavior).[20]

Other ancient records, albeit scant, support a hypothesis for smaller family size long before the Roman Egyptian censuses were taken. Various documents from the first millennium B.C.E. known collectively as the Assyrian Census List show that most people were monogamous, and the statistics give the average of 1.43 children per family. This is so low that the population would decline rapidly. The supposition is that children who were sixteen or so years of age who had left the house were not recorded. With allowances, the estimated size of the ancient Assyrian family was between two and three children, a figure much below Bagnall's and Frier's rate for children born in Roman Egyptian families.[21] Frier rejects my hypothesis of effective family limitation by ancient populations, but his and Bagnall's data are based on a much higher fertility rate than that used by most other investigators.[22]

A rate of 3.5 children per family was not achieved during some periods of the Middle Ages, according to Russell.[23] Russell's work was done before demographers developed family reconstitution techniques, but these analyses are based on data not available in early periods. Early medieval households in central Italy averaged 2.44 children per household, and there were 2.36 children per woman in the German areas during the eighth and ninth centuries.[24] In a later period, the number of children per married couple in Verona was only 0.97 in 1425, doubling to 1.85 in 1502. Moreover, the poorer households in Verona had even fewer children: 0.74 to 0.96 children per couple during the same period.[25] Lower birth rates for the poorer households suggest possible precautions taken by those who could not afford many children. Sim-

ilarly, urban dwellers had fewer children than did their rural counterparts.[26] Historians who believe that the poor could not quite understand the relation between sexual intercourse and childbirth are hard
pressed to explain what the poor in the country and town were doing
to have so few children. One example cited about the knowledge of
sexuality is a hapless young novice from the fourteenth century who
sought the advice of an older monk. When a man and woman make
love, he inquired, which one becomes pregnant? Why the one on the
bottom, the old monk replied. "Woe is me!" lamented the young man.
It seems that the young novice was on bottom, his instructor on top
of him. The novice thought that he would have the baby. "If the abbot notices, how will I live?" he cried.[27]

Despite the amusing, albeit true, story, I doubt there was truly much
befuddlement about the results of intercourse. Even this wretchedly
naive novice knew that intercourse could result in pregnancy. Rural
populations must have employed some means of birth control and, in
order to do that, they had to know that pregnancy was a possible outcome of penis-vaginal intercourse. Between 1248 and 1427, the average household in rural Pistoia, not far from Florence, had only 1.52
children. The documented decline in the Pistoiese population during
the same two centuries is probably related to the shortfall in the replacement rate. A local chronicler observed that Florentine women had
been barren "for a long time," and Dante complained that Florence
was "empty of the family." Much earlier, Greek and Assyrians thought
that the low fertility was the product of deliberate decisions, while others specifically accused the masses of engaging in anal intercourse to
avoid pregnancy.[28]

Many historians and demographers have postulated that infanticide
explains low populations and family sizes in both the classical antiquity and medieval periods.[29] Partly because other explanations did not
appear to be reasonable, they argued that infanticide must have been
widely practiced because it was not illegal in ancient societies. In sharp
contrast to antiquity, however, the Middle Ages censured infanticide.
Despite medieval condemnation of the practice by custom, law, and
religion, some historians have argued that infanticide continued even
then, since the sex ratio of the adult population favored males.[30] The
figures that lead some to see a differential in sex ratios are disputed by
others.[31] On the other hand, surviving records provide some evidence
that infanticide was too rare during the Middle Ages to account for

the gross demographical changes that occurred.[32] As we shall see later, infanticide did become a widespread problem in the sixteenth century.

The demography of antiquity also indicates that people employed birth control and limited family size.[33] J. Lawrence Angel, an American pathologist who has studied skeletons in ancient cemeteries, reported data on life expectancy past early infancy (see Table 2). Although the number of skeletons in each sample varied and very young children were not among them, these data indicate that life expectancy increased during the pre-Christian centuries. Other data suggest that the population of pharaonic Egypt underwent a parallel increase in life span. Life expectancy then began to decline in both Egypt and the European Roman Empire into the Middle Ages. Scholars are uncertain about the accuracy of early population estimates because the data never are as reliable as those from a modern census and almost never include neonatal mortality.[34] Census data from various regions in Egypt during the early Roman Empire indicate that female life expectancy at age 10 was from 34.5 to 37.5 years. The same study postulates that, with infant and early childhood mortality taken into account, female life expectancy would range from the lower to the mid-20s.[35] So much of the argument about ancient family limitation rests on assumptions about infant mortality rates, which are based on modern data applied

Table 2. Longevity of women buried in ancient cemeteries

Date	Site	Average age at death
11,000 B.C.E.	North Africa	31 years
5,800 B.C.E.	Nea Kikomedeia	29.9 years
2,400 B.C.E.	Karatas	29.7 years
1,750 B.C.E.	Lerna	30.8 years
650–350 B.C.E.	Athens and Corinth	36.8 years
100–200 A.C.E.	Roman Empire	34.6 years
100 A.C.E.	Britain	45 years

Sources: John Lawrence Angel, "The Bases of Paleodemography," *American Journal of Physical Anthropology* n.s. 30 (1969): 427–438, at 430–431, and "Ecology and Population in the Eastern Mediterranean," *World Archaeology*
4 (1972): 88–105; Mirko D. Grmek, *Disease in the Ancient Greek World* (Baltimore, 1989), pp. 99–107; Don Brothwell, "Paleodemography and Earlier British Population," *World Archaeology* 4 (1972): 75–87.

to ancient populations. Ancient or classical infant mortality data do not exist. When data are limited, the method should not be rejected, but should they be regarded as conclusive?

Female skeletons provide three possible clues to the number of full-term pregnancies: (1) dorsal pitting of the pubic plate; (2) scarring of the preauricular area of the os coxae; and (3) scarring of the groove for the interosseous ligament of the symphysis pubis.[36] Each time parturition occurs, one or more of these features is produced. Thus, for example, the dorsal pits on a female pubis indicate the number of infants she has delivered. The data compiled by J. Lawrence Angel and Sarah Bisel from various Mediterranean sites (see Table 3) imply that fertility rates had fallen below what was necessary to maintain the population just as the Roman Empire reached its zenith.

The use of skeletal lesions to determine precisely the number of pregnancies is not without controversy. First, as always with premodern populations, neonatal infants are not accorded regular burials and, therefore, important information is omitted from the calculations for estimating life spans. Furthermore, although the number of lesions in modern skeletons has been found to be correlated with the known number of pregnancies experienced, the correlations are not perfect, and the number of lesions can be obscured in old age.[37] At this time

Table 3.   Average births per female

Date	Number of births per adult female
2,000 B.C.E.	5.0
1,500 B.C.E.	4.7
1,150 B.C.E.	4.1
300 B.C.E.	3.6
120 A.C.E.	3.3
79 A.C.E. [Herculaneum]	1.81 [All the women in this sample died simultaneously.]

Sources: Data from Herculaneum reported in Ann Hanson, "Graeco-Roman Gynecology," *Society for Ancient Medicine Newsletter* 17 (1989): 83–92, at 89. Other data from John Lawrence Angel, "Ecology and Population in the Eastern Mediterranean," *World Archaeology* 4 (1972): 88–105, and Mirko D. Grmek, *Disease in the Ancient Greek World* (Baltimore, 1989), p. 97.

in our understanding of the skeletal evidence, we cannot be certain how precise these figures are. Senator Joseph McCarthy once prefaced an assertion with the phrase, "These facts, if true . . ." So must I as well. Whether or not the skeletal data are precisely accurate, the evidence corroborates what we know from other indicators: toward the end of the Roman Empire, women had fewer children than they would have had if there had not been some means to control birth.

Another way of looking at the data is to observe that the life span of adults was increasing at the same time as the number of births was declining. This conclusion is inferred from both the archeological evidence of the physical sizes of cities and from the anecdotal evidence left behind by observers such as Plato and Polybius for the period from the fifth century B.C.E. to the early Roman Empire. Similarly and even more emphatically, the demographic profile of the Middle Ages persuades us that people engaged in some kind of birth or population control, as we shall see in the next two chapters. Peasant families must have had some judgment about how many children they could support with available resources and food supply.

How did they do it? How did they limit family size?[38] Any form of contraception prior to the eighteenth century was, according to Philippe Ariès, *impensabilité* ("unthinkable").[39] When a low family size was desirable, people engaged in perverse practices that could not result in pregnancy, he suggested. To be sure, the obvious postulate is that people simply restrained themselves if they did not wish to have children. Those who have studied the classical literature of the ancient Greeks and Romans know that sexual restraint was not a quality about which the ancients could boast or lament. The official culture of the medieval period, at least in the West as represented by churchmen and fiefholders, stressed sexual constraints even within the marriage bond. The results in both eras were much the same: low birth rates that would not have come about if people satisfied their sexual appetites without using any means of birth control, even if intercourse was confined to married couples. Each period, in other words, had some population controls.

There were several devices, other than medicinal herbs, that people may have used to limit population, such as delayed marriages, prolonged lactation, using the rhythm method, interruption (coitus interruptus), condoms and other barriers, abortions, and infanticide.[40] No one would suggest, however, that any one of the above methods was not employed from time to time. The question is not which possibility may have been an occasional practice but which practices, if any, were employed on a scale large enough to have a significant consequence on gross population size.

We saw that Béatrice's first thought about her lover's claim to have an herb that would prevent conception was to inquire whether it was the herb that cowherds put over a pot to keep milk with rennet from curdling. In revealing this much, she informs us that she had heard of birth control prior to her affair with Pierre. Cowherds in ancient times did put an herb in milk for coagulation. The herb was the fig. A Greek herbalist, Dioscorides (fl. 50–70 A.C.E.), said that fig juice could be a substitute for rennet, this being the process in the manufacture of cheese as it is sometimes done in modern India. Fig juice can dissolve that which has already been coagulated.[41] Modern chemistry confirms that fig juice contains ficin, an enzyme that prevents the coagulation of milk by digesting caseinogen.[42] Béatrice was recorded as saying that the herb was placed over the pot, not in it. Either she may not have known or, equally possible, the scribe missed the detail.

Could she have heard that figs were also used for birth control? This is quite likely. Dioscorides said that figs stimulate menstruation.[43] Again, we need to turn to modern sources for the scientific reports. A survey of drugs taken by the inhabitants of the Hawaiian and other Pacific islands for birth control reveals that figs *(Ficus benjamina; F. pumila)* were eaten for this purpose. In modern tests of fig extracts, it was found that in mice fed the leaf and fruit twice daily there was a 61 percent reduction in the number of litters.[44] It is quite possible that Béatrice had heard from folklore about figs as a birth control agent; however, she did not give the details to the court. Apparently she never tried them, because her lover had a better idea, one that likely was more effective.

Béatrice revealed to the court these details:

When he wished to ravish me, he carried with him the herb wrapped in a linen cloth. It was about an inch wide and long, or about the size of the first joint of my little finger with a long string that he put around my neck and it descended between my breasts. He always placed it like this when he wanted to make love to me and it remained around my neck until he got up. When he wanted to leave, he removed it from around my neck. And if sometimes during the night, this priest wanted to know me carnally two or more times, he asked me, before uniting, where was this herb; I would grab it, finding it by the string that I had around my neck. He would place it in his hand and place it in the opening of my abdomen, the string passing between my breasts. In this way he could unite with me and in no other way.[45]

The historian Emmanuel Le Roy Ladurie speculated that Béatrice could be referring merely to an amulet. Le Roy Ladurie depended on a French translation of Béatrice's testimony, which says "au bout du fil, descendait . . . jusqu'à l'orifice de mon estomac [*sic*]."[46] The original manuscript in Latin which I consulted is less ambiguous because it clearly says "in the opening of my abdomen *(in orificio stomachi ipsius)*."[47] The priest who wrote the account of Béatrice's testimony delicately pointed to the vagina. Béatrice spoke in the vernacular language, known as Occitan, but she was recorded in Latin. We cannot be certain whether Béatrice employed a nice term like "opening in my abdomen" or a common, perhaps nasty name for her genitalia. For that matter, she may have named the herb she used and the scribe omitted the detail.

Le Roy Ladurie could have been correct in believing that Pierre had given her an amulet. During the Middle Ages amulets were thought to protect against childbirth. On that part, Le Roy Ladurie is correct. A bishop of the city of Rennes, Marbode, wrote in the late eleventh century a very popular treatise, called "On stones," in which the orite stone, a black stone, was described:

> Hic facit appensus ne fiat femina praegnans,
> Aut vel in praegnans fuerit, cito fundet abortum.[48]
>
> [Wearing this stone a woman will not become pregnant,
> Or if she is already pregnant, she procures an abortion.]

An amulet, even an herb, is not what Béatrice was describing, however. She said that the herb was placed "in the opening of my abdomen." This would be a pessary, that is, a vaginal insertion.

We are not told in the Latin account what the herb was. Already she had heard about figs, we surmise. Could it be that Béatrice did not know the plant that Pierre provided? "I asked him one day to let me have this herb. He told me that he could not do it because I would be able to give myself to another man without becoming pregnant," she explained. Pierre would not give her the herb "so that I would abstain [from sexual intercourse] for fear of the consequences." In particular, he was "thinking of his cousin, Raymond Clergue, called Pathau, with whom I had maintained company."

It must be kept in mind in reading this remarkable account that Béatrice spoke in the vernacular, but a scribal clerk to the Inquisition took down her words in Latin. The scribe, who was, importantly, a male priest, had to translate her testimony and then record it. He did this without the modern electronic recorders of our time that make the task so much easier and more exact. The scribe may have missed information. The court did not query her about the techniques, just the deeds. The scribal clerk was apparently intrigued with the string descending between her breasts *(inter mamillas);* he repeated the phrase three times in this short account. What visions might have occupied his mind as he dipped his pen in the inkwell?

A woman accused of heresy before the Inquisition should have felt threatened and rightfully fearful. Béatrice was intelligent, literate, and wily, although not well educated. As such she may have avoided the vulgar terms used by villagers for genitalia and resorted to circumlocutions, such as "opening of the abdomen." It is reasonable to conclude, however, that what she was describing is a pessary. That would explain the string, used to retrieve it after each use. Also it clarifies the detail that when a second union was imminent, Pierre first inquired where the herb was and then he would "put it into his hand." Either left unstated by Béatrice or unrecorded by Bishop Fournier's notaries was the detail about what he did next.

If we surmise that she wore a pessary around her neck, what was the herb that is lost in the record? Seemingly the best place to find Béatrice's secret is in the popular literature of her time, specifically a book that was known as *The Secrets of Women (De secretis mulierum).* It was written in the late thirteenth or early fourteenth century, around the time Béatrice was alive. There are eighty-three surviving manuscripts from the Middle Ages, and there were over fifty printed editions in the fifteenth century and over seventy in the sixteenth century.[49] The work was ascribed to Albertus Magnus, the well-known philosopher and theologian from Cologne, although we now know that an unknown author borrowed some material from Albertus's works along with information from other sources to compile this guide to "women's secrets."

The Secrets of Women does indeed reveal information about women but the secrets seem to have come from men. For example, it explains why women menstruate. The menses are nothing more than super-fluous food. By nature women are cold and moist, not like men, who are warm and dry. Unable to assimilate food in the same way by hav-ing a "natural flow" as men do, women's bodies expel the food in the form of menses. When women become pregnant, menstruation ceases so that the excess nutriments normally conveyed in menstrual blood can go to the fetus. During intercourse a woman receives great plea-sure by the rubbing of the penis in the vagina. The pleasure causes an expulsion of the menses, the book explains, apparently confusing the menses with the fluid produced at sexual climax. A man's semen (from Greek for "seed") has the "nature of milk" when deposited in the womb. If the woman's and man's semens (or seeds) are compatible, the womb cooks the man's semen for nine days, during which time the semen changes from milk-like to blood-like qualities. The next twelve days see the beginning of the fetus's formation.[50] We should note that this account indicates no certain time for an event called conception. Nei-ther the high nor the low science of the Middle Ages had our defini-tion of conception as the acceptance of the sperm by the ovum.

The Secrets of Women describes coitus and conception as understood by the age. This work is where we could expect to find information about contraception, but it is not found there, despite the fact that items which promote conception are included. Just the same, a me-dieval commentator on *The Secrets of Women* lets us in on a couple of secrets about contraception. This unknown commentator explained that women who desire frequent sexual intercourse have weak fetuses. Those women who are prudent and abstain from coitus (except upon a rare occasion) have stronger children. Their seed has more "vigor." Some women, the commentator says, have "exceeding sweetness for the male, but I am saying nothing more about these matters at pres-ent."[51] Before he gets off the subject entirely—clearly he was in-trigued—he has some practical advice for those women who do not wish to conceive. "If a woman drinks sage that has been cooked for three days she will not conceive for a year because sage is cold."[52]

Sage is a common plant, and what is referred to here could have been a number of species of *Salvia*, perhaps *S. officinalis* L. Being in widespread use as a culinary herb, sage has been consumed for thou-sands of years by diverse cultural and ethnic groups. Could sage possibly be an antifertility agent, as the commentator said? On the face of it, it seems unlikely. There are no claims about sage as a contraceptive in medical and other sources earlier than Pierre, Béatrice, and the anonymous commentator. And we are inclined to doubt the claim when we read the second and final contraceptive that the commentator prescribes: "Let a woman eat a bee and she will never conceive."[53] This injunction appears to the modern mind to be a superstition and, if the bee were alive when swallowed, just a bit foolish. In light of this and many other of his comments (for example, a woman who drinks a man's urine "impedes conception"),[54] should we not place his "secret" about sage along with "the snips and snails and puppy dog tails" of fairy tales?

We need to probe deeper into the Gothic mysteries of the Middle Ages before we dismiss the idea that sage might have contraceptive properties. In Haiti and Jamaica sage is taken to stimulate menstruation. The technical term for such an agent is *emmenagogue*. Traditional medicine authorities of India consider sage an abortifacient drug.[55] That is to say, sage can cause an abortion or miscarriage. The difference between an abortion and miscarriage in usage here is intention, not results.

Defining Pregnancy and Abortion

As women know all too well, there can be many reasons for a delayed or irregular menstruation, a condition called amenorrhea. Among them are febrile and chronic diseases, malnutrition, overwork, stress, mental depression, and, all too important, mistaken perceptions and memory. Of course, another possible reason for the delay is pregnancy. There is no reliable way for a woman who misses a normal onset by a few days or so to know what the cause may have been. If she takes a drug to stimulate menstruation, she could not possibly know whether she had assisted a natural process or terminated a very early pregnancy. "Early pregnancy" here is defined by modern conventions, by which pregnancy begins at conception or implantation.

Indeed, during the Middle Ages, a woman would not have stated the situation as I just have. As we shall see in the next chapter, pregnancy was not thought to have occurred until the woman so declared it or her pregnancy was so visibly evident that it could not be denied. Neither a medieval woman nor a man would have held the first month or so as a pregnancy. By and large this is true for medieval persons, lay or clerical, noble or peasant. In normal circumstances she who took an emmenagogue was likely guileless. In the Middle Ages and before, there was no suspicion of abortion because there was no suspicion of pregnancy. The cessation of menstruation was not thought to be particularly important, because some women menstruate in early pregnancy.[56]

As we learned from the medieval treatise, there was no single event that instantly produced a declaration of pregnancy. These were the Middle Ages, unfairly known also as the "Dark Ages." Those moderns among us who suspect that medieval people did not connect sexual intercourse with pregnancy are wrong, though. From all indications—and they are numerous—the medieval mind knew the connection all too well. The consequences were very great, greater than today: there was a higher risk of death from complications, and no welfare support was provided except what came from the family. Because a pregnancy out of wedlock violated religious doctrine, support could not always be expected.

The ethics espoused in the Middle Ages permitted sexual intercourse only within a marriage bond and, even then, only for the purposes of procreation. This purpose led to the adoption of the "missionary position" as being the only acceptable position for coitus; it is because the man's seed would be deposited more deeply in the womb and allowed to stay longer if the woman remained on her back. This explanation clarifies why the old monk thought the novice would be in the top position when the novice asked who becomes pregnant after intercourse.

Pregnancy was a process initiated over an indefinite period of days. As we shall see in the next chapter, this concept is embedded in the scriptures. *The Secrets of Women* revealed that there was an interval between the deposit of a man's semen and the uncertain point at which a woman's body turned her seed along with the man's into an embryo. Latin terms for what we call an embryo were *conceptus, embryo,* and *fetus.* In modern speech, we distinquish between an embryo (the fertilized egg in the first three months) and a fetus (the child *in utero* after three months of development). Neither the Middle Ages nor the classical antiquity of the Romans and Greeks made such distinctions. Thus, there was an indefinite but fairly certain time, a window of opportunity as it were, during which a woman could end what we call a pregnancy, and neither she nor her contemporaries regarded the act as an abortion. Taking a drug for delayed menstruation was just that and nothing more.

In stories of folk and even medical usage of a drug that stimulates or produces menstruation, it may not be clear that the same action might be an abortion, depending on the circumstances. People in Haiti are reported to use sage as an emmenagogue, whereas in Jamaica one species of sage (*S. serotina* L.) is taken in pregnancy to abort a fetus.[57] It may be that the recorder or observer of the herb's use did not know what the action was, or perhaps even the women who took sage to encourage menstruation did not know.

A Doctor, a Pope, and a Theologian on Birth Control

In Beátrice's village of Montaillou there were no university graduates. Likely, then, no one was there who had heard the lectures given by Albertus Magnus (1206–1280), who taught at Paris and Cologne. This is the same person who was thought to have authored *The Secrets of Women*. The ideas expressed by Albertus in his lectures on the development of the embryo and the question about when a person has a soul were part of the popular culture.

Uneducated though they were, the inhabitants of Montaillou knew about the soul. At least some of them thought about when the soul enters the body. After the death of her husband, Béatrice had an affair with her steward, Raymond Roussel. At the time she was pregnant. Raymond was of peasant stock but with heretical as well as romantic tendencies. He suggested that he and she run off together to Lombardy, where there was more freedom and they could live together. "I am still young. If I go away with you, Raymond, tongues will start to wag. People will say that we have left the country to satisfy our lust," Béatrice said to him. Not so, replied Raymond. Not to be robbed of her lover, Béatrice agreed to go with him provided there were two chaperons. Raymond readily supplied them.

Raymond enjoyed explaining life to his young lover. He disclosed to her that the souls *(animi)* of men and women leave a person's body at death and go to a new body. The soul of her future child would enter her womb and unite with the fetus so that the child would have a soul before birth. Béatrice was not to be outdone in logic: "If this should be, why don't babies speak when they come from the opening of the abdomen *(os eius ventre)*, since they inherit old souls?" Good question she had asked but Raymond had a reply, "It is because God wills it so."[58] So that explains that.

In his lectures, Albertus Magnus explained much better Raymond's views on when the soul united with the fetus. Raymond represents the opinion of popular culture, but Albertus, after all, had read Aristotle. What is more, Albertus had read Christian and Islamic philosophers on this subject. Albertus joined both the physical aspects of embryo development with a metaphysical definition of the soul's origins.

Neither Albertus nor those whom he read nor practically any one in the Middle Ages thought that the soul originated immediately after intercourse. The event was too ill-defined in the experience of those lacking microscopes and an understanding of cells and mitosis and DNA combinations. Albertus believed that conception took place some time after coitus and then there is an embryo. First, it becomes alive and then for months it develops. He noted that in a fresh abortion or miscarriage the embryo (or fetus) will exhibit a movement of dilation and contraction *(dilitationis et constrictionis)* when it is pricked with a needle: "and, on account of this for certain, the creature *(creatura)* is known to be animated *(esse aninata)*."[59] The embryo had animal character or virtue at this point, but it is not human, because it had not yet received its soul.

Aristotle addressed a question, the answer to which Albertus accepted. Do any parts of the soul develop before the whole body? No, this cannot be because parts cannot preexist the body.[60] "Some of our colleagues," Albertus said, believe that each plant and animal has a soul that is transferred, split off *(ex traducde)*, from its parents. These misguided colleagues argued from the observation of nature that a "spirit" of the parents is embedded in the offspring. Thus, they argued, the "spirit" *(spiritus)* must have been present from the beginning. They may have looked at nature, but God, through nature, supplies the soul, and it does not come from the body's parents, Albertus believed.

Albertus believed, as did Aristotle, that the embryo/fetus developed like other animals until a time came when it connected with the Divine Intellect or, in another way of saying it, God. This connection is the soul as it enters the body. Thus the soul derives from God, not from the child's parents. Aristotle said, "What is alive is not at the same moment sentient, and what is sentient is not at the same moment man *(non est vivum et sentiens simul, et non est sentiens et homo simul)."*[61] The wisdom of these words *(intellectus verborum)* is confirmed, Albertus said, by Avicenna, Averroës, Theophrastus, and "all the peripatetics or philosophers." What Albertus understood this to mean is that the embryo develops life first and only afterward is it endowed with rationality. "Man is a rational animal," Seneca asserted. Albertus agreed when he wrote:

> The rational [i.e., the human] soul is one substance, which is put in place by the vegetative, sensible, and intellectual powers, some of these being affixed to the body, while some are not. Those that are not cannot come from the body; no virtues are there that derive from a material body but rather they [i.e., the virtues] have a certain similarity to the lucid intellectual agent in nature and in the spermatic principle . . . Therefore entirely from outside the matter of the seed *(sperma)*, the rational and intellectual soul is brought into the fetus *(conceptus)* by the light of the intellectual agent.[62]

Thomas Aquinas, Albertus's student, did not always accept what his teacher told him, but on the matter of the soul he did. Even stronger were his words. It is heretical, Thomas said, to argue that the soul comes from the seed *(anima sensitiva traducatur ex semine)*, which is to say from the parents. Like his teacher, Thomas believed that the soul is created by God and not by humans *(sed sit per creationem a Deo)*.[63]

Giles of Rome (1243–1316) restated the Aristotelian-Albertian-Thomistic position in even stronger terms: the early stage of the human embryo is not human but a kind of animal. The logical nail was driven in by Robert Kilwardby, Archbishop of Canterbury (1272–1279), who said that were the embryo to perish before the soul entered the body there would be no soul to have perished because a soul cannot exist without a body. Otherwise, the soul would be denied the opportunity of resurrection since it would never have had a body from which to resurrect.[64]

Medieval theologians provided the interval between intercourse or conception and formation of a human fetus as a period when a woman could terminate what we, but not medieval people, call pregnancy. It was in this period that women took drugs to abort. No one can read Albertus and believe that he thought either contraception or abortion to be sinless. In his works on theology, Albertus agreed with the Church's position that humans should not intervene to prevent conception or a birth. There are, however, varying degrees of sin.

Albertus rejected the assertion made by Regino, abbot of a monastery in Lorraine about 830, when he equated contraception with homicide: "If someone [*Si aliquis*] to satisfy his lust or to make deliberate hatred does something to a man or woman so that no children be born of him or her, or gives them to drink, so that he cannot generate or she conceive, let it be held as homicide."[65]

Early in the eleventh century Burchard cited Regino in his work, *Decretum*, which very much influenced the Church's position on birth control. Without directly citing Regino's position, Albertus plainly said no to Regino's and Burchard's assertion because he thought it was too strong for humans to live by. First, there is no guarantee that neither conception nor a birth will occur, Albertus reasoned. Second, it surely is not the same thing to kill an infant or an adult as it is to prevent birth. Finally, those who cited Genesis 38—where the "sin of Onan" was interpreted as God's wrath for "spilling the seed on the ground"— misunderstood an important distinction. The conduct of God was not necessarily a precedent for human action.

The surprise comes when Albertus relates information about specific contraceptives and abortifacients. Anise (*Pimpinella anisum* L.) "stimulates menstruation" and, more explicitly, birthwort (*Aristolochia clementitis* L. and other species) "stimulates menstruation and expels a fetus."[66] In modern science reports, anise has been found to have abortifacient qualities because it has a substance that blocks progesterone production.[67] Birthwort has even stronger antifertility qualities. It can act both as a contraceptive and as an abortifacient and is known to have done so on humans.[68] Albertus names numerous antifertility agents, seemingly contradicting his theological position. Relevant to what Béatrice may have used under her lover's control, Albertus said that colocynth (*Citrullus coloquinthus* Schrad.) in a "pessary kills the fetus in women."[69] Presumably he added "in women" so that he was clearly not discussing animal populations. In general he believed that procreation was divinely ordained, but that there were circumstances when prevention or termination of pregnancy was an acceptable choice.

Trotula and Marbode

Women physicians were not numerous during the Middle Ages, but there were a few. Perhaps the most famous was Trotula, the doctoress of Salerno. Salerno, in southern Italy, was known for its physicians.

The details of Trotula's life are obscure; she lived in the late twelfth or early thirteenth century, and she supposedly wrote a treatise on gynecology that was famed.[70] Various versions circulated on the medieval equivalent of interlibrary loan. This would be where one would expect to find mention of the birth control drugs that Béatrice did not disclose to the Inquisition. The scholastic theologians and Béatrice's peasant lover all agreed that the early-stage fetus had no soul. Would it not follow, then, that human intervention prior to ensoulment was acceptable? One would believe that medical writers would have no hesitation in revealing the types of herbs that Beátrice used to prevent pregnancy or to produce a timely termination.

Like many medical writers during the Middle Ages, Trotula does not disclose the secrets, at least not openly. She provides no details about birth control devices, either of the contraceptive or abortive variety. Just the same, without saying so she lets her readers and patients know how to produce an abortion. She tells us about emmenagogues or menstrual stimulators. A woman with a delayed menstruation should drink artemisia in wine and take baths. If this combination does not work, there is a stronger combination: take artemisia together with other herbs. Among the other herbs was sage.[71]

Sage was not the central herb in her pharmacy. Artemisia was. *Artemisia* is a genus of plants that are known by common names like mugwort, southernwood, and absinthium. It grows in fields, beside roads, indeed, in many places. Most people regarded it as a weed, but many women did not. The plant was named for the goddess of love, and for good reason. Animal studies over the past twenty years have reported that artemisia delays the onset of estrus and ovulation and interfers with implantation. There is modern scientific support for its doing just what Trotula and her predecessors believed it would: it was both a contraceptive and an abortifacient.

The leading writer on medicinal herbs in the Middle Ages was Marbode of Rennes, Bishop of Rennes (1035–1123). His herbal describes seventy-one plants in verse for easy memorization. The first, most honored of all the herbs, was artemisia, "the mother herb." The Christian bishop explains that the herb was named after Artemis, whom the Romans called Diana, who first discovered its uses. "Mainly," the bishop wrote, "it cures female ailments. It stimulates menstrua and, whether drunk or applied, it produces an abortion."[72] Marbode discussed a number of other herbs that produce abortions and one herb, spearmint, that contracepts.

All this is strange and unexpected. Here we have people in a medieval village who know about birth control drugs and use them. We have the medical writings of a leading female physician on women's problems, but her work skirts the issue by listing only menstrual regulators. In contrast, Albertus Magnus, now Saint Albertus, condemned abortion in his theological works but included in other writings information on practical and, we would say, effective drugs for abortion and contraception. And we find a similar attitude in a prominent bishop, Marbode, who not only relates the same type of information but celebrates it by discussing drugs for abortion as the first of all in his pharmacopoeia.

Pope John XXI

On September 13, 1276, Peter of Spain was elevated to the papacy and assumed his new name, John XXI. He was born in Lisbon. His father was a physician. He studied at the University of Paris and went to Italy to teach medicine at the University of Siena. In his career he moved from dean of a cathedral to the archbishopry in Braga, Portugal. A stormy session of the cardinals that followed Adrian V's death raised him to the popehood. His pontifacy is known as a short but effective attempt to restore unity. An investigation of heresy charges at his alma mater, Paris, resulted in his condemning by a bull some 219 propositions. Among those condemned were nineteen written by St. Thomas Aquinas, Albertus's pupil.

Prior to his papacy, Peter wrote a medical work called *Treasury of Medicines for the Poor*. The new professionalization of medicine increasingly required that practitioners be university graduates. As a result, medical costs rose—after all, their education costs had to be paid. Peter wanted to tell the poor that there were many medicines free in nature that they could use. Perhaps because of his papacy, Peter's book enjoyed great popularity.

The surprise is this: Peter's *Treasury* is the greatest single source of information about the practical means of birth control that exists from the Middle Ages. Peter, the physician, gave no hint that John, the pope, would preside over a giant religious institution that regarded any form of human interference in the areas of fertility, conception, and birth as sinful. The first advice he gave to the poor was how to restrain sexual desire. Not surprisingly, his advice was directed to men: to place a hemlock plaster on the testicles before coitus.[73] The reasoning here is a little shaky, because the remedy is to decrease desire. Unstated is whether this act would diminish desire or the chances for conception. After making a faulty start in listing birth control drugs, Peter provides a long list of herbs found in the ancient Latin sources he had read. Then, however, he gave his own list, those for which in some way he vouched. They included sage but, interestingly, not figs.

Béatrice took the herb as a pessary and not by mouth, the way most drugs in the sources were taken. She never states that she did not have full confidence in the herbs she inserted prior to lovemaking.

How much knowledge was there about birth control during the Middle Ages that a woman like Béatrice could use? What were the attitudes about birth control, ranging from contraception to abortion? Already we know from the Inquisition's records, the philosophers, physicians, popular writers on secrets, and one pope that people in the Middle Ages knew a lot about birth control. In some ways, they knew more than we do today about natural products as antifertility drugs. From whom did they gain this knowledge? They learned from tradition, from those who had died long before they were born.

2

The Herbs Known to the Ancients

When a woman has intercourse, if she is not going to
conceive, then it is her practice to expel the sperm
produced by both partners whenever she wishes to do so.

Hippocrates, *The Sperm*, 5

Found in the sands of Egypt, the Ebers Papyrus is one of the largest
Egyptian papyrus scrolls ever to be found. Its translator, George Ebers
(1837–1898), was excited about the discovery because he believed that
the text might possess information about the pharaohs' lives, the mysteries of the pyramids, or the secrets of the ancient Egyptians. Instead,
he found that it contained medical prescriptions, more mundane than
mysterious.[1] Even more than other papyri, the Ebers Papyrus (published
in 1875) reveals important details about the lives of ancient Egyptians,
even the lives of the pharaohs. And it tells us that they had birth control.

Although the Ebers scroll was written sometime between 1550 and
1500 B.C.E., internal evidence indicates that the scribe writing it had
before him a copy of a much earlier version. The prescriptions date
back to the Old Kingdom, a thousand years or more before the scribe
copied what to take for upset stomachs, headaches, and, yes, abortion.
One of its "recipes that are made for women" reads:

To cause a woman to stop pregnancy in the first, second or third period [trimester]:

Unripe fruit of acacia

Colocynth

Dates

Triturate with 6/7th pint of honey; moisten a pessary of plant fiber and place in the vagina.[2]

It is difficult to translate hieroglyphics for plants into modern plant names for the exact species. But our knowledge of the ancient Egyptian language, as well as clever detective work by modern scholars who match the names with drawings on temples and other ancient evidence, allows us to make reasonably accurate translations. "Acacia" comes from the Greek meaning "thorn," and to the ancient Egyptians it meant one or more species of our *Acacia*, most probably *A. nilotica* Delile.

Another ancient source, the Kahun Papyrus on medical topics compiled around 1900 B.C.E., lists similar contraceptive pessaries.[3] Several also include acacia gum. Pessaries may have originated as quasi-magical attempts to block the birth canal in either direction, but the repeated inclusion of acacia hints that the Egyptians placed confidence in it as at least one satisfactorily contraceptive ingredient. And recent studies indicate they may have been right. Modern researchers have noted that when acacia is compounded, lactic acid anhydride is produced. Lactic acid is used in modern contraceptive jellies; for example it is bonded to vaginal diaphragms to prevent spermatozoa from passing the edges.[4] Whereas Egyptian acacia is probably *Acacia nilotica* Delile, it could be *A. seyal* Delile or other species. In one study, the leaf of *Acacia koa* was fed to rats twice a day for five days, and their litters were reduced by 88 to 100 percent; feeding the rats *A. koa* seeds reduced pregnancy by 100 percent.[5]

The second ingredient is colocynth, almost certainly *Citrullus colocynthis* Schrad. This is the same plant Albertus Magnus named as an abortifacient in a pessary. It is also the same ingredient that modern Arabic women take to induce abortions. Unfortunately, one woman recently took the wrong dosage (120 grains in a powder) and died.[6] This raises a question that is difficult to answer. How would the medieval readers of Albertus Magnus or the Egyptian readers of the Ebers Papyrus know the (safe) amount of each herb needed to produce the desired effect? The Ebers Papyrus is more definite than the writings of Albertus, who did not specify the amounts. The Ebers Papyrus called for the amount that could be absorbed in six-sevenths of a pint of honey and placed on an absorbent pad. The amount delivered by this method would be far less than the fatal dose taken by the hapless experimenter.

Pessaries or Oral-Route Drugs?

Both Béatrice's testimony and the Kahun Papyrus recount that antifertility drugs were administered as pessaries, but in animal experiments done today to test a drug the dose is given orally. Most of the antifertility agents listed in ancient and medieval medical works are taken by mouth.

If we are to compare modern data with historical evidence, we need help in understanding medically how pessary and oral-route drugs work and the degree to which they can be interchanged. Modern science offers some assistance but it is not conclusive. Studies of estrogen hormones in humans show that systemic activity by an agent can be more efficient than the same agent given orally.[7] Many of the antifertility agents have hormonal and pharmacological actions different from those of estrogen production. One cannot conclusively infer that an antifertility agent delivered orally is as good as it is when administered via a pessary.

In some respects the ancients may provide us with quite accurate information. Soranus wrote a treatise on gynecology early in the second century A.C.E. He distinguished between contraceptives and abortifacients in a precise way:

> A contraceptive differs from an abortive, for the first does not let conception take place, while the latter destroys what has been conceived. Let us therefore call the one "abortive" *(phthorion)* and the other "contraceptive" *(atokion)*.[8]

Soranus explains what we wanted to know about comparisons between antifertility pessaries and oral-route drugs with the same action:

> [Pessaries] are styptic, clogging, and cooling [and they] cause the orifice of the uterus to shut before the time of coitus and do not let the seed pass into its fundus. [Some pessaries, however, are hot] and irritating, not only do not allow the seed of the man to remain in the cavity of the uterus, but draw forth as well another fluid from it . . . In our opinion, moreover, the evil from these things is too great, since they damage and upset the stomach, and besides cause congestion of the head and induce sympathetic reactions.[9]

The Hippocratic Oath on Pessaries

The ancients told us that both pessaries and oral-route drugs were given for both contraceptive and abortive purposes and that some preferred to administer drugs orally. In one detail, the "lower status" of pessaries led to great historical consequences—namely, that pessaries are mentioned in the Hippocratic Oath. From Roman times, at least, some Western physicians were reluctant to administer an abortion on the basis that he—occasionally she—was prohibited from doing so by the Hippocratic Oath.[10] What the oath actually had in it concerned only pessaries.

From Roman times through the nineteenth century, the oath was believed to have been composed by Hippocrates, the founder of medicine, who lived about the same time as Socrates and Plato in the late fifth century B.C.E. Sometimes as a direct translation of the ancient Greek oath, more often in one of several revisions incorporating modern values, the oath is still administered to physicians at their graduation from medical school. Even if the oath were omitted, the physician still would be bound to its precepts because these are incorporated in common law and, subsequently, into most of the modern laws of Western nations. One example is the oath's prohibition of disclosing what a physician is told by a patient. What was traditional and customary has attained the status of law in modern society, even though there is little evidence that the custom was widespread during the intervening centuries, not even during the period of Hippocrates' life.

The ancient oath contained a line pertaining to birth control. The actual wording in literal English translation is: "Similarly I will not give to a woman a pessary in order to induce an abortion." The actual Greek words are *pesson phthorion*, meaning "abortive pessary." The word *pesson* unambiguously means a pessary, that is, a vaginal suppository. The earliest manuscripts clearly have this word in the text, so there is little likelihood of text alteration. At some time, most likely during the Roman Empire, the wording was changed in Latin copies. The new wording prohibited a physician from administering an abortion by any means. The consequences of the change were tremendous.

Before we go into the tangled web of texts and who thought what, it should be said that present scholarship on the origins of the Hippocratic Oath has added some important new information. The oath was not written by Hippocrates, and it was not taken in the form we have it by most "Hippocratic" physicians in classical Greek society. Not long after it was written, confusion arose. Most Hippocratic physicians would not have pledged themselves to hold a number of values in the oath, such as not assisting with suicide. Suicide was an acceptable form of behavior among both the Greeks and the Romans. Indeed, what separated the barbarians from civilized people was that the barbarians did not believe in suicide. Modern scholars have come to the conclusion that whoever wrote the oath ascribed to Hippocrates was a member of a fringe group and not representative of those practitioners who traced their tradition through their teachers to Hippocrates.[11] "History" is often what people think the past was. By the Roman period, the oath was regarded as having been written by Hippocrates. Although they did not actually take the oath, physicians regarded it as a set of ethical standards toward which they aspired. From the Roman period through the Middle Ages, a properly trained physician should have based his moral and professional code on the oath's precepts. Therein lay the rub that was to last for over two thousand years: the popular understanding of the text, not the oath's original text, became the historically influential factor.

In the first century of our era Scribonius Largus, a Roman medical writer, said, "Hippocrates, who founded our profession, laid the foundation for our discipline by an oath in which it was proscribed to give to a pregnant woman a kind of medicine that expels the embryo *(conceptus)*."[12] Shortly after Scribonius, Soranus recommended a number of practical prescriptions for birth control, despite believing that the oath by Hippocrates forbade it. Soranus read the oath as saying, "I will give to no one an abortive."[13] Soranus himself was puzzled because he knew that in some Hippocratic works advice was given about contraception and abortion.[14]

The confusion expressed by Soranus was reflected in the discussion by Theodorus Priscianus, a late-fourth-century Roman medical writer. He began a discussion of abortions with the observation that a physician ought not to administer abortions because it was not right to do so. The oath of Hippocrates had forbidden it, an oath that was to be held "in purity and holiness," as the words read. But a simpler phrase was seen as countervailing: the physician also was pledged to act "for the benefit of the sick." There were circumstances in which the life of a woman was put at risk by her pregnancy. As examples Theodorus noted that in some women the opening to the womb was too small for delivery or that an extremely young girl's health might be put in danger by childbirth.

Theodorus developed his argument on the basis of what we would call situational ethics. The health of a tree sometimes depends on skillful pruning. In a storm it might be necessary to throw cargo overboard in order to save a heavily laden ship and its passengers. Remarkably, Theodorus employed the same metaphor as modern debaters of "lifeboat" ethics. For the greater good, the physician needed to know about birth control remedies in order to save lives. Theodorus listed nine prescriptions for abortion, the first using artemisia. The only abortion procedures he discussed were drugs, most of which were given orally, not as pessaries.[15]

As we shall see in forthcoming chapters, the interpretation of the Hippocratic Oath has governed attitudes and at times laws, secular and religious, through the Middle Ages and down to our modern day. We shall look at the ancients' views of contraception and abortion, but first let us look at some of the principal antifertility herbs that they took. Their attitudes toward birth control would be fruitless were it not for the fact that they had the means to control conception and birth.

The Ancient Herbs

Pomegranates

Ancient lore about pomegranates is revealed in Greek mythology. Persephone (or *Kore*, meaning "virgin") was the daughter of Zeus and daughter-in-law (later, daughter) of Demeter, the goddess of fertility and earth-mother. Pluto kidnapped Persephone and brought her to the Underworld. Unable or unwilling to intervene, Zeus instructed Persephone not to eat while in the Underworld. Demeter's distress was manifest on earth: all that was green and fertile died. Facing the laments of Demeter and the wilted earth, the other gods beseeched Zeus to rescue Persephone. Before he did so, however, Persephone ate some pomegranate seeds. For her disobedience she must return for some months each year to the Underworld, and when she does the leaves turn, plants die, and, in Hesiod's description, "the beasts shrink" from the wintry winds.[16]

As this story tells us, pomegranate seeds were associated with a pause in fertility in Greek legend, and they were recognized as antifertility agents in Greek medicine, as well. Hippocrates, Soranus, Dioscorides, and Aetius are among the ancient Greek and Roman medical writers who prescribed pomegranate seeds and rind to prevent conception.[17] Long before the Greeks, even, pomegranate was a prominent symbol of the goddess of love in ancient West Asia. An alabaster cult vase from the temple of Eanna, goddess of love, in Uruk that dates from the third or second quarter of the fourth millennium is decorated with a processional offering on the top relief and pomegranates on the bottom.[18] A magnificent piece of jewelry made of gold-silver alloy was found in a grave from the seventh century B.C.E. in Kamiros. It depicts a naked female figure, likely Astarte or Aphrodite, and from it hang pendants of pomegranates.[19]

From Greece, a picture drawn on a Boeotian plate shows either Demeter or Persephone (some say both in one) seated, enthroned and heavily draped. Her right hand holds a torch while her left hand holds two stalks of grain and two twigs with a pomegranate on each end. She touches the grain and pomegranates to an altar on which there is what appears to be a pomegranate.[20] The goddess holds, and therefore controls, the symbols for fertility *and* sterility. Demeter's symbolism is herculean.[21]

A number of curious discrepancies about the pomegranates in lore and medicine make the story of Persephone's kidnapping incomplete. First, according to the legend, Persephone ate the pomegranate; the medical writings indicate that pomegranate was administered as a suppository. There is only one possible source in which I have found pomegranate taken orally. During the Middle Ages, the Arabic text of Ibn Sīnā (Avicenna, ca. 980–1037) prescribed pomegranate as a postcoital contraceptive, whereas the Latin translation made by Gerard of Cremona (d. 1187) implies that it is orally taken.[22]

Over time, the pomegranate faded in usage, but the story has a second chapter. In 1933 Adolf Butenandt and H. Jacobi announced in a German chemistry journal their discovery of chemicals in plants that were the same as female sex hormones.[23] This possibility was heretofore not suspected. After all, although higher animals, mammals, produce hormones that affect sexual and generative processes, often in endocrine glands, it was believed that plants operate more simply. In 1939 Adolf Butenandt would receive a Nobel Prize in chemistry, but not for the small article he wrote in 1933 on the date palm. The date palm, he and Jacobi reported, contained a compound that they called α-follicle hormone, which was similar in action to human female hormones. What they were describing was an estrogenic compound. The trouble was that others were unsuccessful in duplicating their experiments. It was not until 1966 that their experiments were confirmed.[24]

Animal scientists, not chemists, soon followed Butenandt and Jacobi's lead. They wanted to know, for example, why sheep that grazed on a type of clover (*Trifolium subterraneum*) produced so few lambs. In an article published in the *Australian Veterinary Journal* in 1946, scientists had the hard evidence: plants can reduce fertility, in some cases up to 100 percent.[25]

How did Butenandt and Jacobi come to delve into the chemistry of the date palm, which does not grow in Germany? In their article they describe the samples tested but do not say how these materials came to their laboratory or why they tested them. One story, which I have been unable to confirm, is that the pomegranate and palm samples came from German possessions in southeastern Africa. It may have been that the samples were sent because someone observed that animals eating the plant's fruit had reduced fertility. This same observation has been made by the mountain people of North Carolina. They know that it is difficult to raise sheep because the ubiquitous rhododendron reduces fertility and, when eaten in too large amounts, can have fatal consequences.

The pomegranate is a good example of the way modern science has rediscovered what the ancients knew about birth control drugs. In experiments conducted during the 1970s and 1980s, female rats fed pomegranate (*Punica granatum* L.) and paired with male rats not fed with it had a 72 percent reduction in fertility. The same experiment conducted on guinea pigs resulted in a 100 percent reduction.[26] Forty days after withdrawal from pomegranate, the fertility of both animal groups returned to normal.[27] Still another experiment with rats had a 50 percent reduction in fertility.[28] Many parts of the plant (seed, roots, whole plants) had no appreciable effect on fertility; only the fruit skin around the seed was found to lower it.[29] One test indicated that pomegranate root has substances that inhibit growth by nearly 100 percent.[30]

What may we conclude from these limited results about the effectiveness of pomegranate as a birth control drug in circumstances that may vary widely from experimental models? There are many variables in the "doses" of chemicals produced by plants, as a phytochemist knows all too well. The season, the part extracted, the quality of the soil (acid, alkaline), the climate (desert, moist, warm, cool), and even the time of day can cause differences in the concentration of drugs taken from plants. For example, the effective drug in opium poppy can be harvested only during a period of a few weeks. The method of extraction is also very important; some chemically active compounds are not soluble in water, whereas others may fare poorly when submitted to alcohol.

The ancient sources usually name the seed of the pomegranate as the agent that affects fertility. We have to assume that their term for seed would include what we identify as pulp or seed covering, because in modern experiments the heaviest concentrations of active substances are found in the pulp. In general, there is no absolute, irrefutable evidence that the ancients used pomegranate in precisely the same way as modern researchers have used it. Moreover, different animal populations have different reproductive physiologies, as the experiments on rats and guinea pigs demonstrate. Also, one should not extrapolate results from an animal population and assume that the same reduction in fertility would be obtained in a human population. One can, however, accept that the substances testing strongly positive in smaller animal populations are likely to have a similar result on humans.

With all the variables in the interpretation of data on the historical use of the pomegranate, how can we be led to any conclusions? The answer lies in an overall question: given the historical and scientific information—and the lessons learned from in modern folklore—is it more likely that people in the past were using an effective drug than that they were not? The evidence is never absolute, but the historian must weigh the details as they accumulate to the point where it is reasonable to assume that the substances people used to reduce fertility did have the desired effect.

The pomegranate is not a perfect example because it was not an enduring birth control agent. Reports of its use are mostly from classical antiquity. By the Middle Ages, the pomegranate seldom appears in medical works or in anecdotal accounts as an antifertility agent. One of the most detailed writers on drugs, Serapion the Elder (who lived in the ninth century), said of the pomegranate only that it increased sexual desire.[31] The memory of Persephone and why she ate the fruit in the first place had faded.

Although the pomegranate was not employed extensively in medieval and modern European culture (as judged by references to it), it is used for birth control in modern Indian, East African, and Pacific areas today. A reasonable hypothesis is that the pomegranate was of limited effectiveness for birth control and that over time Western populations abandoned its use as more effective drugs became available. The fact that non-Western peoples consider it an antifertility agent, however, reinforces the evidence that at one time it was perceived as such in the West.

Silphium

Nowadays we have drugs of choice. Often any number of drugs will treat an affliction or injury, though some drugs are better than others. The approval of a drug is now a matter of state policy. The process of certifying drugs began with medieval pharmaceutical guilds and culminated in national pharmacopoeias, official guides to approved drugs. The distribution of medicines was an entirely different story during ancient times. "Let the buyer beware" was a serious warning. Ancient cities were filled with vendors plying their wares, and the countryside had more than our modern communities' share of traveling medicine-show salesmen and saleswomen. Who knew what best to take for this or that? Drugs were chosen on the basis of word-of-mouth information or traditional lore, which itself was based on cumulative experience and reputation. Anecdotal and medical evidence from classical antiquity tells us that the drug of choice for contraception was silphium.

The history of fertility is linked to the history of population movement. We have much to learn about fertility patterns from the study of migrating populations, people leaving crowded cities, for example, and colonizing new territories. In the seventh century B.C.E., colonists from Thera settled in a newly founded city in northern Africa (in what is now Libya) they called Cyrene, and what they found must have made them question the oracle's advice to go there. Unlike most colonists, they had migrated reluctantly, selected by lot. They were surrounded by non-Greeks and were not afforded citizenship rights if they sought to return home. Around them were dry, unfriendly expanses of land, a long way from home. According to Theophrastus, a pupil of Aristotle, the Cyrenian colonists soon discovered a plant which made some of them wealthy and all of them famous for living near where it grew. They called the new plant *silphion*, from which the Romans derived their name *silphium*. On the basis of ancient descriptions and pictures, modern botanists identify *silphium* as a species of giant fennel (genus

Ferula), because of the shape of its leaves. The pungent sap from its stems and roots was used as cough syrup, and it gave food a richer, distinctive taste. Its true value was not as a medicine or a condiment, however. When women took *silphium* by mouth, they supposed that they would not conceive.

A Greek vase of the sixth century B.C.E. shows Arkesilas, King of Cyrene, supervising the weighing and loading of *silphium* for export. Not all investigators believe the picture represents *silphium*, because of the packaging. They suggest instead that the product shown on the vase is wool. Exporting wool from Cyrene to the Greek mainland would truly be a case of taking coals to Newcastle. It was not wool but *silphium* that made the city's reputation. Demand for it drove up prices enough for Aristophanes to write, "Don't you remember when a stalk of *silphium* sold so cheap?"[32] Fortunately for the Cyrenians, attempts to cultivate the plant in Syria and Greece failed.[33]

Cyrene placed pictures of *silphium* on its coins as its distinctive symbol, just as Athens used the owl. Many Cyrenian coins depict a woman beside the plant or on the coin's obverse. One four-drachma series depicts *silphium*'s use more graphically: a seated woman has *silphium* at her feet, while one hand touches the plant and the other points to her reproductive area.

To the reproductive area ancient medical authorities pointed as well. Soranus, after stating that oral contraceptives are better than pessaries, gave as his prescription that women should drink the juice from a small amount of *silphium* about the size of a chick-pea with water once a month. He added that it "not only prevent conception but also destroys any already existing."[34] Similarly, Dioscorides gave it both as a contraceptive and as an abortifacient, whereas Pliny the Elder, who was against abortion, listed it only as a menstrual regulator.[35]

The famous poet Catullus (d. ca. 54 B.C.E.) asks how many kisses he and Lesbia may share. Why, he answers, as many times as there are grains of sand on Cyrene's *silphium* shores. That is, Catullus told his lover that they could make love for as long as they had the plant. Acquiring it soon became difficult. Over the centuries *silphium* became expensive: demand increased while supply of the undomesticated plant declined. In 93 B.C.E. thirty pounds of *silphium* were imported to Rome during the consulship of Gaius Valerius and Marcus Herennius. Within forty years, it had become rare from over-harvesting. Around a century later, Pliny (d. 79) said that *silphium* was worth more than its weight in silver. He reported that in the Emperor Nero's time, "only a single stalk has been found there within our memory."[36] Although he may have exaggerated, the famous remedy for both coughs and pregnancy was scarce. *Silphium* grew only in a thirty-mile band along the dry mountainsides, especially those facing the Mediterranean Sea. By late antiquity it had become extinct, last being mentioned in two fourth-century letters by Synesius of Cyrene, who said that his brother had *silphium* growing on his farm and elsewhere referred to it as a gift.[37]

How we can judge the effectiveness of an extinct plant? There is a way: we can examine what the ancients used when they could not find or afford *silphium*. The most common substitute for it was asafetida *(Ferula assa-foetida* L.), a plant whose root sap we employ to give Worcestershire sauce its distinctive aroma. Crude alcohol extracts of asafetida and a related plant, *F. orientalis* L., were found to inhibit implantation of fertilized ova in rats at rates of 40 percent and 50 percent, respectively.[38] Other *Ferula* species have produced impressive results; one species, *F. jaeschikaena*, was found nearly to be 100 percent effective in preventing pregnancy when administered to adult female rats within three days of coitus.[39] In 1963, asafetida was found to be effective as a contraceptive in humans.[40] The species also acts in humans to induce early abortion.[41] Given the effectiveness of other species of *Ferula*, it is apparent why the ancients valued *silphium* so much.

Long after *silphium* became extinct, during the rule of Charlemagne (ca. 800), medical guides were compiled by the monks of a Benedictine abbey of Lorsch (now in Germany), who had a tradition of treating the sick. Their medical knowledge was based on classical roots but was adapted to the needs of their society. The monks found *silphium* in their texts, and so they noted its substitute: *"Silfio id est radix lasar"* ("Silphium, that is take the root of asafoetida").[42] The bad news was that asafetida, grown in Persia, was an expensive import, like cinnamon and pepper. To fill the supply, then, the brothers cultivated other birth control plants in their monastic garden.

Pennyroyal

Growing most places, especially in herb gardens, is pennyroyal *(Mentha pulegium* L.), a member of the mint family. Contrary to many mints, pennyroyal is not pleasant in salads. Over the centuries, however, pennyroyal appears in home herb gardens for one of two reasons or, possibly, the two together. One use gave pennyroyal its name in Greek, *pulegion*—when smeared on the body, it drives away fleas. For its other use, the reason it is still found in health food stores, it must be prepared as a tea. Not known particularly for its taste (few people like it), pennyroyal tea acts as an abortifacient.

In Aristophanes' play, *Peace*, presented in 421 B.C.E., Hermes gives Trigaius a female companion. Delighted to have her in his arms, Trigaius asks his benefactor if there would be a problem should the woman became pregnant. "Not if you add a dose of pennyroyal," Hermes says. If the use of this member of the mint family to control birth had not been familiar to his Athenian audience, Aristophanes could have expected to elicit no laughter from Hermes' reply. A similar joke in Aristophanes' *Lysistrata* also assumes common knowledge on the part of the audience. Calonice, an Athenian woman and all too pregnant, is told that she should withhold her body from her husband. Onto the stage comes a slim woman from Boeotia who is described as "A very lovely, and Well cropped, and trimmed and spruced with pennyroyal."[43]

Aristophanes was referring to what must have been a well-known drug for antifertility, albeit not to the pregnant Calonice. Pennyroyal was not a "home remedy," either, as Greek physicians knew its power. The nearly contemporary Hippocratic works on gynecology refer to pennyroyal as a birth control agent. In fact, it was so employed in Western medicine until the nineteenth century, when most Western nations made abortion a criminal offense.

Pennyroyal grows wild in many places and would have been generally available to ancient women. Its chief drawback was its toxicity. It had to be taken in precise amounts in a tea. In order to produce the desired effect without harming the woman, the specific directions would have had to be more precise than they are in most ancient and medieval texts. A number of modern animal and human studies show that pennyroyal contains pulegone, which does terminate pregnancies when taken in controlled amounts.[44] In too large amounts it is toxic to the liver.[45] Little wonder, then, that *silphium* commanded such a great price, because it seems to have been safer and, probably, surer.

Artemisia

Artemisia, already mentioned in Chapter 1, is another plant that grows most places. So familiar is it that most of us regard it as a weed. To the ancients this plant was of more noble standing, because it was the plant of Artemis, the goddess of the woodland, forest, childbirth, and fertility to men and beasts. Artemis looked after women in childbirth and, like birthwort (discussed below), her plant was sometimes used to hasten or to assist delivery.[46] Some herbs that were believed to stimulate menstruation were also thought to help in childbirth and, as the ancients expressed it, to remove the afterbirth.

The plant artemisia was associated with the goddess for good reason. Artemisia has been found to be an effective antifertility agent.[47] In one test in 1979 on rats, 10 mg of scoparone, isolated from *Artemisia scoparia*, were fed to rats on days 1 through 7 after coitus; the result was a 100 percent termination of pregnancies.[48] Artemisia also may interfere with spermatogenesis.[49] Little wonder, then, that Artemis and her plant were associated with both fertility (the stimulation of menstruation) and infertility (the reduction of pregnancies) in animals and humans alike.

Rue

Just like artemisia and pennyroyal, rue *(Ruta graveolens* L.) grows over much of Europe and Asia. Unlike artemisia and pennyroyal, rue has a very unpleasant odor and a disagreeable taste. Its most recognized use in classical antiquity and the Middle Ages was as an abortifacient. Today, perhaps, that is its least recognized use.

In *Richard II*, William Shakespeare describes the comments made by gardeners, and overheard by the Queen, as they discuss Richard's reversals and the imminent loss of his kingdom. Why should they "keep law and form and due proportion" in the garden when the kingdom loses its law and order? they ask themselves. Unaware of the news until she overhears their question, the Queen startles them:

> Gardener, for telling me these news of woe,
> Pray God the plants thou graft'st may never grow.

After the distraught Queen exits, a remorseful gardener laments:

> Here did she fall a tear; here in this place
> I'll set a bank of rue, sour herb of grace;
> Rue, even for ruth, here shortly shall be seen,
> In the remembrance of a weeping queen. (ii.3.4)

Ruth in the last line meant pity.[50] Rue was known as the herb of repentance in the Middle Ages, and here to Shakespeare as the "sour herb of grace." The kingdom together with its king and queen are all aborted, and in their place will be a bed of rue for remembrance. How strange is the medieval mind to say that an abortion herb represents repentance, regret, and rue (yes, in its different sense)? The verb *to rue* derives from the Old English *hrēowan*, meaning to grieve or be sorry, but the plant name apparently comes from the verb as well. When one thinks about it, the medieval mind is not so much strange as different from ours. Rue for repentance, "herb of grace," makes sense to one who is in distress and in need of its help.

Ophelia was in distress also. In the scene where she becomes mad, she frenetically expresses her distress to Laertes:

> There's fennel for you, and columbines; there's rue for you; and here's some for me; we may call it herb-grace o'Sundays. O! you wear your rue with a difference.   (*Hamlet*, iv.5)

What did Shakespeare convey to us here? Why was Ophelia's rue different from Laertes'? Ophelia may have been more involved with Hamlet than the modern reader knows. Ophelia's use of the word *rue* may be different, not just a symbol of remorse, as it was for Laertes. She may have been referring to her use of the plant for an abortion, hence we better understand her madness. As we shall see in forthcoming chapters, Shakespeare's contemporary audience would understand this reference better than today's readers, who do not know what a difference rue would have made.

Rue does cause an abortion. Chinese investigators administered chloroform extracts of the whole rue plant in daily oral doses of 0.8 to 1.2 grams per kilogram of body weight to female rats over the first 8 to 10 days of pregnancy. The extracts reduced the number of pregnancies in the experimental group by from 20 percent to 75 percent (depending on the potency of the extract administered). The active ingredient is chalepensin, toxic in high dosages, but this effect may be simply the result of non-selective toxicity.[51]

Rue belongs to a botanical family Rutaceae, which includes several plants that produce antifertility agents. Another related species, a plant named *Murraya paniculata* var. *M. sapientum* L., is reportedly 100 percent effective in preventing pregnancies in rats when administered orally in doses of 2 mg/kg on the first day after coitus.[52] Interestingly, another Rutaceae species, *Pilocarpus jaborandi* Homes, produces a cholinergic agent called pilocarpine, used in modern veterinary medicine to induce abortion in horses.[53]

In addition to having an effect on animals in tests, rue is employed by people in South, Central, and North America as an abortifacient.[54] One report about human usage said that, even though it was widely employed as an abortifacient, its greatest effect may be contraception by preventing implantation.[55] Thus, from the earliest Greek medical records to the present, rue, "sour herb of grace," has been used by people to control their reproductive activity.

Queen Anne's Lace

One of the more potent antifertility agents is also a common plant in many regions of the world, Queen Anne's lace (*Daucus carota* L.), called by some the wild carrot because it is in the carrot family. Its seeds, harvested in the fall, are a strong contraceptive if taken orally immediately after coitus. Extracts of its seeds have been tested on rats, mice, guinea pigs, and rabbits. In mice given the seeds (doses of 80 to 120 mg) on the fourth to sixth days of pregnancy, the pregnancies were terminated. The action is such that the implantation process is disrupted and a fertilized ovum either will not be implanted or, if it has been implanted for only a short period, will be released.[56] In other experiments with rodents, the seeds were found to inhibit implantation and ovarian growth and to disrupt the estrous cycle.[57]

The seeds' antifertility effect is inhibited by progesterone, and recent evidence suggests that terpenoids in the seed block crucial progesterone synthesis in pregnant animals. Even though the active ingredient(s) have yet to be isolated, Chinese investigators see Queen Anne's lace as a promising post-coital antifertility agent. Folklore reports indicate that its seeds are regularly employed by modern women in rural areas of the Appalachians and India. One woman in Watauga County in the North Carolina mountains reported that she took a tablespoon of the seeds with a glass of water immediately after intercourse. For over ten years she did not become pregnant until she went on a trip with her husband and forgot the mason jar of seeds. The lapse caused her undesired pregnancy.[58]

Queen Anne's lace may have been what women relied upon in ancient times. We cannot know how many. The earliest reference to it appears in a work ascribed to Hippocrates that dates back to the late fifth or fourth century B.C.E.,[59] where it is described as an abortifacient. Similar uses were recorded by Dioscorides, Scribonius Largus, Marcellius Empiricus, and Pliny the Elder.[60] Pliny was not a medical person, only a collector of information. Influenced by the Stoics, Pliny was against contraception and abortion.[61] Loath to transmit its lore, he said only that Queen Anne's lace was an emmenagogue (the common circumlocution). In a bit of intriguing, and no doubt related, folklore, elsewhere in his work Pliny said that four-footed animals will not eat any kind of wild carrot, including Queen Anne's lace, "except after a miscarriage."[62] Pliny did not make the connection but the message lived on in folklore, because it was an accepted tradition in folk medicine that the plant caused infertility.

If judged by the number of references to it, Queen Anne's lace was not in frequent use for birth control. But here is a perplexing point to ponder: to what degree can usage be determined by the frequency of appearance in the historical documents, which are themselves scattered over the centuries? It is not difficult to accept as a working hypothesis that there is a link between the women in antiquity who knew the effect of Queen Anne's lace and those in modern India who chew its seeds and those in North Carolina who take the seeds with a glass of water. My hypothesis is that generally the information about the drug's usage was transmitted orally. The documentary evidence, whether in medical works or otherwise, simply records the know-how available at a point in time. Modern women in North Carolina neither read the ancient works nor learned from great-grandparents who read them. The chain of learning about antifertility drugs was forged by vocal cords.

Myrrh

Myrrh was known to Greek mythology before it appeared in Greek medical records. Famed in our day as one of the three gifts—gold, frankincense, and myrrh—of the Magi to the baby Jesus (Matthew 2:11), it was also familiar to the ancients. Myrrha was the daughter of Theias, also called Cinyras, a legendary king of Assyria. A great misfortune befell the innocent girl because of her father's impiety. When he angered Aphrodite, the goddess of love, Aphrodite caused him to lust after his daughter. As a result of incest, Myrrha bore a son, Adonis. But Theias continued to assault her, until at length she fled and Theias pursued. When Myrrha called upon the gods to help her escape from her father, they transformed her into the plant known by her name. Her tears, the plant's sap, became the rescuer of daughters victimized by a father's lust. "Even the tears have fame," Ovid wrote in his *Metamorphoses* (10.500–5022), "and that which distills from the tree trunk keeps the name of its mistress and will be remembered through all the ages."[63]

The sap was highly fragrant and valued for that reason by the people of ancient Greece and Rome, who believed in smelling good. To most Greeks and Romans, "myrrh" was this precious scent, for the plant itself grew only in East Africa, a shrub of the genus *Commiphora*. Whatever was intended by the Magi's gift to baby Jesus, however, myrrh was recognized in the ancient world as an antifertility drug.[64] For example, Dioscorides recommended that myrrh be used in a prescription along with a kind of artemisia (*Artemisia absinthium* L.), lupine, and rue to expel either or both the menses and a fetus.[65] The actions of artemisia and rue have already been discussed, and experiments have shown that lupanine, found in lupine (a bean), produces contractions in isolated pig uteri and, when administered to guinea pigs, is "very effective" in the interruption of the second half of pregnancy.[66] If lupanine is given in doses of 200 mg injected into the muscles, there are no known unsafe side effects.[67] Many ancient physicians included myrrh among the antifertility agents, usually as an abortifacient.[68] Later, Muslim physicians also valued myrrh, but often as an oral contraceptive.[69] In the western Middle Ages, the famed female gynecologist Trotula recommended it,[70] and a work allegedly by Arnald of Villanova prescribed myrrh as an ingredient in a pessary to induce an abortion.[71]

On the other hand, Platearius (d. ca. 1161), the author of a popular herbal, saw myrrh as an aid to conception. Possibly Platearius was ill-informed about gynecology, but it is at least equally possible that myrrh's action may have been estrogenic. If given in the appropriate amounts and at the right time, estrogen assists conception, just as estrogen ingested at the wrong time or in the wrong amount can impede the same. The action, if any, of myrrh is scientifically speculative. I have found no scientific tests of its action in the laboratory or the clinic. Myrrh was found in one study to have pharmacologically active substances, but it was not tested for fertility effects.[72] Even so, its usage as an antifertility drug persists in the modern world. Myrrha's tears were shed to save daughters from the consequences of incest. Myrrha's sacrifice, however, was not available to everyone. Her tears were far too dear to reach all the victims of this madness.

Squirting Cucumber

The people of the eastern Mediterranean, notably modern-day Turkey and Greece, would probably be familiar with another ancient plant, the wild gourd called appropriately the *sikos agrios* ("wild cucumber") by the Greeks. The English common name, "squirting cucumber," is also appropriate, because its fruit (shorter than a garden cucumber) squirts out seeds when it dries. Carolus Linnaeus gave the plant its modern scientific name, *Ecballium elaterium*. *Elaterium* is a name of the drug taken from its sap, and *ekballios* is Greek for abortion. Thus, the Linnean name is "abortion drug." The ancients knew this, but for a long while the purpose of this drug was lost to modern medical lore, despite the meaning embedded in its name.

A Hippocratic treatise on women's problems claimed that the squirting cucumber was good as "an abortive pessary for the uterus" and, the author(s) added, "there is nothing that is better."[73] By indicating that it was the abortion drug of choice, the author did something that was very rarely done in classical or medieval medical sources. Normally a drug's properties were defined but not ranked in respect to drugs with similar actions.

A number of classical sources that followed the Hippocratic writers, Dioscorides and Galen among them, testified to the squirting cucumber's abortive properties, but none spoke of it as a contraceptive.[74] Authors of the late Roman Empire and early Middle Ages were more circumspect: they referred to it only as an emmenagogue[75] Even so the author called Apuleius, who lived around the fifth century, was more precise in his treatise on herbs: the squirting cucumber is "for an abortion."[76] The name is seldom found in medieval sources, however, probably because the plant is not found in northern Europe. Why, when exotic abortifacient drugs were traded across continents, there was not a market for this plant of such apparent effectiveness is left unexplained.

Only "apparent" effectiveness can be determined. Recent animal tests support the notion that squirting cucumber has a contraceptive effect. When mice were given daily doses of 20 to 100 mg per kilogram of extracts from the whole plant or from the flower alone, they failed to ovulate.[77] The abortifacient effect has not been confirmed.

Juniper

"Gossip records a miracle," states Pliny the Elder: "that to rub it [crushed juniper berries] all over the male part before coition prevents conception."[78] Another source near the same time had much nearly the same message, except that the directions were for the crushed berries to be placed on the vulva prior to insertion.[79] One way or the other, juniper is inserted in the woman's vagina, and there it will act either as a contraceptive or an abortifacient, as Galen stated.[80] Juniper was also taken orally.

Juniper is a shrub or small tree of the cypress family that grows primarily in mountainous regions but is found all over Europe. One common species, probably one known to Dioscorides and Galen, is *Juniperus communis* L. The habitat of another species, *J. sabina* L., is the Alps and central Europe. This is the species probably mentioned in most documents during the Middle Ages. Often its name was *sabine* or *savin*.

The abortive qualities of juniper generally are attributed to its essential oil (1 to 3 percent of plant), more precisely to the major component of the oil, sabinyl acetate (more than 50 percent).[81] The oils have caused relaxation and inhibited uterine movement to an extent that could lead to an abortion in tests conducted on isolated human uteri and Fallopian tubes. Abortion by juniper in humans is attested to in our time.[82] The evidence available would indicate a systemic action for the drug, as would be the consequence of its use in a pessary. Furthermore, animal tests show that juniper can act when taken orally.[83] One recent study demonstrated that *J. sabina* oil subcutaneously injected during organogenesis had a dramatic effect in interrupting pregnancy. The percentage of interrupted pregnancies was correlated with the dosage.

Juniper, then, was demonstrably employed as an antifertility agent both as a systemic drug—that is, a drug absorbed through an organ membrane (not through the digestive system), in this case by vaginal insertion—and as an oral drug. While it had a degree of effectiveness,

Table 4. Effect of *Juniperus sabina* essential oil (S.E.O.) subcutaneously injected, during organogenesis, on pregnant dams and their fetuses

	S.E.O. dose (mg/kg body weight)			
	0	15	45	135
Maternal parameters				
Mated	22	22	22	22
Pregnant	19	20	20	22
Unaffected	12	5*	3*	1*
Affected	7	15*	17*	21*
Effect				
Resorbed fetuses[e]	6	12	16	18
Abnormal fetuses[e]	0	0	0	0
Resorbed and abnormal fetuses[e]	1	3	1	3

*Significance at $p < 0.05$; e = exclusively.

Source: N. Pages, G. Fournier, G. Chamorro, M. Salayar, M. Paris, and C. Bondene,
"Teratological Evaluation of *Juniperus sabina*. Essential Oil in Mice," *Planta Medica* 55
(1989): 144–146.

it may also have had some toxic side effects. As will be noted in the
coming chapters, however, juniper is found often in documents from
classical antiquity down to our day.

Aloe

If you were to go into a drug store today and ask for aloe, you would
most likely be directed to the cosmetic section. But aloe (*Aloe vera* L.
and other species) is also sold as an over-the-counter medicine, because of its numerous therapeutic qualities. The ancients recognized
in aloe more than thirty medicinal usages, most related to its digestive
and dermatological actions.[84] Aloe was sometimes used in compound
prescriptions for abortion and contraception.[85] For example, Theodore
Priscianus put aloe with opopanax roots (a species of *Ferula*, related to
silphium) and myrrh to induce an abortion.[86] Aëtius of Amida (fl.
502–525) put aloe with wallflower (or stock) seeds, pepper, and saffron
in a recipe for contraception.[87] Tests on guinea pigs show that aloe has

abortifacient qualities.[88] When aloe in an alcohol extract of 100 mg was administered to rats from one to seven days post-coitus, the rats had a 50 percent reduction in implantation. When the dosage was increased to 200 mg, the reduction was 100 percent.[89] With both contraceptive and abortive effects, it is likely that at least some of the ancients knew of aloe's antifertility properties. This use for aloe is found seldom in ancient documents, however, so we must assume that it was not widespread. Aloe's popularity increased in time, though, as the use of other agents, such as pomegranate, decreased.

Dittany

Of all the emmenagogic drugs, dittany has the greatest efficacy, said Pliny the Elder. While Pliny did not support abortion, he said it could be used to "force out the fetus when dead or lying transversely— [for this] an obolus of leaves is taken in water." He, among others not advocating abortion, resorted to saying that women could take menstruation-inducing drugs if the fetus was dead or imperiled. It was left unstated who was to determine if the fetus was dead, especially if the time was before "quickening" or perceived fetal movement. Just the same, Pliny knew that dittany ought not be taken by pregnant women: "so powerful [it is] that it shall not be in a room with a pregnant woman."[90]

Dittany is an herb of the mint family, but little research has been conducted on its alleged antifertility effects. One modern report says that dittany is an abortifacient.[91] A 1987 report of an animal test said that administering the root up to ten days after coitus reduced fertility in rats. Further study showed that estrogenicity was not indicated, but the action of the drug appears to be the inhibition of implantation.[92]

The amount of dittany taken is often stated in the ancient documents, more often than is done for other drugs. I know of no reason for this. A Hippocratic work said that one *obol*, the same amount as Pliny gave, is taken with leek juice and a large shell of oil of bitter almonds.[93] Both Dioscorides and an old English herbal resorted to the same round-about expression about dittany expelling a dead fetus.[94] Aspasia, the gynecologist who lived around the second century, gave more detail. One drachma (approximately six *obols* or three grams) of dittany seeds is given to terminate a pregnancy in the third month.[95]

It makes sense to us that the dosage for terminating a very early pregnancy would have to be less than the dosage needed to terminate in the third month. Dittany was one of the means for an abortion chosen by women. Just the same, Serapion the Younger (fl. ca. 1070?), an Arabic writer, placed dittany in the second class of "menstrual movers."[96]

Chaste Tree

Long before Hippocrates and the earliest Greek medical writings, Greek women celebrated a festival for Demeter, whom we encountered in connection with pomegranate. During the festival days women put boughs from the chaste tree beneath their pallets so that they might be chaste during the celebration. This is strange because it is an antifertility plant. *Vitex agnus-castus* L. is called the "chaste tree" in English because of some connection, I presume, with the Greek name for the small tree: *agnos* means "chaste."

Galen said that an athletic trainer required his men to sleep on a "botanical" bed of chaste-tree twigs, and a pseudo-Galenic treatise disclosed that priests eat the chaste tree, presumably to prevent an erection.[97] The tree was also considered a cure for priapism.[98] At the festival of Thesmophoria, the symbols for the chaste tree indicate that, paradoxically, it suppresses sexual desire and promotes fertility.[99] In the Homeric *Hymn to Hermes*, the connection is made for us: Hermes is the manager of livestock who fences in the cows, isolates them, leads them to the chaste tree, and conducts them to the bulls.[100] In other words, the chaste tree symbolizes regulated, orderly reproduction.[101]

Greek, Roman, and medieval medical sources say that the chaste tree "destroys generation" (in the words of Dioscorides) and is an abortifacient.[102] Often, the seeds are specified. Several modern animal studies show that the chaste tree does have abortifacient qualities.[103] The flavonoids in one species (*Vitex nehundo* L.) inhibited all (100 percent) implantations in mice at doses of 60 to 120 mg per mouse on days 4 to 6 of pregnancy. If they were administered on days 8 to 10, however, the pregnancy continued in 50 percent of the mice.[104] Even more interesting is a study, published in 1989, that indicates the seeds act on the male reproductive system by disrupting sperm production in adult dogs. The conclusion was that the seeds may "work either as an antiandrogen or as an antagonist of spermatogenesis."[105] Again, there may be a connection with Greek ritual. The switches with which adolescent boys were whipped at the annual flogging at Sparta were probably chaste-tree twigs.[106]

In the light of modern scientific data, we might speculate that during the Thesmophoria festival the chaste tree was required not under the bed but on top of it. As was true of pomegranate and myrrh, knowledge of the chaste tree's antifertility action was passed on through myth, religion, and ritual long before it was recorded in medical writings. The connection is strong: at the festival of Demeter, when woman slept on the chaste tree they also ate pomegranate seeds.[107] As a postscript, Leo the African (ca. 1485–1554), presumably referring to folk beliefs of his time, remarked that the chaste tree was so powerful that when men urinate on its roots, they acquire an erection, and when women do the same, they lose their virginity. For both genders, it seems, the tree is connected to sexual intercourse.[108]

Birthwort

A very ancient depiction of the connection between childbirth and the plant known in English as the "birthwort" is found on an Egyptian vase from the city of Thebes: a woman nursing a baby is portrayed with birthwort leaves in the background. A strand of the climbing birthwort vine also is depicted on a tomb in Thebes. The birthwort or Aristolochiceae family includes *Aristolochia sempervirens* L., *A. clematitis* L., and *A. rotunda* L. In North America birthwort often is called "snake root," for example, *A. serpentaria* L. or Virginia snake root. The reference was not to the plant's climbing, twining characteristics but to its ability to counteract the poisons of snake bites.

The plant may be used today as a cure for snakebite, but that was not the usage suggested in Thebes. Birthwort was taken to ease a difficult childbirth, but it could also prevent the difficulty altogether through its contraceptive or abortive action. There are cases in modern times where birthwort was shown to be effective in humans as a contraceptive[109] and as an abortifacient.[110] In laboratory testing of aristolochic acid, the active substance, a *p*-coumaric acid, was found to be 100 percent effective in blocking pregnancy in mice after a single oral dose (100 mg/kg) on the sixth or seventh day after coitus.[111] There are no toxic side effects.[112] Doses of 20–90 mg/kg were sufficient to block implantation, and a dose of 30 mg/kg interrupted midterm pregnancy.[113]

The ancients knew what the plant would do. Dioscorides said that it could be drunk or placed in a suppository with pepper and myrrh to provoke menstruation or to expel a fetus.[114] Galen put it in a recipe for an oral-route abortifacient.[115] It was also used during the Middle Ages, and a Cairo hospital formulary (ca. 1200) listed it as an ingredient in a pessary to expel a "dead fetus."[116]

Asarum

Very closely connected botanically to birthwort and in the same family is asarum, *Asarum europaeum* L. As we who know the chemistry of plants expect, asarum has similar medicinal qualities to birthwort: it contracepts and aborts. The North American counterpart *(A. canadense)* appears in folk medicine: a recipe made by boiling its roots down and is taken orally as a contraceptive.[117] Without knowledge of chemistry or botany, ancient peoples learned asarum's uses and put it to work. Dioscorides mentioned it as an emmenagogue but said that it was good to administer after childbirth, as birthwort was sometimes employed.[118] Writing in her convent, the Abbess Hildegard of Bingen (d. 1117) said of it: "A pregnant woman will eat it, either on account she languishes or she aborts an infant with a danger to her body or if she has not had a menstrual period for a time period so that it hurts."[119] Interestingly, Serapion the Younger (ca. 1070) placed both asarum and birthwort in the second class of menstrual movers.[120]

The Male Fern for Females

A number of ferns were employed both as contraceptives and abortifacients, more often as the former. Dioscorides named three ferns *(asplenon, thelupteris, agaricon)*, but it is difficult to identify them by their proper scientific names. *Asplenon* is probably *Adiantum capillus veneris* L. or *Asplendium adiantum nigrum* L.; it "causes sterility," as Dioscorides called contraception.[121] The first of the possibilities, the one named by Linnaeus as *capillus veneris*, meaning "hair of love," was found by modern investigators to be an active inhibitor of implantation when taken after coitus.[122]

The fern called *thelupteris* in Greek is the same as the fern called *felix* or *filix* in Latin. It may refer to *Pteris aquilina* L., *Dryopteris filix-mas* (L.) Schott, or, just possibly, both and maybe another species or two as well. Sometimes it is called the "male fern," a term presently applied only to the *Dryopteris*. Dioscorides and al-Rhasis said that it was both a contraceptive and an abortifacient, whereas Pliny noted only its contraceptive effects.[123] A species of the *Pteris* fern is employed in traditional Chinese medicine as a contraceptive.[124] The *Dryopteris* is taken in modern Hungary as a contraceptive.[125] Rats given a dosage of 2–3 mg injected subcutaneously on pregnancy days 7 through 9 experienced 100 percent termination.[126]

The last fern, the one Dioscorides called *agaricon*, is either *Formes officinalis* Bradasola or *Polyporus offficinales* Fries or both. The *Formes* fern is used in New Guinea as both a contraceptive and an abortifacient.[127] Some research indicates that all these ferns have filicic acid, better yet *crude* filicic acid, which may be the active substance.[128] These ferns are distributed over much of Europe and Asia, even in Greenland, so it may not have mattered very much which exact species was being referred to within the range described. Unquestionably, the "male fern" was employed from ancient times through modern times over a wide area, from New Guinea to Hungary to China, as both an abortifacient and a contraceptive.

In the Middle Ages, for example, William of Saliceto called the fern *scolopendrum* and said it was a contraceptive to be given with juniper.[129] Curiously, Hildegard of Bingen called it merely *Farn* (German for "fern") and noted only its use as an amulet for childbirth.[130]

Willow

Often in the history of science, discoveries come about almost simultaneously, enough so that historians have difficulty determining which was first. The modern rediscovery that plants have sex hormones that affect mammals began in 1933, as discussed earlier with reference to the Butenandt-Jacobi article on the date palm. In the same year, before the Polish Academy of Sciences, Boleslaw Skarzynski reported that willow contained a substance (trihydroxyoestrin) that was similar to a female hormone.[131] Subsequent laboratory tests published in 1974 and 1985 confirmed Skarzynski's findings by showing that the estriol interferes with ovulation and implantation.[132]

Before the uncanny feats of the chemists, ancient writers reported what women had long known: that willow bark or leaves prevent conception.[133] Aetius' contraceptive recipe was given in the sixth century: boil willow bark down and drink it "continually" with honey "to temper its bitterness."[134] A later medieval writer, Constantine the African (d. ca. 1085), related only one contraceptive in his book of pharmacy, which was adapted from a earlier work in Arabic: "juice of willow leaves so that a woman will not conceive."[135] Oribasius (fl. 360) suggested combining fern root with willow leaves as a contraceptive to be drunk after coitus.[136]

Willow belongs to the Salicaceae family, the same as another tree, poplar (*Populus alba* L. and other species). Occasionally, older sources named the poplar as having contraceptive qualities also,[137] but no modern testing of poplar has been done. Willow and possibly poplar were contraceptives but, as judged by the frequency of their appearance in the early documents, their use may have been less widespread than that of the other antifertility drugs already mentioned. The eminent physician Galen mentioned willow only in a recipe for stimulating menstruation, and Pliny said only that it depressed sexual desire.[138] Neither Galen nor Pliny was a true expert in what women were doing.

Cypress

Cypress is closely related to juniper. The ancients knew of this relationship pharmaceutically, not botanically. Curiously, ancient sources called cypress a menstrual stimulator (for example, Dioscorides and Oribasius), whereas medieval sources were more direct by calling it an abortifacient (for example, Marbode and William of Saliceto).[139] Modern science has found that it has estrogenic qualities with a number of pharmacologically active coumarins.[140] Paraguayan Indians make a juice by macerating the stalks and roots of the tree and drink the juice every five days.[141] And in Peru the aerial parts are used for birth control.[142]

The Mint Family

"Parsley, sage, rosemary, and thyme"—familiar to us as a line from a song—have more in common than a popular melody. They are culinary herbs, to be sure; they are all members of the mint family; they are all contraceptives and abortifacients. Although they are antifertility agents, probably they are less strong than the herbs discussed earlier. A captain and "whorish" lad in Aretino's sixteenth-century novel, *Dialogues*, said of a woman whose bed he had visited that her ass smelled of mint.[143] It may have, and for two probable reasons: the aromatic enticement and the protection from pregnancy. Of course, we do not know what he meant by "ass," either. Aretino was likely referring to the same thing that Macer did in his late-eleventh-century herbal when he wrote that, if spearmint is "applied to the womb before the coitus, the woman will not conceive."[144]

Sage and pennyroyal, both mints, have been discussed already for their antifertility qualities. One effect that sage, marjoram, thyme, rosemary, and hyssop are known to induce in animal testing is the inhibition of gonadotrophin or prolactin secretion.[145] The term sometimes used is *antigonadotropic.*

The writer of a treatise ascribed to Hippocrates knew the actions of mints and the combinations that were appropriate. He gave one recipe for a "potent uterine abortifacient": "A small handful of mint [*minthe*], rue, coriander [*Coriander sativum* L.], juniper or cypress chips, boiled down in a sweet wine and drunk."[146] This recipe tells us much more than what ingredients were used for birth control; it tells us that the ancients probably made drug substitutes on the basis of similarities in taste and smell.

The "mint" may have been generic mint or some species, such as pennyroyal. If it were corn mint (*Mentha arvensis* L.), for example, its effects would be pronounced. A daily administration of 10 mg/kg from day 7 through day 10 of pregnancy in rats resulted in a 90 to 100 percent loss.[147] In another test also using rats, an alcohol extract of 500 mg of *M. arvensis* was given on days 1 through 7 post-coitus and there was a 100 percent reduction in implantation.[148] In any case, most plants of the mint family have that effect in some proportions, pennyroyal being one of the more effective.

Coriander is not tested or known for being an antifertility agent, but it is a member of the Apiaceae (old umbellifer family), the same as giant fennel (*Ferula*, the ancients' *silphium*), Queen Anne's lace, and celery. As an oral contraceptive celery seed (from *Apium graveolens* L.) is found in a recipe written in the Berlin Papyrus from Egypt's Nineteenth Dynasty (ca. 1300 B.C.E.).[149] From the Hippocratic corpus through the Middle Ages, celery seeds were occasionally found in antifertility recipes. They are employed in various traditional medical systems of India and Africa, but scientific reports are mixed.[150] One test that employed different extract procedures indicated no inhibition of implantation on days 1–7 of pregnancy with a dose amount of 100 mg/kg.[151] Later tests, however, involving a higher dosage (250 mg/kg) and extracts from the whole plant, resulted in a reduction of 33.3 percent of the pregnancies for the same pregnancy periods.[152]

Juniper or cypress chips were mentioned last. Both are members of the same family, Cupressaceae. Thus, this prescription in the Hippocratic work has five plants—"mint," rue, coriander, and either juniper or cypress—from the three families in which most of the antifertility agents appear: mints, cypress, and celeries (Apiaceae). The ancients probably were capable of making associations of like qualities found in species within these families. These similarities, however, were identified on the basis of smell, taste, and effect. The ancients may not have observed the botanical similarities that determine *our* classifications.

3

Ancient and Medieval Beliefs

They [midwives] cause miscarriages if they think them
desirable.

Socrates, quoted by Plato, *Theaetetus*, 149d

Socrates, the barefoot stone cutter from Athens, knew that women had
some control over reproduction. His mother, Phaenarete, was a midwife, so he probably knew more than most men about such matters.
Plato quotes Socrates' conversation with a student, Theaetetus:

SOCRATES: Is it not, then, also more likely and even necessary that
midwives should know better than anyone else who are pregnant and
who are not?
THEAETETUS: Certainly.
SOCRATES: And furthermore the midwives, by means of drugs *(pharmakia)* and incantations *(epadousai)*, are able to arouse the pangs of
labor and, if they wish, to bear who have difficulty in bearing, and
they cause miscarriages if they think them desirable?[1]

Predictably, Theaetetus replied, "True." Socrates' point was made and
understood as true.

Living at the same time as Socrates was Hippocrates, known as the
Founder of Medicine. In *On Generation*, a work attributed to him, there
is this line: "When a woman has intercourse, if she is not going to conceive, then it is her practice to expel the sperm from both partners
whenever she wishes to do so."[2] In this Hippocratic work, there was

no straight man to declare the statement "true." Would a typical man of the time know this, or at least ascribe to women an ability to regulate reproduction?

Ancient beliefs concerning biology and sex are strange to us. Greek males did not accept the testimony of women in court; women were too emotional to ascertain truth objectively. After all, women were imperfectly formed human beings. According to Greek lore, a person's sex was determined by fetal development. Women are the product of weak seed and are, in Aristotle's generalization, "softer, more vicious, less simple, more impulsive."[3] Men formed from good seed are "brilliant in soul and strong in body," according to a Hippocratic writer.[4] Some Greeks, among them Aristotle, believed that women did not have any seed and contributed only nourishment to their offspring. Man's semen is concentrated blood (warm and moist) and composites of all parts of the body (so that it can reproduce all the organs and features). Female bodies attempted but were unable to complete this process: they produced only the menses (cold and dry), for fetal nourishment.

This belief is even more strange: although women were thought to be inferior biologically and psychologically, it was accepted that they determined reproduction and that they did so deliberately. To have or not to have children was a woman's decision: these passages from Plato and Hippocrates say this is the case, and there is nothing in Greek literature to say otherwise. The number of children in a family could be a matter of public policy. Plato said that if too few children were being born for the welfare of the city, incentives or marks of disgrace—carrots and sticks—could be given to encourage more children. This statement may not have been just a theory: during Plato's lifetime, a man was allowed to "have children by another" than his wife, because the Peloponnesian War had so reduced the population.[5] But, if too many were being born, Plato said, "There are many devices available."[6] In the words attributed to Socrates in a different context, the devices were "drugs (*pharmakia*) and incantations."[7] Aristotle spoke similarly but specified only drugs to prevent children "before sense and life have begun in the embryo."[8]

We now know what the drugs were. If we believe Plato and Aristotle on antifertility drugs (and we should), what are we to make of the prescription for "incantations"? To us the drugs are rational, the incantations irrational. In the dialogue *Charmides* Plato explained through Socrates. If one took a certain leaf as a drug (*pharmakon*) to cure a headache, there would be a charm *(epoda)* to go with it. "The remedy made one perfectly well; but without the charm there was no efficacy in the leaf."[9] Charms and incantations affected the soul, whereas the leaf affected the body. Many illnesses were a result of maladies both in the soul and the body, therefore the cure must treat both. These sentiments led an Arabic writer in the tenth century, Qusṭā ibn Lūqā, to adduce that the efficacy of some drugs derived from the *belief* in their efficacy and not from anything intrinsic to the medicine itself. Whether or not Plato recognized the placebo effect the way Qusṭā did is one topic for thought, but let a discussion of that be postponed for now. Our concern is what influence psychological factors might have had on people taking antifertility drugs they perceived as "working"? This was Plato's question in *Charmides*.

Magic, Psychological Factors, and Pregnancy

Full-term pregnancies are neither psychosomatic nor psychological. They are real, and no placebo can alter them. If a woman takes an antifertility drug to prevent conception or to terminate one already thought to exist and she becomes pregnant, she knows that the drug did not work. False, so-called hysterical pregnancies do exist, but although they result in various physical manifestations, including bloated abdomens, none result in childbirth.

Just as there were antifertility agents throughout history, there also were aphrodisiacs and conception stimulators. A study of aphrodisiacs concluded that these agents did not work pharmaceutically, as best we can tell.[10] What effect they had was either psychological or beyond the knowledge of modern science today. In contrast, the conception enhancers present more difficulty. Today there is substantial anecdotal evidence of couples unable to conceive, for no detectable medical reasons, who decide on or complete an adoption only to learn that the woman has become pregnant. For this phenomenon there is no adequate scientific explanation, other than an obvious stress factor—and that explanation really does not provide a mechanism for the action.

The placebo effect is very real in medicine, and it possible that it accounts for much of the positive benefit that ancient peoples received from taking drugs. For that matter, the same effect is still very important today. Just the same, a placebo effect would be discounted entirely by a woman who was relying on a drug to prevent or end pregnancy, if the pregnancy occurred or did not end. In a real way, as real as reality can be, she would know that it had failed if she became or remained pregnant.

Drugs that have come to be known as antifertility agents have been subjected, in modern jargon, to millions of efficacy trials. In the past contraceptives and abortifacients were known for what they could and could not do. No medical writings, no literary or anecdotal references appear in the ancient period as to what we would consider a scientific test of contraceptives. We postulate that they worked because (1) generations in the past were confident about them; (2) reproduction rates show that people were able to influence population increase; (3) modern anthropology studies document that some traditional peoples continue to rely on herbal contraceptives and early-term abortifacients; and, finally (4), scientific studies confirm the antifertility actions of some of the herbs used. For these reasons we believe that the contraceptive and abortifacient drugs did work. But the fact that ancient records also stress the role of magic causes us concern.

Something made of brass "worn on the finger is an abortifacient; if suspended on the neck of a woman she will not conceive while it is worn." Or, "if a woman takes a frog and spits into its open mouth three times, she will not conceive for a year." These were medical recipes of Qusṭā ibn Lūqā.[11] By our accounts, these are examples of magic and superstition. The question we must answer, then, is how we are to distinguish between what *to us* is magic and what *to us* is science. Consider, first, that many ancient medical accounts distinguished between magic and rational medicine and express scorn for things magical. Some learned, classical science writers, Galen and Dioscorides among them, included magic in their discussions. Galen mixed magic and prescriptions in his medical reports—for example, he recorded the use of amulets in pharmaceutical discussions. In contrast, Dioscorides' practice was not to embrace magic but to report it. His method was to begin such reports with phrases like "It is told that . . ." or "Some people say . . ." Thus, he began a report on the hawthorn, "It is told that the property of its roots is such that it causes abortion if [the root is] hit three times on the abdomen or anointed thereon."[12] On the face of it, this is magic.

We must probe deeper. Crategolic acid taken from the hawthorn (*Crataegus oxycantha* L.) is used in modern medicine to treat elderly patients with heart disease and patients with mitral stenosis.[13] The plant depresses respiration, affects the heart, relaxes the uterus and intestines, and constricts the bronchi and coronary artery. Modern Chinese medicine employs it for menstrual problems, primarily for pain associated with menstruation and for postpartum distension.[14] Given such pronounced effects, it is quite possible, although still unknown, that hawthorn root could produce an abortion, even if only because it can be toxic. Likely, too, there would be a systemic action through dermal absorption when anointed on the skin. In other words, today we would accept as true some of the lore about hawthorn that has come to us through the ages, but we would reject accounts of "superstitious" acts, such as hitting the abdomen three times with a hawthorn root to induce abortion.

As might be expected, the earliest record of a contraceptive presents us with the same kind of interpretive problem. The recipe is found in the Kahun Papyrus, which dates to around 1850 B.C.E. but was based on an ancient prototype that may go back to the Old Kingdom, roughly 3000 B.C.E. Prescription Number 21, "Recipe Not to Become Pregnant," calls for crocodile feces to be mixed with fermented dough and, it would appear, inserted into the vagina.[15] Possibly the crocodile feces could alter the chemistry in the womb, or perhaps it mechanically blocked the cervical opening or acted as a spermicide, or . . . We just do not know. Is it relevant that the god associated with abortion is Seth, represented by a crocodile head on ancient Egyptian uterine amulets? There is too much distance, and too many imponderables, for us to judge today whether the Kahun Papyrus recipe is "scientifically plausible" or "religious and/or magical."

A Sumerian tablet that was written earlier than the Kahun Papyrus has only a fragment of what appears to be a recipe for an abortifacient. Unfortunately, the instructions are lost, but the recipe was for a woman who wished to abort her fetus.[16] A cuneiform recipe from Assur gives pomegranate on wool in the uterus for what surely was intended as a contraceptive.[17] These examples attest to the fact that not only the Greeks but also the ancient Egyptians and Sumerians had knowledge of contraception and abortion.

Another reason we may conclude that ancient peoples had what we would consider reliable information about fertility is that they were able to identify certain diseases and toxins as the cause of *inadvertent* reductions in births. Ergot, for example, is a toxin derived from a fungus that grows on various plants, most readily on types of rye. As we shall see in the modern period, it produces chemicals that, if ingested, may cause an abortion. Ancient peoples also knew of its devastating effects. When it contaminated bread supplies, entire communities suffered: besides the toxins that cause various physical symptoms, including miscarriage, ergot produces contains acid, which, like the synthetic LSD, has dramatic psychological effects. Pre-modern populations probably did not deliberately ingest ergot, except possibly in some rituals.[18]

Because ergot flourishes during cold winters, outbreaks of ergotism often follow seasonal patterns. Robert Biggs found passages in cuneiform texts that indicate that ancient peoples, by keeping records of weather conditions, predicted plagues or infestations, as well as recovery periods. A chief characteristic of these periods was miscarriages. A seventh-century (B.C.E.) text foretold: "there will be recovery for sick people in the land, pregnant women will carry their fetuses full term."[19] More ominously: "there will be an epidemic of *li'bu*-disease in the country, pregnant women will not carry their fetuses full term."[20] In Greek literature there are many allusions to a disease of sterility.[21] The lesson here is that, even without the benefit of modern medicine, ancient peoples knew the difference between birth control and unintentional infertility.

In exploring the question of the ancients having effective birth control drugs, however, we come across an ancillary problem. The fact is that some of the same sources where we find drugs that appear reasonably pharmaceutically effective also contain magical and religious formulas.

Some insight into the relationship between magic and medicine may be gained from a cuneiform tablet of the Assyrian period. Sickness that accompanies pregnancy is discussed. Drugs of vegetable origin whose names we cannot translate were heated over a fire and mixed with oil and beer, soaked in a woolen pad, and inserted into the vagina, twice daily. In case this procedure did not work, various magical devices were prescribed.[22]

Our purpose is to evaluate those recipes for which modern scientific knowledge may help us assess efficacy. By not evaluating the magical formulas, I am not discounting the possibility that psychological factors may have affected the body's reproductive system. We know that we do not know all there is to know about reproduction, and we must realize that another day may come when judgments about what appears magical to us now will have a reasonable explanation. Truly, to us, spitting three times into a frog's mouth to prevent conception is irrational. For now nothing more can be said.

The Soul, the Fetus, and Property

The Egyptians believed that a person had two souls, named *ka* and *ba*. *Ba* stayed with the body, even after death, whereas the *ka* departed at life's end and journeyed across the celestial Nile to an uncertain future in an afterlife. *Ka*'s position in the afterlife is strengthened if the *ba* remains intact, hence the importance in Egyptian custom of preserving the body. But what about when life begins? When did the *ba* and *ka* begin?

From all indications, the ancient peoples of West Asia and Egypt believed that life began at birth. There is not even a hint that the ancients regarded a fetus as a human persona. Quite the contrary. In fact, the property rights of a fetus were recognized and ascribed to the father of the family. A Sumerian law (ca. 1800 B.C.E.) reads:

> If (a man accidentally) buffeted a woman of free-citizen class and caused her to have a miscarriage, he must pay ten shekels of silver. If (a man deliberately) struck a woman of free-citizen class and caused her to have a miscarriage, he must pay one-third mina of silver.[23]

One-third mina is twice the value of ten shekels, thus a deliberate act is a doubly egregious offense. Hammurabi's laws (1728–1686 B.C.E.) permitted the same recovery (ten shekels) for one causing a miscarriage, and five shekels for a commoner's daughter. If a slave's owner caused a slave to lose a fetus through a miscarriage, he was fined two shekels.[24]

According to Middle Assyrian law, a citizen who caused a wife of another citizen to miscarry would be required to give up a fetus (thereby indicating, incidentally, that a miscarriage can be deliberately induced). If the blow was fatal to the woman (and not to the fetus), the penalty was death to the perpetrator.[25] When the husband of the woman who loses a fetus because of a blow has no son, then the deliverer of the blow will forfeit his life regardless of the gender of the fetus.[26] This provision clearly indicates that what is being protected is not the fetus or the woman but the male's right to have a child.

A later Assyrian law prescribed a penalty of impalement to a woman for procuring her own abortion.[27] Unstated is who would bring claim, but, from our understanding of later laws and practices, it is clear that what the law protected was the asserted right of the husband to receive a child he sired.[28]

Sumerian, Lipit-ištar, and Middle Assyrian laws maintain the same principles as those in the Hammurabic code (except that the penalty in the Middle Assyrian law is death for taking the life of a fetus by delivering a blow to the mother).[29] The latter is the only law that could be said to protect the fetus itself, but that interpretation would be inconsistent with the practice of exposure or infanticide. A deformed, abnormal, or even unwanted child could be killed without legal sanction. The law's purpose may have been to protect a community from being robbed of a healthy child.[30] More likely, the laws protected a male's right to have a child he sired.

A Hittite law made another distinction, one that will underlie later law: the fine for causing a miscarriage after the fifth month of pregnancy is five shekels of silver but if the fetus is lost during the tenth month the fine is twenty shekels.[31] The Hittite principle acknowledges two principles that will last for thousands of years: (1) there are progressive stages of fetal development, with more value placed on the about-to-be born than the long-to-be born; (2) no crime or infraction is committed if a pregnancy is terminated earlier than five months. One can easily imagine (because the court records themselves do not exist to confirm) the contentions in the law courts over which stage of pregnancy had been reached. Not only was the monetary fine based on its determination, but also there was the need to determine whether a crime was committed in the first place.

Hebrew Ideals and Practices

Hebrew religious laws have guiding principles similar to those of other cultures in western Asia. Hebrew religion categorically rejected prostitution, temple or otherwise,[32] and it offered little protection to the fetus itself, and then not for its own sake. Exodus 21:22 says that "If two men fight, and they hurt a woman with child and her child comes out and yet no harm *('āsôn)* ensues, he [the one causing the blow] will be seized by the woman's husband and [brought before the judges] forced to pay a fine as the judges determine." The usual interpretation is that this passage embodies the same principle as that which prevailed in Babylonian and other ancient legal traditions. Because the harm (*'āsôn*) to the woman was not great, the penalty is not very severe. There was no protection of the fetus. The male was robbed of a child, thus an appropriate fine was levied.[33]

Some modern scholars have advanced the idea that because the blow (in Exodus 21:22) did not injure the baby (though it arrived prematurely), the harm was not great.[34] This interpretation is entirely modern and contrary to ancient practices throughout the Mediterranean world. Nothing in the Hebrew language or mores leads us to assume that a premature but healthy birth was implied. A passage in the *Mishnah Oholoth* (7:6) deals with dismemberment of a fetus during in a breech birth; it permits the procedure provided the fetus has not over half emerged and disallows the procedure if it has.[35] The fetus was recognized as being protected for its sake at birth, not prior to it, in a fairly precise way. In a number of places the Talmud refers to the fetus as *ubar yerekh imo* ("part of the mother"), in the same meaning as the Latin *pars viscerum matris*.[36]

The next passage is clearer. Exodus 21:23 addresses the situation where a woman is harmed and loses her fetus: "If harm follows, then you shall give life for life, foot for foot, burn for burn, wound for wound, stripe for stripe." A transgression or harm has occurred, but the harm was to the woman. Still the passage reads "life [in Hebrew, *nefesh*] for life." Could this statement declare that the fetus has a life, that of a human, as some modern scholars have argued?[37] The position those scholars hold is without precedent in ancient thought.

When taken in the context of Hebrew and other contemporary cultures, the argument that Exodus 22:21–25 represented a recognition of human life before birth is not tenable.[38] The fetus is not "a viable, living thing" (in Hebrew, *bar kayyama*).[39] The Exodus passage did not apply to homicide, because homicide means killing a *person*, not a fetus.[40] If the harm done to the woman was fatal, then "life for life." As in Babylonian law, deliberate abortion in the Old Testament is not mentioned, only injury by a third party resulting once again in a man being denied progeny he sired. And, in keeping with the same principles, no compensation is due the women injured. Hebrew law protected the family and the position of the father as its ruling head. According to Talmudic interpretation, the fetus was the property of the father.[41]

The very fact that none of the ancient codes mention a deliberate abortion performed by a woman on herself argues that the act was not illegal. A fetus who is threatening the life of a mother during childbirth may be dismembered until which time as its head emerges, so said the Talmud.[42] The implication is clear: the fetus is not a person until birth. Because the evidence is certain that abortifacient drugs were known to the ancients, and because in some circumstances a third party was held responsible for administering them, one would have to be naive in the extreme to believe that women did not take these drugs to end a pregnancy (as defined by our age).

Be Fruitful and Multiply

In the words of John Noonan, the Hebrews had a "mistrust of sex."[43] There was God's injunction: "increase and multiply; fill the earth" (Genesis 1:27–28). The Talmud (*Yevamot* 63b) and Mishnah (*Yevamot* 6:6) amplify the meaning.[44] Many scriptural passages advance pronatal positions.[45] Sexual intercourse had a purpose, and that was procreation; sex was not intended for satisfying lusts, although mutual pleasure was an acceptable motive among married couples.[46]

While there is no mention of intentional abortion or contraception in the Old Testament, both practices are in the Talmud, Tosefta, and Mishnah. Both were acceptable in some situations according to rabbinical writings.[47] An important Talmudic statement delineated the acceptable circumstances for contraception in the "*Baraita* of the Three Women":

Three [categories of] women may use an absorbent *(mokh)* in their marital intercourse: a minor, a pregnant woman and a nursing woman. The minor, because [otherwise] she might become pregnant and as a result might die. A pregnant woman because [otherwise] she might cause her fetus to become a *sandal* [a flat, fish-shaped abortion due to superfetation]. A nursing woman, because [otherwise] she might have to wean her child prematurely [owing to her second conception], and he would die. And what is a minor: From the age of eleven years and one day. One who is under [this age when conception is not possible] or over this age [when pregnancy involves no fatal consequences] must carry on her marital intercourse in the usual manner.[48]

The "absorbent" was hackled wool or flax used as a pessary, similar, I presume, to those pessaries mentioned in the Egyptian papyri.[49] Rabbinic opinion differed on whether the three examples were an exclusive and exhaustive list of the conditions for permissible contraception or merely illustrations. In the sixteenth century Rabbi Solomon Luria interpreted the passage as meaning a woman could use a contraceptive pessary if pregnancy would be dangerous.[50]

A more controversial interpretation is made of another mention of *mokh*, the pessary, in this instance a Talmudic passage on preventing pregnancy (*Niddah* 3a–b).[51] In a discussion of the exact beginning of the period of impurity (onset of menstruation as detected by the presence of menstrual blood), the question arose as to what happens if absorption by a *mokh* delays by days the perception of impurity. In this context the presumption is that use of the contraceptive pessary was routine.

The Talmud also has passages that speak of "root medicines" that cause sterility. The Hebrew *'qr*, meaning sterility, is the equivalent of the Latin *sterilis* (adjective) or *sterilitas* (noun). In the Babylonian Talmud, a woman inquired whether she could take a root poison to prevent having a child. Rabbi Hiyya replied that God's injunction to be fruitful applied to men but, because men were the aggressors in sexual union, the charge did not apply to women.[52] The Tosefta says, "A man is not permitted to drink a cup of roots *(ikarin)* in order not to beget, and a woman is not permitted to drink a cup of roots *(ikarim)* in order not to give birth."[53]

Not surprisingly, Jewish rabbinic opinion was divided on this issue. Rabbi Johana ben Beroka asserted that God's injunction applied to both sexes.[54] The Mishnah added a different perspective: a man was excused from propagation after "he already has children." One rabbi said that the Mishnah meant two male children, another, a boy and a girl. Maimonides and Caro interpreted the passage as a reference to roots that would cause permanent sterility, not temporary; in other words, a male could not be excused for a life from his responsibility to propagate the race.[55]

Explicit in these passages is the notion that males could continue sexual unions but that they too could practice birth control. How? The only clear reference is to root drugs for males and females. One male contraceptive was specified in the classical medical literature: the seeds of a plant called *periklymenon* are drunk by men who become sterile, according to Dioscorides.[56] The problem is that we cannot identify the plant. Later, in the Renaissance, Dioscorides' Greek plant name was identified as honeysuckle (*Locerna periclymenun* L.), but there is doubt that the translation is correct. Medieval sources do not continue a tradition for male antifertility agents, so what began in antiquity ended there, as best we can learn. Earlier, I mentioned that the chaste tree that was used for antifertility purposes has an effect on male dogs, but there is no evidence that men took it for that purpose.

The real identity of the root drugs mentioned in the Hebrew sources is not known, but some clues are provided. The possession of antifertility drugs is confirmed by a passage in the Book of Jasher (*Sefer ha Yashar*, "The Book of Righteousness"), a Jewish account of the Creation composed in the thirteenth century. A recounting of the generations that came from Canaan (based on Midrash Genesis Rabba 23:3 explaining Genesis 4:19–22) contains this passage:

> And they gave some of their wives to drink a potion of barrenness, in order that they might retain their figures and *whereby* their beautiful appearance might not fade.[57]

This is startling. Here it is confirmed that the oral drugs were used for birth control, and also that occasionally the purpose was cosmetic, not merely for family planning. Such actions were disapproved in the Book of Jasher, and implicitly in Talmudic commentaries, but there was no absolute prohibition of birth control. The reasons for these traditions were all-important. No one can read the Hebrew accounts and believe that contraception and abortion were encouraged, but neither were they banned altogether. There were circumstances in which each was appropriate.

The Greeks on Birth Control

The ancient Greeks were at least as receptive to birth control as the peoples of ancient Egypt and West Asia. The records of the Greeks' thinking are more abundant than those of earlier peoples of antiquity. Some Greeks advocated the rational ordering of family size, although the only city-state known to enact actual policies was Sparta, which pressed hard for pro-natal goals. A woman in Plato's ideal city would be permitted to bear children during the twentieth through fortieth years of her life.[58] Hesiod advised fathers to have only one son lest the family's property be divided beyond its capacity over succeeding generations.[59] These passages show that family planning was an accepted idea.

A Greek man had the power to declare the legitimacy of a child on his own. If he accepted the child (usually within a week of birth), the child was made a member of the family and community by the ceremony known as *amphidromia*. We suppose that the Greeks "exposed" a fair number of babies for reasons varying from illegitimacy, frailty, or deformity to the inability of a family to care for it.[60] Some, perhaps many, of these children were not literally wasted on the mountainsides but sold or given away. Slavery was common, after all, and one source of slaves was exposed children. Aelian, however, records one Theban law that prohibits a father from exposing a child, but the same law provides a mechanism by which a magistrate can sell a deformed child.[61]

How widespread was the practice of exposure? The answer is debated by scholars, but the skeletal evidence presented in the first chapter indicates that the declining population of the Hellenic world was due to one factor: women were having fewer babies. They were not exposing them, they were simply not having as many. Finally, there is the contrast with the Middle Ages, when infanticide was strictly forbidden; records show that the practice was rare.[62] Yet the same phenomenon as in classical Greek times was present in medieval Europe— stable or declining birth rates.

Greek medical texts contain specific information about how to induce an abortion.[63] In a case history of an abortion recorded in a Hippocratic treatise, a physician is called to the wife of Simon after she had "drunk something, or it was spontaneous?"[64] Implicitly, abortions were women's secrets, the physician dealing only with those that went awry.[65]

In addition to the texts, Greek surgical instrument for abortion have survived.[66] The Christian Church Father Tertullian accused Hippocrates of possessing one of the brutal instruments designed to dismember a fetus in a breech birth.[67] Although no surviving Hippocratic treatise has instructions on this procedure, it was performed in those years to save the life of the mother.

One Hippocratic work, *Nature of the Child*, describes the procedure of abortion by manipulation (if this is the correct word), or the so-called Lacedamonian leap in the case of a six-day-old embryo: "jump up and down, touching her buttocks with her heels at each leap [for] ... seven times"; after this, "there was a noise; the seed fell out on the ground" ... "as though someone had removed the shell from a raw egg."[68] Aristotle said that induced abortion was a means "to limit the size of each family ... if children are then conceived in excess of the limit so fixed."[69]

The Greek medical concept of the "wandering uterus" may have increased birth rates, at least to the extent that women believed the male physicians who told them that cramping and other troubles were caused by the womb moving around in the abdominal cavity. The condition was relieved by intercourse and pregnancy.[70] All of the evidence makes it certain that the Greeks practiced abortion and that little restricted it.[71] A statement in Roman times, falsely attributed to Galen, claims that the early lawmakers of Sparta and Athens, Lycurgus and Solon, had laws that protected the fetus.[72] The statement is an invention, perhaps a Christian one.[73] Also, Lysias ("On Abortion") records a legal case in which a man named Antigene accuses his wife of "homicide, the woman having voluntarily aborted, and he says that she had, by aborting, impeded his being called the father of a son."[74] Even though the act was called homicide, it is clear from the short fragment of the discourse that it was not the fetus's right to life that was at stake but Antigene's right to have a son. Nancy Demand, who studies ancient Greek women, concludes, "The issue is not the sanctity of life or the rights of the fetus, but the rights of the (lawfully married) father."[75] Again, the same principle is operative among the Greeks that existed among the cultures of West Asia and Egypt. Slowly, other considerations entered the human picture.

The Soul and the Fetus

Three conceptional changes took place over hundreds of years that led to the question about the fetus and the soul. First, the Greeks developed the concept of the soul; second, the question arose as to whether the fetus had "life"; third, the Greek translation of Exodus 21:22–23 took on an added meaning that implied that the fetus had a soul at some point in its development.

Like the Egyptians, the Greeks believed that people had a soul (*psychē*). The word is used once by Homer (*Odyssey* 14.426): when a pig was killed, "*psychē* left it."[76] Homer did not mean that the swine went to pig heaven; he meant that "life left it," as in the early meaning of the word. Gradually, Greek philosophers altered the meaning. According to Plato, the soul was an incorporeal substance that moved the body.[77] In addition to the soul there is the spirit, which has the power to animate the body. The physical spirit *(pneuma physicon)* is made in the heart from the nutriments received by the liver from the small intestine and carried from there in the pulsating veins or arteries. The spirit in the liver is called the "vital spirit" *(pneuma zōtikon)*. Some of the animal spirit is taken from the heart to the brain, where there is a substantial transformation into the psychical spirit *(pneuma psychikon)*.[78]

Aristotle made two observations on the soul, one of which was of critical importance historically, the other ignored by history. We have already discussed his observation that the fetus develops *psychē*, meaning "life" in the old sense of the word, after it has assumed human form. The ancients, Aristotle possibly among them, said that the "life" comes to a male fetus about forty days after conception and to a female after ninety days.[79] The gender differential apparently was based in part on some conventional wisdom of the ancients, because it is reflected in Leviticus 12:1–5. Aristotle knew a fetus had life prior to birth because an accident or a caesarean could bring forth a live infant before the natural time was up. Thus, life occurred prior to delivery, the discerning ancients concluded.

When prior to birth did life begin? Aristotle's hint that a male fetus has life after forty days and a female fetus after ninety days is the answer that survived through the succeeding ages. It survived because it was believed. But elsewhere in his work Aristotle said that animals develop "by such small steps that, because of the continuity, we fail to see to which side the boundary and the middle between them belongs."[80] On this point he was not believed, until the development of modern embryology was made possible by the microscope. So Aristotle was on both sides of what was later to become a crucial debate: on the one hand, he pointed to a dividing line, albeit different for males and females, marking the point at which "animation" occurs; on the other, he said there was only incremental or gradual development from seed to personhood.

The course of history would have been different, perhaps, had not the Stoics changed the meaning of *psychē*. The Greek poet Pindar spoke of the *psychē* as being non-material and immortal.[81] Gradually, the philosophers broadened the meaning of the term from its original sense of "life" to "life and consciousness."[82] The Stoic philosophers held that life and consciousness come at birth with the first breath of cold air. The Greek language accounts for these associations: *psychē* for "life/soul" is related to *psycha*, meaning "cool"; *psychos*, meaning "cold" or "winter"; and *psychō*, meaning "breathe" or "blow." The Stoics were aware of the biology of fetal development, and so they asserted that the potential for life, not life itself but its capacity, began with conception.

As used by the Stoics and later philosophers, *psychē* came to mean "soul," that which is non-material and survives after death. Later medical writers were concerned about where the "soul" resided in the body. Galen asserted that the soul's psychic functions were controlled by the brain.[83] The soul (in Latin, *anima*) survives death and is immortal; the spirit (or *spiritus*) perishes with the body.

The Septuagint and the Two-Staged Fetus

After the conquests of Alexander the Great, there were more Greeks living in Alexandria in Egypt than in any city on the Greek mainland. Alexandria also had more Jews than did Jerusalem. Here, in a city far from Palestine, Hebrew came less and less to be learned by the young. Alexandrian Jews spoke only Greek, so there was a need for a Greek translation of the religious writings, the "Bible" as it was later to be called by Christians, if they were to learn their religious legacy. During the third century, seventy scholars—hence the name "Septuagint"—made a translation so that the works of Moses and the songs of David could be recited and sung in Greek. In respect to birth control, the translators—intentionally or unwittingly—added to the Hebrew meaning in a way that altered history. Exodus 21:22–23 was translated to mean (with italics added for emphasis):

> If two men fight and they strike a woman who is pregnant, and her child comes out *while not fully formed*, he will be forced to pay a fine; ... But *if it is fully formed*, he will give life *[psychē]* for life, eye for eye ...

In the Greek, the passage is far different from the Hebrew. In the Septuagint translation a distinction is made between a "formed" fetus and an "unformed" fetus, the same as that made by Aristotle. The idea was added to the Hebrew text by the Greek translators. And the new meaning had another subtlety. The Greek word selected for the Hebrew word *nefesh*, meaning "life," was *psychē*. We have seen how that early meaning of *psychē* was "life," but, by the third century B.C.E., *psychē* also meant "soul." The implication to those who read the passage in Greek was that the formed fetus had a soul, and anyone causing the death of a fully formed fetus was guilty of killing something with a soul; therefore, the deed was a homicide. Aristotle had expressed what must have been a common attitude among the ancients, the Greeks among them. Another example is an inscription found at Cyrene (dating 331–326 B.C.E.) declaring that a woman who aborted a fetus with distinct features has incurred an impurity whereas a woman who aborted one whose features were indistinct or unformed incurred no pollution.[84]

Writing in commentary to the Exodus passage, Philo of Alexandria (25 B.C.E.–41 A.C.E.) said that "if the fetus already shaped and all the limbs have their proper qualities, he [who delivered the blow] must die." If the fetus is not yet formed, then a lesser crime has been committed, because the person who strikes the blow has deprived nature of bringing a human being into existence.[85]

Philo's views were more Hellenistic than Jewish and do not represent all Jewish thought in the Hellenistic and Roman world.[86] For instance, Josephus, the Jewish historian, expressed two contradictory opinions on the Exodus passage. Reading the Hebrew, not the Greek, he concentrated on the Hebrew '*āsôn* for "harm" and argued that the meaning applied to the woman, not the fetus. If the woman was not harmed, there was harm done in depriving society of another person, and a fine would be assessed. If the woman was fatally harmed from the blow, the crime was punishable by death.[87] This much he wrote in his history.

In another work on Judaism, Josephus wrote: "The Law orders all of the offspring to be brought up and forbids women either to abort or to do away with a fetus, but if she is convicted, she is viewed [as guilty of] an infanticide because she destroys a soul and diminishes the race."[88] This last statement shows that Josephus' views were clearly influenced by the Greek translation.

Pagan, Christian, and Judaic Views Altered

In the period between approximately 300 B.C.E. and 200 A.C.E., there were changes in the attitudes of some toward birth control, albeit not dramatic ones. Prior to then, the evidence is clear that birth control was acceptable so long as a man's asserted right to have a child sired in wedlock was protected. A Greek inscription dated in the first century B.C.E. above a sanctuary in Lydia (North Africa) infers that those who "employ or advise others" to use "love-charms *(philtron)*, abortives *(phthoreion)*, contraceptives *(atokeion)*, or other means of infanticide" are "polluted." The implied methods here are drugs and not surgical procedures. The practitioners of this cult regarded any restraint or interference with the reproductive processes as religiously wrong.[89] Already discussed was the modification to the Hippocratic Oath, which, by the first century A.C.E., was interpreted to prohibit all abortions, not merely abortive pessaries. Whoever modified the oath, whenever he lived, was a pagan Greek, because this version of the oath is still taken to Apollo and other Hellenic pagan deities. Before Christianity and seemingly separate from the tradition of the Stoic philosophers, some minorities in the Greek communities came to regard sexual activity with more distrust and birth control as wrong.

The changed pagan attitude toward birth control is thoughtfully expressed by the philosopher Porphyry (d. ca. 305 A.C.E.) in a letter to his friend, Gauros:

> The doctrine relating to the entry of souls into bodies in view of the production of a living being has filled us with an extreme uncertainty . . . Well then, supposing one has shown that the embryo is neither a living thing in reality . . . nor a living thing in potentiality [i.e., having the soul within, awaiting "activation"], then it becomes easy . . . to establish the entry of the soul and the precise moment of that entry: namely that which must happen after the child is born outside the womb. On the other hand, if the embryo is potentially a living thing, in the sense that it has received the soul, or, moreover, if it is not at least without a great deal of mistrust that one will accept this moment . . . so that should the occasion arise, one should note with precision what it was. For one may well define it as that moment when the sperm has been injected into the womb, as if the sperm could not be retained in the womb and become fertile unless the soul having come from the outside had been realized . . . Or one may place

the moment of the entry of the soul at the first formation of the embryo ... or one may assign the entry to the moment at which the
embryo has begun to move.[90]

In revealing his thoughts about birth control to his friend, Porphyry
raised some questions for the first time in the surviving records. In this
he was ahead of his time. In the centuries ahead new mystic religions
would arise and the Roman Empire would decline and fall, and the answers to the questions he posed were a long time in the making. This
early example, however, is a sign that at the beginning of the Christian era some pagans were beginning to change their thoughts about
the nature of fetal life. And, as we shall see, the question was an issue
of importance among some early Christians.[91]

Christian Views on Birth Control

The nuances of Paul, the zeal of Tertullian, and the sagacity of Clement
need not be explored in detail here in respect to sexuality and birth
control.[92] The Christians took the lessons attributed to Jesus and mixed
them with ideas from the Stoics to arrive at beliefs not much different
from prevailing Judaic, Hellenic, and Roman values. Some statements
by the Christians indicate that they did not approve of drugs employed
for birth control.

In Galatians 5:20 Paul provides us with a list of sins of the flesh, and
among them is the sin of *pharmakeia*, often translated into English as
"sorcery" or "magic" (as we shall see in Chapter 4). This is the same
word that Socrates through Plato had used in reference to birth control: "drugs *(pharmakia)* and incantations."[93] Revelation 9:21, 21:8, and
22.15 denounce those who employ *pharmakon*, translated "magic,"
"sorcery," or "drug."

There is likely a direct connection between the *pharmakia* of the New
Testament and the "root poisons" of Hebrew literature. In the *Didache*,
or *Teaching of the Twelve Apostles*, (5:1), *pharmakia* is a sin labeled "Way
of Death," one of several loathsome things done by "murderers of children" (*Didache* 5:2).[94] The *Epistle of Barnabas* (20:1) speaks of the Way
of the Black One, who uses "things that destroy their soul *(psychē)*: ...
pharmakeia," and condemns those who are "murderers of children"
(20:2). The same work placed the abortion issue within the context of

loving one's neighbors: "Love your neighbor more than yourself. Do not kill a fetus by abortion, or commit infanticide" (19:5). The *Apocalypse of Peter* (26) spoke unfavorably about those women who "produced children outside marriage and who procured abortions." The *Gospel According to Egyptian* has Salome saying: "I will have done better had I never given birth to a child." To her the Lord replied: "Eat of every plant, but do not eat a plant whose content is bitter."[95] Since many birth control plants are bitter, among them artemisia and willow bark, the obvious inference is that God prohibited birth control drugs in this unaccepted Gospel. These passages indicate that among some Christians there had developed a notion that the fetus should be protected and that abortion, at any point, was religiously wrong.[96]

In Elvira (now in Spain), a church synod was held in the year 309. This was just after the Diocletian persecutions, and one would expect the Christians assembled from around Spain to be most concerned with political issues, as the Church was moving toward victory over the pagans. As judged by the number of synodal resolutions, however, the primary concern was sexuality. Sexual behavior was a focus of attention because it was a means by which the Church, at least in Spain, sought control and definition.[97] All sexual activity outside of marriage was forbidden and in marriage discouraged. In numerous synodal acts abortion was regarded as a sin without forgiveness, but contraception was not mentioned in the acts.[98] No means were stated for birth control and, when sexual acts were discussed, the point of view was that of the male.

Four Christians of the second and third century who were very much opposed to both abortion and contraception were Athenagoras, Marcus Minucius Felix, Tertullian, and Clement. In relating their attitudes, they left a record of antifertility methods. All but Athenagoras revealed the means by which birth control was accomplished. And Athenagoras asserted unambiguously that abortions were homicides and that the fetus should not be regarded as an animal, stopping just short of saying it was a person:

> How can we kill a man when we are those who say that all who use abortifacients are homicides and will account to God for their abortions as for the killing of men. For the fetus in the womb is not an animal, and it is God's providence that he exist.[99]

Minucius contrasted Christian women with pagan women who "by drinking drugs extinguish the beginning of a future man, and, before they bear, commit parricide [i.e., the murder of one's father]."[100] Tertullian said that "we [Christians] may not destroy even the fetus in the womb."[101] In the same vein Clement denounced women "who, in order to hide their immorality, use abortive drugs which expel the matter completely dead, abort at the same time their human feelings."[102] Tertullian may have been the first Christian writer who connected abortion with the Scriptures.[103] He cites God's words to Jeremiah (1:4): "Before I formed you in the womb I knew you." To which Tertullian rhetorically asks, "Was it, then, a dead body at that early stage? Certainly not. For God is not the God of the dead, but of living."[104]

Irrespective of Tertullian and Clement, Augustine of Hippo was the Church Father who handed down most later Church interpretations regarding abortion. In elucidating Exodus 21:22, Augustine wrote:

> If what is brought forth is unformed *(informe)*, but at this stage some sort of living, shapeless thing *(informiter)*, then the law of homicide would not apply, for it could not be said that there was a living soul in that body, for it lacks all sense, if it be such as is not yet formed *(nondum formata)* and therefore not yet endowed with its senses."[105]

The Greek Church Father Gregory of Nyssa (ca. 330–395) expressed similar sentiments.[106] Augustine and Gregory shared the same view as held by Aristotle and central Jewish thought.[107]

Augustine and Gregory set the prevailing opinion on abortion, but other voices arose among the Christians. Basel (ca. 330–379) spoke harshly against women who "destroyed a fetus" . . . "whether the fetus was formed or unformed." Such women have sinned doubly; first, they risk their own lives and, second, they rob the fetus of life to come.[108] The observation that abortion was fatal to a person-in-the-making raises the question of whether Basel was primarily referring to late-term, surgical abortions. Most of the written evidence does not indicate that early-term drug abortions were potentially dangerous, much less fatal. Even though he said that abortion was the equivalent of murder, he mitigated the penance required of the sinner because it ought not extend to death. Roughly ten years' repentance was appropriate, although "the manner of repentance" was more important than the time of the term.[109]

Roman Attitudes toward Birth Control

If the Hebrews viewed sexuality with distrust, the Romans regarded it "with some anxiety."[110] The image of the Roman family permeated the ancient Romans' view of themselves. Even though women could marry shortly after menarche,[111] Roman women managed to have fewer children than one would expect, considering that the life span probably extended to the age of menopause. Tombstone inscriptions show that families typically had one or two children. A large family with three or more children was rare.[112] Some modern historians believe that, in the first century of our era, a shift in attitudes occurred that idealized the marriage partner as a source of affection. Prior to then and to some extent afterwards, marriage was valued for procreation.[113]

The question has to be raised: why, if marriage was for children, did the Romans fail so miserably in living up to their ideals? In 131 B.C.E. Metellus Macedonius may have proposed making marriage compulsory.[114] He was reflecting the same sentiments as Polybius, the Greek historian, who was in Rome earlier and who lamented that Greek city-states were declining in population. Families produced only one or two children, he said.[115]

About a century after Metellus' proposal (which was never enacted), Roman lawyers revived a "law of Romulus," the legendary founder of the city, that forbade exposure of sons and first daughters.[116] Our judgment today is that this law was not a revival, as proclaimed, but an invention probably of the first century B.C.E. Invention or not, the alleged law demonstrates more a concern that patriotic Romans had for population size and less a concern for children as children. Were the concern for children, it would be for all of them, including daughters after the first.

Through the Senate, Augustus Caesar (31 B.C.E.–14 A.C.E.) enacted a number of measures designed to encourage family life and increase family size. They included laws against adultery, incentives for widows to remarry, "sin" taxes on bachelors thirty years and older, and incentives for fathers of three or more children. The laws' success was limited, to say the least. By the second century, Roman emperors, alarmed that the hordes of barbarians on the frontier would overrun the Romans facing them, devised elaborate public welfare schemes to encourage families to raise children. To encourage child-rearing they offered "alimentary payments, named after the word for bread or grain.

Monthly allowances for children in the town of Veleia about the year 100 were as follows:

16 sestrices per male born in wedlock;
12 sestrices per male born out of wedlock;
12 sestrices per female born in wedlock;
12 sestrices per female born out of wedlock.[117]

The amounts of money were small and approximate the cost of raising a child. The differences due to wedlock and gender were values of the age. The need for more population was recognized as a matter of self-interest. One way or another, most of the factors that caused the fall of the Roman Empire in the West were related to a decline in population, especially relative to the Germans and Goths, and the attendant repercussions in the economic and social domains.[118] The government had less revenue and fewer soldiers. Increased burdens were placed on citizens to maintain support for the government and its defenses. Agricultural estates tended to become self-sufficient, which weakened their ties to central authority. There were too few Romans facing too many Germans and Goths, Picts, and Persians.

Musonius Rufus (ca. 30–100 A.C.E.) observed that the Augustan legislation was enacted because the lawmakers believed that small families hurt the city and large ones helped it. "Therefore," he wrote, "they forbade the women to abort and attached a penalty to those who disobeyed; secondly, they forbade them to use contraceptives on themselves and to prevent pregnancy."[119] Musonius Rufus was wrong, because the legislation did not prohibit contraceptives or abortifacients. But his words are important because it reveals the assumption that the laws had done so. He likely reasoned as follows: There were too few children, and the legislators recognized this problem. Contraceptives and abortifacients were the means that families used to limit size; therefore, the legislators forbade their use. Writing about the same time as Musonius, Juvenal said that "we've so many sure-fire drugs (*medicamina*) for contraception or killing an embryo."[120] The poet Lucretius wrote of a woman who "forbids herself to conceive."[121]

Whether it is literary works with chance anecdotal evidence or the medical writings with more precise information, the message is always the same. Whenever the means to limit population were either specified or indicated, drugs were named for birth control. We must admit, therefore, that drugs must have been the primary means. Jerome, the Latin Church Father, spoke plainly by condemning those who "drink sterility [*sterilitas*] and murder those not yet conceived," while others use poison to destroy those yet to be born.[122] Jerome's sterility drinks and poisons are direct descendants of the roots and drinks named in the Talmud and the Bible. These drugs were the same that Juvenal boasted of as being so sure and reliable.

Roman Law on Abortion

Neither Roman nor later medieval law regulated contraception. Abortion was different in the eyes of legislators, but the same principles held from the more ancient civilizations: the right of the father to have a child was protected. Nowhere in Roman law is there a hint that the fetus itself was protected. Only those who lived were protected by law, and a fetus was not yet a person in law. In the late second or early third century, Roman law modified a principle that afforded protection for women who were victims of either maleficent or beneficent abortions. The celebrated jurist Paulus stated the principle as follows:

> Those who administer a beverage for the purpose of producing abortion, or of causing affection, although they may not do so with malicious intent, still, because their act offers a bad example, shall, if of humble rank, be sent to the mines; or, if higher in degree, shall be relegated to an island, with the loss of a portion of their property. If a man or woman should lose his or her life through such an act, the guilty party shall undergo the extreme penalty.[123]

First, note that, once again, the means specified was a drink. Furthermore, it is clear from this quote that the drugs were not always safe. Although the possibility of harm is not mentioned in the medical literature of the time, we know both from sources like these and from modern knowledge of the toxicity of some of these drugs that some deaths were caused by antifertility drugs.

Second, what, one might ask, recourse was available to women and husbands or fathers when harm resulted to the women from abortionists who employed surgical or manipulative procedures not covered by this law? We assume that surgical abortions were employed and that they were, as always, perilous in the late term, when drugs were less effective. Presumably a general suit for malpractice was an available redress, but it is not mentioned in this law.

Third, the law was prohibiting both abortifacients and aphrodisiacs and applied to both women and men. The intent of the drug administrator was irrelevant, because the crime was committed whenever the harm was done. It would be literally true that one who administered antifertility measures to a male would have similar liability, but it is not clear whether male contraception was practiced.

Finally, the law provided recourse neither for a self- administered birth control drug that resulted in harm nor for the result when a husband administered the drug. A woman was prohibited from denying a child,[124] but for a woman to be blamed for an abortion the pregnancy would have to have been visible. There was no practical way that the court could probe that an early-term pregnancy had ended.

The Middle Ages and Birth Control

"Have you drunk any *maleficium*, that is herbs or other agents, so that you could not have children?" This question was asked in early medieval penitentials during confession.[125] If the woman (assuming it was a woman) answered affirmatively, she was directed to do penance for forty days. Most legal codes of the early Middle Ages adopted the Roman principles concerning abortion and did not mention contraception, but there were a few significant modifications. Late Roman law made infanticide a criminal offense.[126]

Some recognition was given to the fetus, not as a person but as a value. A Merovingian law (ca. 590) assessed a fine of 700 *solidi* for administering a substance that resulted in a woman's death and a fine of 200 *solidi* if the fetus was killed.[127] An Allemanian law of about the same time levied a fine for killing a fetus that increased with the stage of development. If the sex of the fetus was recognizable (corresponding to Aristotle's "formed fetus"), the fine was double that for the killing of a fetus with unrecognizable features.[128] Astronomy contributed to the medieval notion of staged fetal development. During each period of gestation a new mix of heavenly bodies was believed to press their power on the developing fetus. Hermetic and Arabic astronomical works influenced Christian beliefs. After Jupiter had congealed the blood of the fetus, the sun (or God) breathes in its soul in the fourth month, just before Venus helps its limbs to form and move.[129] Thus medieval canonists and lawyers had every reason to believe that a bad sin or crime occurs only if a fetus is killed after it received its soul from outside the womb.

Neither the Church pronouncements nor the legal codes named a physician as the person who assisted in the act of killing a fetus. A Bavarian code of the seventh century specifically stated its law: "If a woman gives to another a drink *(potionem)* so that it makes an abortion . . ." and gives the fine.[130] A similar Westgothic law does not specify a woman, only a person, although it might be expected to refer to (female) midwives.[131]

The medieval ecclesiastical pronouncements were not consistent— some condemned abortion, others contraception and abortion, and they meted out penances for each that were about the same as the penalty for stealing an ox. Some penitentials and canonists noted that the motive for birth control was significant. If a woman desired no more children because she was poor and could not feed them, the sin was less than that for a woman who sought "to conceal a crime of fornication."[132] A fourteenth-century canonist, Johannes Andreae (1270–1348), observed that there were many reasons why a woman would take a contraceptive: she might not want to bear a child because of her relations with the father; she might not want an heir to his estate; she might not want a child.[133]

Both the confessional questions and the various law codes make clear that contraception and abortion were associated with black magic *(maleficia, veneficii)*. Sometimes there was confusion over the word *sterilitas*, the same word used by Jerome for contraceptives (and possibly also abortifacients). Evidence from the law codes indicates that not (male) physicians but women were expected to administer the "drinks" and other antifertility agents. They knew the secrets, but, as we saw in the first chapter, so did some medieval men. Medical writings by physicians had information less explicit about birth control than did the writings of people like Marbode and Hildegard, who were not themselves physicians.

Medieval women and some physicians were the possessors of much of the knowledge about birth control. One reason the use of effective pre-modern birth control escaped detection is that, by and large, it was a woman's secret. A glimpse of a manuscript from a male religious community informs us what medieval men knew and how they knew it.

About the year 800 in the Benedictine abbey at Lorsch in what is now Germany, medieval monks composed a medical treatise that contained cures for common illnesses and afflictions. Much of the information in this medical manuscript that has survived to this day dates back to classical antiquity. Some, however, was derived from medieval discoveries. A monastery for men would not be a likely place to find information about birth control.

Folio 19 *verso* of the Lorsch manuscript has the title, "A Cure for All Kinds of Stomach Aches."[134] The prescription consisted of eleven ingredients, all but one (opium poppy) being abortifacients, according to modern studies. The medicinal purpose is further specified: "For women who cannot purge themselves, it moves the menses." In other words, the prescription would cause an abortion. Embedded in this beautiful early ninth-century Carolingian script was a practical prescription for abortion, only it did not say that is what it was.

The Middle Ages present us with an increasingly confused picture. On the one hand, the classical legacy of medical data about birth control was transmitted, copied, and even modified. One example is the text of Dioscorides' first-century herbal (which did not say that rue caused an abortion). A manuscript of his text that was written in the tenth century included the comment that rue "brings forth the menstrua and aborts an embryo."[135]

Furthermore, medieval authors of medical tracts wrote about contraceptives and even more about abortifacients. Presumably, therefore, they had some experience with these antifertility agents. There was no other way for new abortifacients to have been discovered. For us to know of medical discoveries, medieval authors—such as Hildegard, who said tansy caused an abortion—had to record the finding.

The Middle Ages is presented by the sources as a period in which people were actively engaged in birth control. In contrast comes an increasingly strong stance by the Christian Church against any form of birth control. Thus it is to be that Pierre and Béatrice will stand before the Inquisition in Montaillou and reveal their contraceptive practices.

4

From Womancraft to Witchcraft, 1200–1500

Who knows how to heal knows how to destroy.

A woman's testimony before the Inquisition,
Modena, 1499

In the beautiful Italian poetry of Dante's *Divine Comedy*, medicines that are for "cures" are virtuous, but there are other medicines, "poison of Venus (di Venere ... il tosco)," that the laws of marriage reject.[1] Chaucer's no less beautiful English was more direct: if a man makes a woman barren "by drinkinge venemous herbes," thus causing her not to conceive or to kill a child in the womb, that person is guilty of "homicyde."[2] About the same time an English herbal gave a recipe for "sickness which is in the womb" that specifies: "Take rue [*ruw*] and sage [*sawge*] and drink it with water."[3] The sickness is a guise.

Dante and Chaucer reflect a changed attitude toward birth control: that it is wrong to use contraceptives or abortifacients. The recipes contained in a Middle English herbal reveals that information about birth control was available, only disguised.

It was disguised because the church and, to a lesser degree, the law increased opposition to birth control. Thomas of Aquinas expressed what became the church's stance: sexual intercourse was for procreation in animals and humans. Anything that violated this principle of natural law was wrong because it violated "right reason." Thus, con-

91

traceptives—what Augustine called poisons of sterility (*sterilitatis venena*)—were wrong, just as abortifacients, before and after the fetus had "formed," were wrong.[4] Thomas's position was different from that of Augustine, who did not explicitly disapprove of early-term abortifacients and, conversely, did not say that they were right. Thomas was definite: abortions are wrong. For that matter, Thomas also was condemning drugs that promoted lovemaking and fertility. God, not drugs, determines rightly the outcome of sexual liaisons. Thomas, however, gave no new definition of abortion, because he held to the convention of the age and those before it: abortion was the termination of pregnancy after the fetus was formed. So had said Augustine.

The Church's Hardening Stand

Eastern and Western church doctrine alike disapproved of birth control drugs. By the thirteenth century, the position was clear: there should be no human interference with "natural" procreation.[5] Unwittingly, the church misread Genesis 38:8–10, the passage that describes Onan incurring the wrath of God for "spilling his seed upon the ground." In our modern scholarly interpretation of Genesis, based on Hebrew and Aramaic readings, God was displeased because Onan by his act refused to sire a child in the name of his brother. As early as the fourth century, Epiphanius construed the passage's meaning as a prohibition against coitus interruptus.[6] Later the interpretation will be extended to prohibit masturbation.

A statement by Regino, an abbot at Prüm about 830, was destined to be incorporated into canon law as a doctrinal directive:

> If someone [*Si aliquis*] to satisfy his lust or in deliberate hatred does something to a man or woman so that no children be born of him or her, or gives them to drink, so that he cannot generate or she conceive, let it be held as homicide.[7]

The critical motives here are "to satisfy lust" and "deliberate hatred." Sexual intercourse's purpose was procreation, the church canonists concluded from Corinthians I 7:3–6 and other passages.[8] Lust was wrong. The question not raised is: what if the motive for termination of pregnancy was different, not lust or "hatred"? Could a motive be worthy?

Later, as we shall shortly see, Regino's rule was canonized, although in modified form, by the Catholic Church through its incorporation with Burchard's *Decretum* about 1010. Burchard referred to the "fetus *(conceptus)* being excluded from the uterus by *maleficia* and by herbs."[9] By this he evidently was extending contraception as a prohibited practice. Why would he say "by *maleficia* and by herbs"? Again we see the association of birth control with "black" or "evil" magic, but Burchard explicitly mentioned herbs as well. His addition appears superfluous, inasmuch as in earlier usage *maleficia* encompassed the use of herbs.[10] Surmising his motives, I speculate that Burchard wanted no ambiguity: he knew that most contraception was achieved through herbs but did not want a wayward soul to suppose that, because it was an herb, it was not a *maleficium.*

Regino's association of contraception and abortion with homicide was not to stand. We saw this in the discussion of the views of Albertus Magnus in Chapter 1. Ivo of Chartres (Bishop, 1091–1116) wrote an opinion—called by its first word *Aliquando,* "at any time"—that became part of canon law. Ivo's rule is like Thomas's and, to some degree, Augustine's principle that what was wrong about contraception and abortion was that they were unnatural acts. God, not herbs, should decide who is born. In Ivo's position, abortion was not wrong after the fetus formed—it was wrong, period. It was *contra naturam.* Regino's and Ivo's positions were adopted by Peter Lombard (ca. 1150) as the prevailing theological position on the subject and by Gratian in canon law (ca. 1140).[11] Let it not be lost that the late medieval position on birth control derived from beliefs in right actions and not from a concept that the fetus was alive and needed protection for its own sake.[12]

Peter's Hypothetical Case

The impact of the church's position is illustrated by a case that was used for scholastic disputation in late-twelfth-century Paris. Hypothesis: A woman has a rupture that would result in her death should she become pregnant and come to deliver. May she "procure sterility" for herself in order to save her life? As stated, the question involves contraception, but the case is similar to those identified in the medical literature as justifications for a therapeutic abortion. The vocabulary was different, however; in the medical literature it was "drugs" that were given not, as stated here, "sterility."

Peter Cantor's answer to his question was as firm in spirit as it was weak in reason: "This last thing is not at all lawful, because this would be to procure poisons of sterility; that is prohibited in every case."[13] Reason, begone; it's against the (church) law, that's all. Peter's failure to cite the specific rule, be it from Augustine, Regino, Ivo, Burchard, Peter Lombard, or Gratian, reflects the acceptance of the position against birth control by the late twelfth century. He was unaware of any intersection between motives and acts. Drugs for birth control are wrong, just as Dante declared later in the *Divine Comedy* in referring to drugs of marriage.

Not all theologians were as rigid as Peter was on contraception. Around 1315 John of Naples asked: Could a physician give a medicine to cause an abortion if the act saved the life of a mother? His answer is based on the familiar two-stage fetal development. If ensoulment has occurred, then the answer is "no," because when "one cannot help one without hurting the other, it is more appropriate to help neither."[14] If the fetus has not received the soul, the answer is "yes," because, although a potential soul will not come into being, the act will "not cause the death of any man." Then, the physician "ought to give such medicine."[15] Again, one should note the means for an abortion, taking a medicine.

Common Law, Feticide, and Drugs

In the mid-thirteenth century, during the reign of Henry III (1216–72), Henri de Bracton wrote a summary of the laws and customs of England. Now considered a compilation by various authors, the work will be referred to here as his. It mixed Roman law from the recovered *Corpus Iuris Civilis* with English common (or customary) law, which is primarily based on cases decided in the 1220s and 1230s.[16] It is for that reason that it is unclear what Bracton was describing when he said: "If one strikes a pregnant woman or gives her poison *(venenum)* in order to procure an abortion, if the fetus is already formed or quickened *(formatum vel animatum)* especially if it is quickened, he commits homicide."[17]

Much the same language was used to describe law under the English king Edward I (1271–1307) that declared a person guilty of homicide who oppressed a woman, gave her a poison, or struck her, thus "not allowing conception" *(non concipiat)* or causing an abortion *(faciat abortivum)* after the fetus shall have "already formed and animated *(for-matus et animatus)*."[18] This rule extends the ancient, legal principle by declaring guilty of homicide one who gives to a pregnant woman a "drink *(potationem)* or similar things in the stomach," thus preventing "an animated [formed] child" from having life. And a woman who takes a drink to destroy a "quickened child" in her womb *(puerum animatus per potacionem et huiusmodi in ventre)* is a murderer.[19] So also was one who took a contraceptive a murderer. These comments on the law came from an anonymous writer, called Fleta, during Edward's reign but, in large part, the writer borrowed from Bracton. The Fleta principle appears to have been based on an application of the interpretation of passages from Exodus (21:22–25) as translated into Greek, then Latin.

As we shall see, other medieval legal principles either followed or preceded law in Edward I's reign, according to Fleta. On one hand, the Bracton principle (not a statute) is in keeping with the old principles of protecting a man's right to have a child whom he fathered, but there is no mention of an aggrieved party. The act itself is criminal. Nothing was said about a woman who took a drug prior to the "forming" of the fetus, a principle known in the English vernacular as "quickening."[20] Quickening was the observance of fetal movement, which is experienced first from the fourth through sixth months of pregnancy.

The Fleta principle contained two other unprecedented and probably ignored provisions. It was not until 1861 that English law charged a woman with homicide for procuring her own abortion. This principle appears to be an extension of the Roman law that gave a family head the right to have a child. It should not be interpreted as a criminalization of contraception, despite the words to that effect.

Doubt exists about the standing of the law—whether it followed Bracton and Fleta—under Henry III and Edward I. No cases are found prosecuting contraception as a crime. Two later cases, frequently cited for precedent, imply that abortion may not have been a felony. The first case was near the beginning of Edward III's reign (1327–1377) and was known as the "Twinslayer's Case." It was tried under Chief Justice Scrope of the King's Bench. A writ was issued to the Sheriff of Gloucestershire to apprehend Richard de Bourton, who was accused of beating an unnamed woman in advanced pregnancy. In subsequent documents we learn her name was Alice. Shortly afterward, Alice delivered one dead fetus and one alive. Two days later the surviving child was baptized, named Jane (or John?), and died, it was claimed, from injuries sustained during the mother's beating. Richard pleaded not guilty before Judge Scrope, but "the justices were unwilling to adjudge this thing a felony *(justices ne fuet en volunte de agard cest chose felone)*." Richard was released to mainpernors ("mainprisne")—similar to a surety in American law—and argument was adjourned "sans tour" *(sine die)*.[21] In other words, even though the case involved both a fetal death and a death of an infant after baptism from injuries suffered by an assault prior to birth, no felony was found. On May 29, 1327, Richard's name was on a list of pardons granted by King Edward III.[22]

Two modern legal experts disagree on the meaning of the Twinslayer case. Cyril Means argues that common law did not regard abortion as a felony (a high crime).[23] On the same evidence, Robert Destro believes that Richard de Bourton was indicted on homicide, because he was released in the hands of mainpernors. The procedure indicates that the justices considered abortion a felony. The mainpernor to whom Richard was released was responsible for delivering him to the court. In effect, the case indicates to Destro that abortion was regarded as a homicide.[24] Richard was not tried on the charge because at a later proceeding in York, Richard was also on trail in Bristol for another charge. A record in a Gloucestershire court, 1328, shows that the indictment against Richard was dismissed because he received a pardon from the king.[25] Therefore, Destro's interpretation is correct, namely that Richard was indicted for a felony, probably homicide, but he was never tried. The offense was indictable for a felony but, given the facts of the case, it is not clear whether the criminal act was the killing of the fetus or the killing of the infant who lived a few days. In some strange twists, however, the case will be employed as a common law precedent for interpretations not supported by the documentary evidence, as will be seen in the next chapter.

In 1348, during the reign of the same king, another precedent, called the "Abortionist's Case," was established. The details are even more sketchy than the Twinslayer's Case because the manuscript is lost, but a summary is found in a sixteenth century abridgement. The case's result is more certain, however. A person (name unspecified) was indicted for killing a child in the womb, the means being also unspecified. The person was not arrested on the grounds that the child had received no baptismal name and that, in the words of the court record, "also it is difficult to know whether he killed the child or not."[26]

The two specific cases, the Twinslayer's Case and the Abortionist's Case, raise doubt about the law as pronounced by the jurists, Bracton and the anonymous author of Fleta. The jurists were commenting on principles as they should exist and not necessarily as they did exist at common law. Case precedent is paramount over texts written by jurists. Jurists and courts from the sixteenth through the nineteenth centuries had different opinions about whether these two cases established abortion as a felony (see next chapter).

Other Common Law Cases

A review of other common law cases reinforces our conclusion that the dividing line for a convictable, felonious crime when harm was done to a fetus *in utero* was the fact of live birth. A woman who aborts a dead fetus has not been harmed unless she herself is bodily injured. The case of John of Wyntercote (Eyre of Hereford in 1292) illustrates the particulars of a dispute in which no crime was determined:

> The jurors present that John of Wyntercote, accused of beating Christine, the wife of William Treweman, whereby she gave birth to a certain abortive child, was taken by Hugh Carpenter the under-bailiff of William Shereman, then farmer of the vill of Leominster, and he escaped from the custody of the same Hugh. Therefore to judgment upon the aforesaid William Shereman, the farmer concerning the aforesaid escape. And the jurors, being asked whether the aforesaid abortive child ever had life *(vitam)* in his mother's womb before she gave birth, or whether he was suspected of wrong; but because he previously ran away from it let his chattels be confiscated for fleeing; and let him come back if he wishes.[27]

In this case the jurors' concern was "life" in the womb, which could be interpreted as the distinction between a formed and an unformed fetus, pre-quickening and quickening, but the meaning appears to be birth.

Some people charged with killing a fetus born dead were acquitted, but the fact that they were brought before justice's bar shows that killing a fetus presumed to have quickened was considered a felony. This is demonstrated by the case of John de Rechich' of a town in Somersetshire (1242–1243), who fled when accused of beating Juliana and causing her to lose a boy baby in the womb. Outlawed, he came to the township of Stoke Curcy and was tried. Twelve jurors and the town failed in their collective responsibility to enforce the law and were placed "in mercy" for the failure to aid in the enforcement of a criminal law.[28]

I have been able to find but one case, however, where a jury may have convicted a person for killing a fetus in the womb, and its details are unclear.[29] In contrast, the reign of Edward I has at least eight cases of homicide for fetal death that were tried but in every case the accused was acquitted.[30] Were the act not considered wrong, however, no one would have been brought to justice ("appealed").

In all the medieval common law cases that I found, the cause of harm was specified as either a blow, a fall, or, in a few instances, the manipulation of a stick or similar instrument. Many instances were assaults that resulted in pregnancy termination. An illustrative case is that against John Cokkes (Somerset, ca. 1415), who was found guilty of a number of offenses, *except* the jurors "in no wise know whether or not he beat and wounded the said Elizabeth," whose child was born prematurely, wounded grievously, and subsequently died.[31] In Kent in 1279 William de Pekkeringe was allegedly robbed by several men. They also beat his wife, Agnes, who aborted her child. The accused men were acquitted of robbery and homicide but punished for trespass.[32]

In a few cases there is a hint that a blow was deliberately aimed at the fetus and, possibly, with permission from the mother to induce an abortion. In one case in Kent in 1279, a Master Thomas, a surgeon, struck Agnes le Deyster so that she aborted a female fetus.[33] In another case, Devonshire Eyre in 1281, Richard de Brente, a clerk, hit his wife with a stick so that she not only aborted but died herself a month thereafter. Richard fled before a trial and was outlawed.[34] Perhaps it was because a blow was the illustration used in Exodus 21:22–23 that the law seems to be limited to those cases; perhaps it was the more common method of abortion; more likely, chemical abortion was attempted early in the pregnancy by the women themselves, and these were not indictable offenses in common law. The church courts would have jurisdiction.

In 1281, Alice was assaulted by four men and in consequence she aborted an *abortivum* about (*quasi*) the age of one month, whose gender was undeterminable. The estimate of one month likely highly understated the fetal age. Indicted and tried, one of perpetrators was found not guilty but the others were imprisoned for trespass. The punishment appears to be for the assault, not the loss of the fetus.[35] In 1284, Rochester in Cornwall, Mabel of Trethyas was assaulted allegedly by John Hobba and "aborted a male child *(masculinum abortit)*" for which John Boleheved called *(appellat)* Hobba to justice. The case, however, was dismissed because "in cases of this kind one ought not to call to justice unless [it is] by a woman."[36] The court in this case was not expressing a general rule, although so it appears to claim, because in other cases charges were brought by third parties. In Mabel's case, it is not clear whether she was married to John Boleheved or not.

In one case a person who caused an abortion was found guilty and hanged. In Middlesex in 1320 or 1321, Maud de Haule pushed Joan de Hallynghurst and caused her to fall and to abort. Maud was hanged, presumably for this deed—it is not for certain because other crimes may have been involved.[37] The significance of Maud's case is that it may indicate that second-party termination of pregnancies was considered a felony by the common law. The paucity of such cases discloses that juries seldom convicted those accused, even when assaults and other crimes were a part of the deed.

In contrast, there are seven cases, five from the year 1321 alone and one from 1285, in which an act, either a blow or a push, caused a woman to deliver a live child before its time. The child was baptized and died shortly thereafter from injuries sustained in the womb. Those causing the early but live birth followed by death all fled and were declared outlaws.[38] In two other cases, however, the person accused of wrongdoing stood trial and was acquitted.[39]

On the basis of cases, it is difficult to discern the principles on which jurors acted. Comments by contemporary jurists clarify matters, but only to a degree. Around the 1290s Andrew Horne (d. ca. 1328), alleged author of *Mirror of Justices*, wrote:

> Of infants killed ye are to distinguish, whether they be killed in their mothers womb or after their births; in the first case it is not adjudged murder; for that none can judge whether it be a child before it be seen, and known whether it be a monster or not.[40]

Even more clear was Britton, writing about 1290:

> As to women, our will is, that no woman shall bring an appeal of felony for the death of any man, except for the death of her husband

killed within her arms within the year and day. For an infant killed within her womb, she may not bring any appeal, no one being bound to answer an appeal of felony, where the plaintiff cannot set forth the name of the person against whom the felony was committed.[41]

On the basis of case law it would appear that English judges and juries were mindful to some degree of the formed-unformed distinction. For this reason the Twinslayer's Case is noteworthy, inasmuch as both factual circumstances were demonstrated. If the child that lived a short time after an injury to the mother (even if the other child was born dead), the offense was indictable; but it was also indictable if the injury resulted in the fetus being born dead or killed in the uterus. Curiously, however, I found no cases where a child was found guilty of delivering a blow that caused a child born alive to die later of the injury. A simple liability for the killing a fetus *may* have resulted in only one conviction (that I have found). Notably that one person was hapless Maud, a woman, but the circumstances are uncertain.[42]

A case as early as 1221 in Gloucester demonstrates that termination of a pregnancy was indictable as a crime. In this case Andrew de Gerur beat Wymark, wife of another man, and as a result of the beating she gave birth to a dead child *(peperit infantem mortuum)*.[43] We must distinguish between legal principles as known by jurists and the principles of fact on which juries were willing to find people guilty. English medieval common law probably did regard abortion induced through physical means by a second party as a crime, if the abortion occurred after quickening, but juries did not convict them. English legal principles may not have been different from those on the continent, where secular courts may have been more willing to be guided by canon law in regard to abortion after fetal formation (as will be seen below). No cases being found where chemical means were used to induce abortion, or where a pregnant woman was even indicted, indicates that most abortions were not criminal offenses.

Islamic Medicine and Birth Control

By and large the Islamic writers, such as Mesue the Younger (ca. 925–ca. 1015), followed the same line of reasoning on abortion that Theodorus Priscianus had.[44] Although abortion may have been wrong to Hippocrates, a physician is faced with difficult problems, where the better course for the love of humanity is to opt for abortion rather than lose the life of a woman. No discussion of fetal life entered Islamic texts.

The Islamic religion was relatively clear about abortion (nearly acceptable) and unambiguous about contraception (acceptable). What we would call abortion was acceptable during the early period of pregnancy. This was on the authority of Aristotle, whom the Arabs regarded as a supreme philosopher. Hanafi jurists said that a woman could abort even without her husband's permission, but, they added, she ought to have good reason. The supreme prophet, Muhammad, said that there were three stages by which "each of you is constituted in your mother's womb." Only in the last stage does God "breathe the soul into it."[45] Ibn Quyyim al-Jawziyya (d. 1350) wrote a Quranic commentary on generation that was thorough in rejecting Aristotle's one-seed thesis and built on Hippocratic-Galenic anatomy interpreted through the Quran and *Ḥadīth*. The fetus is formed by semen from both parents. Had Muslim jurists found uniqueness in male semen, contraception would not have been doctrinally permitted.[46]

Islamic authorities accepted abortion but differed about the length of each stage. Only a small minority of Muslims, called Malikis, prohibited abortion at any time, because of the potentiality for ensoulment. Without religious constraints about at least some forms of birth control, Islamic writers wrote about techniques and agents to the fullest degree that their knowledge allowed them.[47] And their knowledge was elaborate: it was based primarily on Greek authorities, but they added their own experiences and those they borrowed from Indic or Vedic medicine.

Transmission of Birth Control Information

In the Latin West, knowledge of contraception and abortion drugs continued to be recorded, albeit at a level lower than in the classical works. "Books of secrets," similar to the one allegedly by Albertus Magnus, were popular, but if they contained birth control information it was well hidden. "The Secrets of Nature" allegedly by the thirteenth-century Michael Scot said that there are things that women can take to prevent generation and, for this reason, pregnant women ought not to take these things in their food.[48] The very popular book of secrets by Raymond Lull (d. 1315) discussed drugs but in a general, theoret-

CARL A. RUDISILL LIBRARY
LENOIR-RHYNE UNIVERSITY

ical way. For example, he gave a list of purgatives and said that some purge blood but gave no more detail. Among them were thyme, colocynth, squirting cucumber, and savin (juniper).[49] We know that these were given to induce the onset of menstruation, hence blood, but the secret is not spelled out. And there were drugs that dissolve "warmness" and "separate parts" that include artemisia, cinnamon, birthwort, asafetida, garlic, rue, cypress, celery, gentian, and opopanax (a species of *Ferula*).[50] Were those warmnesses and separated parts fetuses? The secrets in the book of secrets remained secret.

The newly written herbals of the late Middle Ages have fewer discussions of birth control. Generally those same herbs were listed as emmenagogues or menstrual regulators, not explicitly for abortion. The contraceptive plants were mentioned in the herbals even less. Just the same, the knowledge was in the books young men read or had available for their education. By the thirteenth century, and from then on, increasingly physicians-in-training resided in universities. Once they passed their examinations and established practices, they joined medical guilds that attempted in every way, every day, to exclude the herbalist, the empiric, the spicer, the drug salesman, and other hawkers of cures. These "irregular" medical providers were in the marketplaces and resided in almost every neighborhood and village.[51]

In the newly established universities, the young men who learned medicine were acquainted with various Galenic and Hippocratic works. They knew the nuances of humoral balance, how to treat a wound, how to explain a four-day fever to a worried family, and when a cataract had to be cut. What they learned about women's health probably was less than what earlier physicians had learned. Unusual and chronic problems stretched a midwife's or "old woman's" knowledge, so they remained within a physician's domain. On the other hand, a typical physician may not have known things that to women were common knowledge.

Soranus's work was not known in medieval Europe, and the birth control data from Dioscorides was learned mostly through Arabic writers on pharmacy, who had taken Dioscorides' learning and extended it. The works of Haly-Abbas, Mesue the Younger and Mesue the Elder, Serapion, and Al-Rhasis were more often consulted, we judge from the medical curriculum, references to their works, and the number of copies that are extant.

In some instances the subject of abortion was carefully circum-scribed. In the mid-eleventh century, Constantine the African trans-lated the medical works of Haly-Abbas (al-Majūsī, d. 994). In the pro-logue the ethics of a physician are discussed, as are familiar points derived from the Hippocratic Oath, such as that one should not ad-minister a deadly poison or even teach its use. Similarly "one ought not teach how to make an abortion."[52] The author clearly understood the oath to restrict abortion but, it appears, only to a degree. Under medical practice, medicines to be taken by mouth that "provoke the menses" are named, such as myrrh, wild calamint, domestic dittany, juniper, asarum.[53] No precaution is included about giving them to pregnant women. In the pharmacy section even more menstrual reg-ulators ("menstrua provocat") are named, such as parsley and Queen Anne's lace seeds, but the direct subject of abortion is avoided.[54] More direct, however, was the comment that opopanax "provokes menstru-ation and expels a dead fetus."[55]

Avicenna (Ibn Sīnā, 980–1037) was supreme among those Islamic writers whose texts were studied in medical schools. He discussed the details of contraception and abortion, but the text is very long and the section on birth control may not have been recommended reading.

In a section faithfully translated into Latin, Avicenna noted that the physician finds circumstances where it is necessary, to protect the life of the woman, to advise contraception and abortion. Examples he gave were women with diseased wombs or other health problems whose lives would be risked by a protracted pregnancy. A physician had avail-able a number of strategies to deal with such examples. He could ad-vise on the favorable periods in the menstrual cycle to avoid fertile in-tercourse, on the practice of withdrawal before male climax, or the following methods: to "jump backwards from seven to nine times force-fully so that the sperm may come out . . . or to sneeze," or to take var-ious contraceptives. Among those Avicenna prescribed were pome-granate pulp, willow leaves, colocynth, and pennyroyal.[56] He included a long list of abortifacients about as complete as was known at the time.[57] What we do not know is how well this section in Avicenna's text was taught and studied in the medieval universities.

Because Avicenna's works were so central in medical education, we must expect that some physicians knew to a degree what he and oth-ers said about birth control. One physician who surely did know Avicenna was William of Saliceto (ca. 1210–1280), who extended Avicenna's knowledge on the subject.[58] First, he gave Avicenna's justification for contraception and abortion, but he added to the reasons for abortion the protection of girls of extreme youth who might conceive but would be in danger of dying during delivery. Like Avicenna, William added his own list of drugs that caused an abortion. Among them were juniper, rue, pennyroyal, and cypress. He added a new word, *mentastri*, which was a generic term meaning a variety of wild mints.

In addition to Avicenna's works, numerous Arabic medical writings were translated into Latin. The translations began appearing in the second half of the eleventh century and reached an apogee in the twelfth and thirteenth centuries. What the Arabs wrote was largely known also in the Latin West. Thus by the thirteenth century the knowledge about birth control in the West was greater than it ever had been, and that includes classical antiquity. The existence of written records, however, tells us neither how well read medical practitioners were on the subject of birth control nor how available the knowledge was to the masses.

Church attitudes must have had some effect on the transmission of information. Even though Western physicians were restricted in practice by conventions—social, religious, legal—the increasing number of those who were educated in universities had access to texts with ample data on birth control agents. We do not know if the relevant sections of the texts were taught, however.

Islamic Medicine in the West

Western physicians had the advantage of reading these texts, preserved by Islamic scholars, newly translated into Latin. Around the late thirteenth century a Western writer, the anonymous author of *Breviarium practice*, went beyond the convention of his age. In introducing the subject of contraceptives, following a rather complete discussion of abortive drugs, he provided a startling justification for their use. Contraceptives are needed by single women who do not wish to conceive in order to maintain their suitability for marriage.[59] This work was rarely, not normally, included among the texts required in Western medical schools. The sentiments expressed by this author were rare and, for the idea that contraception protected the unmarried, they were unprecedented. As a generalization, medical practitioners in the medieval West maintained some knowledge of birth control agents. They learned through classical and Islamic texts as well as personal experiences. The question is how much experience medical authorities had with birth control.

The inclusion in medical writings of new discoveries of birth control agents, such as those by Hildegard of Bingen and William of Saliceto, demonstrates that people continued, in the Middle Ages, to pass along and try new folk remedies. The "scholars" in whose works the discoveries are first mentioned were not responsible for creating the new prescriptions. In William's case, the discovery was the observation that plants of the mint family had the common attribute of causing an abortion. In Hildegard's case, it was the use of tansy for the same. But few birth control agents were discussed in other writings of the late Middle Ages. The popular herbal by pseudo-Platearius, who allegedly was Trotula's son, lists only menstrual stimulators, again the familiar ones.[60]

Another indicator of innovations in and continuous usage of folk knowledge in the Middle Ages concerns *silphium*, the giant fennel plant from Cyrenia, which was so popular in antiquity as to have been harvested out of existence.[61] In the Middle Ages drug-substitute lists, known as *Quid pro quo*, were compiled. People had read in ancient texts about *silphium*, but they did not know it because it no longer existed, but they knew to substitute a familiar and more common plant, asafetida, for the unknown one in the same family.

Nicholaus's Antidotarium

A collection of recipes produced in the twelfth century is attributed to Nicholaus of Salerno, who probably contributed to the recipe list but did not start it (that person is not known). Nicholaus's name became attached to the list at some point, but each time it was copied scribes added and deleted recipes. By the thirteenth century Nicholaus's *Antidotarium*, as it was called, circulated widely in Europe. Through the fourteenth century, the work became as close to a standard "handbook" as medieval pharmacy allowed. Apothecary guilds expected its members to be acquainted with it. For certain, recipes that appear in it were known. Many manuscripts of it exist today. Like their modern counterparts, medieval apothecaries knew their customers already had expectations about the drugs they purchased.

The Antidotarium lists a number of abortifacients, but no contraceptives. Of course, abortion was only one of many things for which the medicinal recipes were given. Most recipes *(antidotaria)* were like some of our old-fashioned tonics that had multiple uses. The recipes are given in large proportion so that an apothecary or physician could mix a large amount and then package smaller doses for sale. These prescriptions would be in most apothecary shops. Thus, we know that apothecary shops throughout Europe possessed the *antidotum* that was for the "passions of the womb."

Some women have difficulty with menstruation, the text explains, and purgatives do not work for this problem. This mixture "miraculously *(mirabiliter)* stimulates the menses and it kills a fetus in the womb and afterwards extracts it." Like so many other drugs, it had many other uses, such as removing the afterbirth and stimulating urination. This *antidotum*, with some thirty-one ingredients, included practically every known abortifacient: asarum, *Ferula*, birthwort, artemisia, century plant (both the greater one and the lesser one), lupine, pepper, Queen Anne's lace, myrrh, licorice, pennyroyal, rue, peony, parsley, and cypress. If a woman had a fever, she should take this draught while bathing; if no fever, she should take it with wine or honey water.[62]

Another version of the Antidotarium has around eight recipes for expelling the menstrua, each of which contains a number of abortifacient drugs.[63] The closest the work comes to being explicit about an abortion is a recipe claimed "to expel a dead fetus"—which is hardly explicit at all.[64] This recipe was a "stictica," an astringent salve for external use, that contained pepper, squill, two species of *Ferula*, celery leaves, Queen Anne's lace, and the lesser century plant. This same recipe ends, however, with a discussion of different preparation methods and a statement that together with warm wine the concoction expels "poisons, menstrua, and a fetus," this time dropping the word "dead."[65]

The unknown factor here is not whether these compound recipes would work, because they probably would. We know that the ingredients put in the compounds acted in various ways to produce abortions. What we do not know is the effect the combinations would have. On this there has been no modern experimentation—all testing has been on single, crude drugs or isolated chemicals taken from the plants. Another truly unknown question is what directions were given concerning dosage. Neither the amounts nor the frequency are specified, and this information is all important. Such involved and complex recipes as appear in Nicholaus' work would not be mixed by an ordinary housewife for herself. Some ingredients, such as pepper, were exotica, that is, they were derived from plants that had to be imported from great distances. The "simples" (single-ingredient prescriptions) are not to be found in the gardens, fields, and woods around European housewives. Nicholaus's work marks a change in medical practice that became more apparent during the late Middle Ages—namely that simple drugs became less important than complex compounds.

The pharmaceutical works of the late Middle Ages reflect a movement toward "polypharmacy," the use of many ingredients in a single mixture. To some degree the change occurred because of the complex pharmaceutical theory taught in the universities (and hence prescribed by physicians). There is a baser motivation for the change, however: the complex mixtures had to be purchased, as they could not be made readily in the home. The movement was away from home remedies and toward bottles and pills from stores. Whether the tactic was deliberately calculated or not, one result of polypharmacy was to cause people to be dependent on apothecaries and to lose the ability to prepare their own remedies. Where Gothic spires of the new cathedrals cast shadows over workshops and markets, people began to rely more and more on apothecaries. The apothecary guilds set standards, regulated who could become an apothecary, and established fair prices. Rules were established periodically that sought to govern overly close relations between physicians and apothecaries.

Until modern times, we have ample evidence to believe that apothecaries sold contraceptive and abortifacient drugs. What we do not know is what was sold because of a physician's prescription. The drug store sold drugs, but the circumstances of their purchase and of their use are difficult to establish. All we have is the general data about population. That the people who built those medieval cathedrals were doing something to limit family size is very likely. Their homes were usually closer to the neighborhood apothecary shops than to the local rectory.

The Dead Fetus as Loophole

The records reveal an established pattern in late-medieval reasoning about abortion. Religious doctrine and canon law increasingly denounced birth control. At the same time, medical writings contained the practical information needed to induce abortion but in increasingly disguised and circumspect form. Meanwhile, university-trained physicians were exposed to less gynecology and other topics in women's health in their curriculum. With the incidental exception of Avicenna's and a few other writers' pharmacy texts, birth control was not included in what they learned. The appearance of new drugs evidenced continuous folk usage and experimentation with antifertility agents, of which some writers included a mention. Finally, as we shall see shortly, birth control came to be associated with witchcraft. These trends caused changes in the openness with which birth control was approached.

The impediments to abortion resulted in increasing use of the phrase "expels a dead fetus," wording that, to be sure, dated back to the Hippocratic works. A German translation of the *Compendium* by Gilbertus Anglicus brought the phrases together in one sequence: juniper "drunk with water or honey provokes the menstrua and urine, expels a dead fetus, stops the bleeding after childbirth, and causes an abortion."[66] The fifteenth-century translator put all these phrases together because, with the exception of postpartum bleeding, they all referred to the same thing. When a fetus died, the body naturally expelled it, and menstrual bleeding begins again.

When a woman declared her fetus dead, a medieval physician did not examine her and, even should he do so, he lacked a stethoscope to hear a heart beat. No medieval records that I have found alert a physician to be aware that a woman might lie about her condition. If we can generalize on this discrete evidence, it appears that when a woman said "dead," dead the fetus was thought to be. Thus, a medicine that assisted its expulsion could appropriately be given. Still, this conclusion might be simplistic, because people always were held responsible when they helped a pregnant women (one whose fetus was formed or "quick") terminate her pregnancy.

Poor Uge, Poor Isaac

A rare glimpse into private lives is found in the archives from the town of Manosque (Manuasca), in the Provençal region of France. The incident demonstrates that jurisdictions on the continent treated abortion differently than English courts did. On November 17, 1298, Isaac the Jew, son of Resplande and a surgeon, was accused of preparing and administering a poisonous drink *(medicamenta venenosa)* to Uge (Huga).

She drank the potion and an infant was born dead ("ex dicta potatione sue medicamento venenoso infans predictus natus fuit mortuus").

It is interesting the way the court records capture the event. In the first statement the drug was called a "drink" and in the second statement a "medicine," the court apparently not being interested enough in this detail to be exact. Also, the court said that the "infant that was expected to be born was dead." The court was not saying that the fetus had life but that there was an expectation that a living person would eventually have been born but for human intervention. Apparently Uge did not indicate that her fetus was dead prior to the doctor's visit.

The next day "Magister" Guillelmus Rocensus (Guilhem Pelegrin) testified that Uge had been pregnant. This determination was based on what he had heard. From his title we surmise that Guillelmus had gone to a university, but he was not said to be a physician. Some of his testimony is lost in the record, but Uge was described only as the daughter of Petri de Dia (Peire de Die) and, to judge from what was said and not said, she was single.

Testimony was taken from others in the community, among them the elder Guillelmus and Beatrix, wife of Guillelmus Gaudridus. Denying any complicity, Isaac said that the baby had been born alive and that Uge's grandmother had "carried the infant to Lurius," presumably to be buried. Disbelieving Isaac, the court wanted to establish whether Uge was known by those in the community to be pregnant at the time that Isaac treated her. After the court heard these testimonies, Isaac was found guilty, fined fifty livres, and jailed, "but not in chains," the length of the sentence being lost in the record.[67]

If we can generalize on this incomplete evidence, we come to the conclusion that medieval communities did not accept lightly the termination of pregnancies. Medieval towns on the continent appear to have been ready to supplement ecclesiastic courts on abortion, which was not the case in England. In 1474 (two centuries after Isaac's trial), the Bavarians had a law making abortion manslaughter, and the Tyrolians in Hals punished abortion by pillorying in 1499.[68]

The Manosque court took three days to receive testimony to establish whether Uge was pregnant or not, when she took Isaac's medicine. He, not she, was on trial. The fact that Isaac was a Jew does not appear to have been an important factor. Only his deed was the court's concern. Presumably, had he been Christian, the results would have been the same. The court's business was whether Uge's pregnancy was advanced enough to have been known and, therefore, whether or not an abortion had taken place. The court did not record what the actual medicine was or whether it was the cause. Uge was given the "medicine/drink" and she aborted. That part was accepted as a matter of fact.

The Midwife and the Witch

Uge's plight was disclosed before a civil court. Three years after her abortion, Béatrice (see Chapter 1) faced Pierre's proposal to have an affair in a village not very far from Uge's home. When it came time to pay the consequences, however, there was a big difference: Béatrice and Pierre stood before the Inquisition. They were among the first of many who faced the dreaded proceedings, which often resulted in torture and, increasingly, burning at the stake. Initially, the Inquisition was an inquiry among Christians who deliberately, stubbornly, and publicly denied the doctrines of the church. By 1215 the Inquisition was recognized by the papacy as a means of combating heresy, then widespread in many regions of Europe.

In 1252 the use of torture to obtain confessions was approved, on the reasoning that since heretics will suffer eternally, the better part of kindness is to subject them to temporary torture in the hope that they may be reconciled to the church and receive eternal salvation. By the fifteenth century, the Inquisition had become an instrument of terror. As many as half a million witches are estimated to have been burned at the stake during the centuries of heresy repression.

Most of those who died were women. In twelfth-century Russia a witch hunt was accomplished first by rounding up all the women.[69] In 1580 Jean Bodin said that fifty women were tried as witches to every one man.[70] Synonyms for witches were *Gifft-Köche*, or "poison cooks" (feminine), *Nachtfrawen*, or "night women," and *Feld-Frawen*, or "country women."[71] The vocabulary betrays the bias.

In the suppression of witchcraft three separate and distinct things—witchcraft, midwifery, and birth control—were joined in an unfortunate, unholy marriage. Witchcraft was the ritualized worship of Satan, or so said their accusers. Historians today believe that there actually were some people who practiced at least some of the things they were accused of and who invoked the devil in the process. But many people today think of witchcraft as a kind of hysteria, an outbreak of bizarre behavior that claimed numerous innocent victims. In addition to being blamed for raising damaging hail storms, causing droughts, and casting evil spells, witches were accused of tying an invisible string (called a ligature) around men's penises so they could not have erections and of causing them to have intercourse that could not be fertile. A seventeenth-century friar said that ligatures were not the only way to prevent men from impregnating women; another method was "the application of certain natural drugs which in some way deprive a woman of the power to conceive."[72]

Henry Boguet's *Examen of Witches* observed that many witches also were midwives:

> those midwives and wise women who are witches are in the habit of offering to Satan the little children which they deliver, and then of killing them . . . They do even worse; for they kill them while they are yet in their mothers' wombs. This practice is common to all witches.[73]

Boguet wrote in the 1580s, long after witchcraft was regarded as an intolerable practice. It also was after midwifery became a separate occupation. Prior to the fourteenth century, there were women medical practitioners of various sorts, but the term midwifery is a fourteenth-century designation, with antecedents as old as classical antiquity.

The Dominican authors of a treatise in 1484 explored the question of why women were more prone to witchcraft. They attributed the answer to three reasons: (1) women had "a kind of perfidy . . . found more in so fragile a sex than in men"; (2) women were more inclined to "superstition and witchcraft"; and (3) some women became "midwives, who surpass all others in wickedness."[74] "Sevenfold witchcraft," the seven things that witches could do, were: (1) practicing fornication and adultery; (2) "obstructing the generative act" by rendering men impotent; (3) performing castration and sterilization; (4) engaging in bestiality and homosexuality; (5) "destroying the generative force in women"; (6) "procuring abortion"; and (7) "offering children to devils."[75] All are related to sexuality and all but the first, fornication and adultery, to birth control.[76] People believed that witches did these things, and Jean Bodin—French rationalist, philosopher, and demonologist—declared in 1580 that the charges were true.[77] In one way or another, many of these things were either practiced or advised by midwives, said their accusers. Even bestiality and homosexuality were said to be a part of satanic rituals. A historian of witchcraft, Margaret Murray, says that midwives, like witches, claimed they could "cause and prevent pregnancy, [and were able] to cause and to prevent an easy delivery, to cast the labour-pains on an animal or a human being . . . and in every way to have power over the generative organs of both sexes."[78]

Sexual offenses were, by far, the leading offenses of which witches were accused in three Essex villages between 1560 and 1599.[79] By the mid-fourteenth century, sexual immorality and witchcraft were connected in the proclamations of secular authorities.[80] Witchcraft has been described as being a projection of women's suppressed sexual wishes.[81] Whatever it was, witchcraft involved sexuality, real or imagined, by man or by woman or by both.[82] In order to remove an obstacle for her lover to marry her, Appolonia Mayr, a servantwoman, confessed that she killed her newborn baby, born while she was in the field by herself. There the Devil came to her as a midwife, she said, and for this reason she burned as a witch in 1686.[83] What we relegate to psychotic stress, the early modern age assigned to witchcraft, itself associated with sexuality, reproduction, and midwifery.

During the Middle Ages, before they had a distinctive name, midwives were already practicing their craft. Much earlier, Plato (as cited above) said that midwives caused abortions by drugs and incantations. The association of midwives with magic was attested by Soranus in the second century.[84] This association appears to have survived through the Middle Ages. A priest in Breslau said in 1494: "In childbirth the midwives are busy with a thousand of devilish things as well as with the women in travail."[85]

Why did midwives—the women who, by and large, delivered the population skillfully and knowledgeably into the world—come to be seen as witches? In the ancient world there were those who deplored the use of magic by midwives, but midwives did no intentional harm. In the late Middle Ages and early modern period, what harm was done was inflicted on the midwives. H. C. Erik Midelfort's study of witchcraft surmised that midwives were singled out as victims because they were well-known in communities.[86] This thesis is questionable. More likely, the primary reason witches were persecuted was the same as that for which a woman in Hamburg was burnt to death in 1477: "because she had instructed young females how to use abortion medicines."[87]

At least some women knew what to take for birth control in the late Middle Ages. Why were these women, having been accepted for millennia, suppressed, relatively suddenly, so forcefully? That which was once accepted became intolerable in the fourteenth century. Jean Bodin stated why midwives and witches were a threat: both the security of the state and the prosperity of the community depended on a flourishing population. In his *Six Books of a Commonwealth* (Paris, 1576), Bodin said midwives employ medical procedures and magical acts to abort fetuses before live birth or to kill them once born. "In my opinion," he wrote, "they err much which doubt of scarcity by the multitude of children and citizens, when as no cities are more rich nor more famous in arts and disciplines than those which abound most with citizens."[88] Believing that witches operating through midwives were a genuine threat to society, Bodin wrote *The Demonology of Sorcery* to forewarn that their forces could topple Christendom and European prosperity just as once classical Greece was destroyed by inflation and underpopulation.[89]

The connection between witchcraft and midwifery, however, has been exaggerated by some modern scholars. In the witch trials in Scotland, for example, a number of those tried were midwives, but most were not. In contrast, between 1627 and 1630 one in three of the persons executed as witches in Cologne were midwives, and this figure probably masks a even larger number, given that many were executed who did not have an occupation listed.[90] Again, the question is how firm was the connection?[91] I argue, with the qualifications just stated, that midwifery and witchcraft were often associate but were never the same thing. An illustration is available in American history. One of the last and most famous witches was Anne Hutchinson, a woman in the household of the governor of the Massachusetts Bay Colony who was also a skilled midwife and a practitioner of medicine.[92] Of the nearly 200 witches accused at Salem in the seventeenth century, twenty-two were identified as midwife/healers, but the occupations of many of the others are unknown.[93]

In reading witchcraft confessions and other documents collected by such famous historians as Henry Lea and J. Hansen, one finds the constant reference to incubi and succubi, forms of devils that seduced men and women.[94] These beings were thought to have arisen in the earliest days of Creation, when Lilith, a wife of Adam, was banished because she insisted on full equality with her husband. By tradition the first witch, Lilith, in the words of the legend, "takes her revenge by injuring babies—baby boys during the first night of their life, while baby girls are exposed to her wicked designs until they are twenty days old."[95]

A fifteenth-century source said that witches have four means of working evil: (1) they cause a man to be unable to "perform the carnal act"; (2) they can prevent a woman from conceiving; (3) they can cause a miscarriage; and (4) they "devour the child [once born] or offer it to a devil." The source adds:

> There is no doubt concerning the first two methods, since, without the help of devils, a man can by natural means, such as herbs, savin [juniper] for example, or other emmangogues, procure that a woman cannot generate or conceive.[96]

Witches could cause people not to conceive (*sterilitas*) or to abort or, if babies were born, they could remove them from their cribs and kill them before baptism.[97] Witches knew poisons ("savin, for example").[98] They "can obstruct the generative powers by means of frigid herbs," said a fifteenth-century account.[99] These were some of the reasons that witches and midwives were associated.

In June 1335, at Toulouse, a young woman, Anne-Marie de Georgel, told a story that is typical in confessions of witchcraft. She said that, years before, "a tall, dark man with fiery eyes and clothed in skins appeared to her while she was washing and asked if she would give herself to him, to which she assented."[100] In the days that followed he would appear to her and, by breathing into her ear, cause her to be transported to the Sabbath, the devil's ritual and counterpart to the Lord's Mass. The details that followed are similar in most confessions, perhaps because there actually were people who participated in such rituals or thought they did. Possibly, too, innocent people admitted to well-known "offenses" because of the torture and hysteria of the Inquisition.

Most witches, or those so alleged, described ritualized dances and sexual orgies and often the killing of babies. An ointment or powder was made of the babies' intestines, bones, and other parts. This medicine/poison was used for evil deeds.[101] Reginald Scot in 1584 gave this gruesome description: "They [witches] boile infants (after they have murdered them unbaptized) untill their flesh be made potable."[102] In the words of a modern historian, Richard Trexler: "Infanticide was far and away the most common social crime imputed to the aged witches of Europe by the demonologists."[103]

Anne-Marie confessed that during the years she was a witch it was her habit to boil together in a cauldron poisonous herbs and substances taken from the bodies of animals and humans. She robbed cemeteries and gallows-trees at night to find ingredients for her medicines. In the end, however, after being denounced and exposed, she saw the error of her ways. She asked for reconciliation with the church, a plea that was granted.[104]

Jerome Cardan, a physician, explained in 1554 about the ointment of the type that Anne-Marie was supposed to have used:

> It was smear[ed] all over themselves. It consists, if it is to be believed, of the fat of infants torn from graves and the juices of parsley and nightshade, as well as of cinquefoil and soot. Incredibly they [the witches] may persuade themselves that they have seen large areas, theaters, green gardens, fishing, garments, adornments, dancing, handsome young men, and lovemaking of whatever kind they most desire.[105]

A contemporary gave a more detailed description:

> They [the witches] take the fat of infants from a watery decoction in a brazen vessel, [fat] which is left after the final boiling off and settling of the mixture, whereupon they collect and preserve it for their continuing benefit: with this they mix eleoselinum [celery], aconitum, poplar leaves, and soot. Or, another [formula] is thus: sium [a kind of parsley], common sweet flag, cinquefoil, bat's blood, deadly nightshade, and grease, and they mix these diverse ingredients.[106]

There are other accounts of the witches' ointment, but all have these common features: fat of infants, often specified as unbaptized babies, various contraceptive and abortifacient plants, and a number of plants of the Solanaceae family (hemlock, nightshade, mandrake, jimson weed).[107] From a pharmaceutical viewpoint, the fat would be a suitable vehicle to deliver the active substances from the other ingredients and assist in absorption. Solanaceae plants contain strong alkaloids, many being atropines (including hyoscymine, hyoscyamus, scopolamine, stramonium). Aconite is a similarly strong alkaloid. The cinquefoil was thought to counter poisons, which is a fair description of the actions of the alkaloids from the Solanaceae and aconite plants.[108] Today medical science uses atropine taken from many of these plants to increase the heart rate. In the Middle Ages and early modern periods, witches allegedly used it for hallucinations, which we know it causes.

Another ingredient said to be in the witches' ointment was acanthus, the same plant as appeared in the early Egyptian papyrus. In Middleton's play *The Witch*, Hecate says:

> Give me *Mar maritin*, some *Beare-breech* [acanthus]; when?
> FIRE: Here's *Beare-breech* and Lizard's braine, forsooth.
> HECATE: Into the vessell;
> And fetch three ounces of the red-haird Girle
> I killed last midnight.[109]

Mar maritin (or manumartis) was cinquefoil. Bear-breech or acanthus was the plant that adorned the capital of Corinthian columns.[110] The classical Corinthian columns stood in time almost midway between the Egyptian recipe for contraception containing colocynth and the witches' brew, a span of around 4,500 years. The Egyptian papyrus, the Corinthian columns, and the witches' brew are connected.

Modern experimentation shows that a person who applies the alkaloids in the witches' brew to the skin may enter a deep sleep. The subjects report that when they wake up they recall wild, exotic fantasies similar to those reported in witchcraft confessions.[111] In the words of Porta, a colleague of Galileo, their memories are "full of . . . [visions of] being borne off through the air to banquets, sounds [of music], dancing and lovemaking of handsome young people."[112] A sixteenth-century Spanish physician, Andreas De Laguna, made an ointment from herbs found in Book Four of Dioscorides' *Materia medica*, but the instructions for compounding the witches' brew he found elsewhere. De Laguna tested the ointment on a woman of Metz, who went into a deep sleep. After he revived her following thirty-six hours of sleep: "Her first words were 'Why did you awaken me, badness to you, at such an inauspicious moment? Why I was surrounded by all the delights in the world.' "[113] The details she related are similar to the descriptions of the witches' sabbath. Women who apply the ointment to the groin with a stick report the vision of flying through the air on a stick, another detail from the witch confessions. As described by Friar Franceso (1608): "so anointed they are carried away on a cowl-staff, or a broom, or a reed, a cleft stick or a distaff, or even a shovel, which thing they ride."[114]

Johann Weyer (1583) tested these herbs by taking some himself and argued from the experience that witches should be excused their delirious fantasies because they were caused by drugs.[115] A modern white, female patient given a dose of atropine sulfate reported, "I never had a delusion or hallucination in my life until that treatment."[116] Because atropine drugs are regularly employed in modern medicine for treatment of heart attacks, we are familiar with their toxicity. We know that they can cause a coma compatible with the descriptions provided by women accused of witchcraft. In addition, modern medicine adds another detail that enriches our understanding of witchcraft. The plants in the witches' brew significantly reduce seminal emissions and penile erections.[117] In other words, the deeds described in the fifteenth century as the sevenfold traits of witchcraft are all creditable, according to modern medicine (with the exception of bestiality and homosexuality). Midwives and witches, whether one and the same, knew the drugs to take to reduce fertility.

Pity, however, the midwife who cared for women and who did not consider herself a witch, a worshipper of the devil, or anything but a poor woman who helped others. In the Middle Ages the "wise woman," the equivalent of a midwife, was fairly well regarded and probably worked closely with physicians. These women passed under various names, such as *vetula, mulier, obstetrix, saga, saga matrona,* and *sage-femme.* As male physicians increased in number and advanced in education and professional organization, they came to regard the irregular women practitioners as *vulgares, illiterati mulieres, indocti, vetulae empiricii,* and *rustica,* all terms of derision or, at the very least, inferiority. The wise women practiced but they did not, in the words of the thirteenth-century surgeon Henri de Mondeville, "know the causes of things" that they treated empirically.[118] One modern interpreter, E. Mansell Pattison, sees the phenomenon of demonic possession and exorcism as a widening gap into a two-world view: henceforth, some would seek cures through science and others who would seek relief through folk healers.[119] The former became dominant, while the latter faltered under the burden of persecution. The burgeoning disregard for the power of relics was not so much the development of a rational, scientific outlook as it was the elites' disdain for the popular beliefs of the masses—the liars, illiterates, and idiots (*mendacos mendaces, illiterati,* and *idiotae*).[120]

By the sixteenth century some of the "wise women" had become professionals in guilds of midwives, but others, especially those who remained "wise women," kept to the old ways and were suspected and persecuted.[121] In order to help women, a midwife had to know drugs or, in the words of Reginald Scot (1584), "those secret mysteries."[122] The problem was that those secrets were the same as those known by witches, "poisoners," and, again in Scot's words, "anie other kind of murther."[123] Through poisons witches "killed the child in the mothers wombe."[124] Midwives were the victims of a vicious syllogism: to know the secrets was to be a witch; it was necessary to know the secrets to be a midwife; therefore, a midwife is a witch. The secrets were not necessarily the so-called witches' ointment; they were the formulas needed for the care of women, including, in some cases, contraceptives and abortifacients. Herbs that had been employed in the popular culture for millennia moved from medical lore to magic lore known only to those with malevolent motives. Those evil intentions were often held by women, so the dominant culture held in the early modern period.[125]

The shift away from the practice of midwifery was a part of broader societal changes, but the persecutions of midwives were not delusions. These events were, in the words of Keith Thomas, "anchored in culturally acceptable view of reality."[126] A woman who testified at an inquisition in Modena in 1499 said it all too well: "Who knows how to heal knows how to destroy *(qui scit sanare scit destruere)*."[127] The magical poisons were real, but to us they are not magic. By the sixteenth century, a woman who knew the "empirical remedies" *(remedia empirica)* was a suspect in any case of a perceived wrongdoing because she also knew "magical remedies" *(remedia magica)*.[128] Jean Sprot, a sixteenth-century witch, caused animals to die but also knew of drinks that heal. She practiced a ritual known to promote fertility when done in the sun, but she went "against the sun" when performing the ritual, an indication of evil intention.[129] A woman and her daughter in Scotland in 1654 went to a king's minister to "get a potion from him to kill the cats." The young woman was denied the request because she was deemed to be with child. She and her mother believed that she had cats in her womb because it was commonly held that a woman who ate food that had been stepped over by a male cat emitting semen would become pregnant with cats. Herbs were the means to expell the cats.[130]

Not all witches were women, and not all witches were accused of interfering with fertility, either to promote or to thwart it. One case was Peter from Bern, who, according to a story told around 1434, confessed that in his home he had caused seven women to miscarry by killing their fetuses and, moreover, that he regularly did the same thing to cattle.[131] The details are not provided but, from ancillary evidence explored in these chapters, we may assume Peter employed drugs, not surgical procedures. We do not know how typical was the case of Walpurga, a licensed midwife for nineteen years who was executed in 1587 for causing the death of forty-three unbaptized children by using a demonic salve.[132]

Midwifery Today

In sorting out the differences between midwifery and witchcraft in centuries past, we have as a resource the example of midwifery as it is currently practiced. According to a 1975 study, midwifery practices in early modern Europe appear similar to midwifery practices in modern Asia. In India, Pakistan, Indonesia, Malaysia, the Philippines, and Thailand, (1) almost all midwives were female; (2) most were illiterate; (3) they learned their midwifery skills from their grandmothers, mothers, or other female relatives; (4) most midwives saw no conflict in serving as advisors to women on matters of family planning and childbirth; (5) they provided other medical services, including herbal medicines.[133] Another study (1980) of midwifery in the rural Philippines found that women whose menstrual periods were delayed took either a pill or an herb to bring on menstruation. In this circumstance most recognized the possibility of pregnancy. About a third of the women (35.6 percent) took an herb, and 43.3% obtained a birth control drug from a drugstore or a physician. Of those using herbs, forty-two (approximately 80 percent of the sample group) obtained them from traditional midwives *(hilot)* and the remaining 20 percent collected the herbs themselves. None obtained the herbs from a drugstore or a physician.[134]

A greater percentage of medieval and early modern women than today's women would rely on midwives, other women, or their own knowledge rather than consult an apothecary or a physician.[135] The difference in the practice of midwifery in Asia today and in Europe in the late Middle Ages and the early modern period, however, is probably only one of degree. Yet modern midwives are not generally accused of witchcraft. In the past, many witches were persecuted for actions having nothing to do with fertility, and when the accusation did concern birth control a particular deed, real or imagined, was usually specified. Witches were accused of 233 deaths in civil courts in Essex in the late sixteenth and early seventeenth century, but only seven of the victims are known have been infants under three months old.[136] Most charges of witchcraft involved sorcery in its various forms. There is not much evidence suggesting that midwifery and witchcraft were synonymous. It is just that midwives were at high risk of attracting an accusation, possibly not entirely for innocent reasons. As late as 1907 a nurse and investigator of midwives in New York City said that some believe that "the two terms 'midwife' and 'abortionist' are synonymous."[137] That was true also in the past, and it may be that the connection with abortion earned the midwife the label of "witch" even if she were never actually accused of killing a fetus or child.

The Do-Gooders vs. the Witches

In regions of central Europe in the late Middle Ages, practitioners of a fertility sect performed their rituals, which may go back to antiquity, in woods connected to their fields. Those around Friuli, now in northern Italy, called themselves the "I Benandanti" or "do-gooders." They were not witches but their opposite. Among the things the "do-gooders" did was to guard the cribs of infants, thereby preventing witches from snatching them before baptism.[138]

Carolo Ginzburg, who studied this sect, interprets these rituals as attempts to guarantee the fertility of the fields. Some of the members' testimony indicates their ultimate plight. Returning at night from their rituals, they said, they encountered witches returning from their sabbaths. Fights occurred, with the "do-gooders" employing weapons of fennel and the witches using weapons of sorghum.

How strange! Both fennel and sorghum, a type of millet, are so flimsy as to be virtually harmless: as weapons they would be as effective as the proverbial ten lashes with a wet noodle. The fennel became the symbol of the do-gooders, probably because this herb was thought to ward off witches and witchcraft. Fennel, too, was thought to hinder abortions.[139] In the Lorsch manuscript (ca. 800 A.C.E.), however, it was used to cause an abortion, and in Macer's herbal (ca. 1070) fennel was listed as a "menstrual purgative."[140] Also, fennel was used in eye medicines; perhaps it came to be believed that it could help one see a witch.[141]

The sorghum's significance is even more difficult to guess. A parish priest of Brazzano quoted Gasparutto, a "do-gooder," as saying: "He begged me not to sow sorghum in my field, and whenever he finds any growing he pulls it up, and he curses whoever plants it; and when I said that I wanted to sow it, he began to swear."[142] Sorghum contains certain alkaloids that can cause an abortion, according to modern science, but it was not found in the texts of ancient or medieval medicine for that effect.[143] Many testimonies have survived that provide us with these details because the Inquisition mistook the "do-gooders" for witches, rooted them out, and burned them in a great suppression that began about 1575. The campaign ended about 1620, when there were no more do-gooders left to persecute.

Ginzburg marveled at the image of fighting between the two groups that the Inquisition had decided were the same: "The essence of these gatherings was an obscure rite: witches and warlocks armed with sorghum stalks jousting and battling with benandanti [do-gooders] armed with fennel stalks."[144] The choice of weapons was interpreted in terms of fertility, as witchcraft rituals are thought to be traced back to ancient pagan rituals.[145] In northern Europe, too, the sagas suggest the magical powers of female helpers who assisted in childbirth. These women knew the magic formulas and songs to invoke the protection of the goddesses.[146] These sagas helped to explain the association of fertility cults, midwifery, and witchcraft.

What Do the Simple Folk Do?

A line in the Broadway play *Camelot* goes, "What do the simple folk do?" The penetration of the church's stance on birth control in the consciousness of the common folk in the late Middle Ages was slow, not sudden. Increasing professionalization of the elite of medical practice meant that those who were not accepted by the profession were beginning to be banned, or at least discouraged, from providing medical care. At the top were the physicians (*phisici* or *medici*), who were expected to be university-educated. In monasteries there were the *infirmarii*, who were learned in medicine. There were surgeons (*cirurgici*), whose prestige varied but some of whom had some university education. Below them were the guilds of apothecaries (*apothecarius, aromatarii, pigmentarii, speciarius, herbolarius*, etc.), whose members were tradesmen and usually literate to some degree. Among those organized and recognized for health care were barbers *(barberius, barbitonsor)*.

By the fourteenth century, many regions of Europe required licenses to practice any of these health professions. Increasingly under attack were the "other" practitioners, many of whom were provided services only part-time. They were unorganized. Many were uneducated. They were variously called rustics *(rustici)* or "old women" *(vetulae)*. It probably was not so much old as post-menopausal women who were under attack.[147] Women were increasingly excluded from medical practice because of the requirement for a university education and guild restrictions. Not all "old women" were midwives: for example, Henri di Mondeville (ca. 1260–1320) defined "old women" *(vetulae)* as a term of derision against all bad women, such as prostitutes, fortune tellers, barbers, *insidatores,* converted Jews, and midwives.[148] The point is that the application of the term was negative and contemptible, and midwives were included in the category. Still, even by the eighteenth century, one word for midwife in French was *sage-femme,* "wise woman."[149]

Also pushed to the border areas of health care were Jewish physicians, because university students were expected to be Christian.[150] A French law in 1336, affirmed in 1353, sought to regulate the distribution of drugs by prohibiting apothecaries from selling "poisonous medicines, dangerous things or other things that cause an abortion" unless directed by a master who is licensed in the science of medicine.[151] There is no indication that the law had an impact or could have been enforced. Just the same, its existence indicates an awareness of a problem, even if the solution was delayed five hundred years before the modern state could enforce it.

The medical curriculum included the writings of Avicenna and, rarely, *Brevarium practice,* with their discussions of birth control. But Avicenna's *Canon of Medicine* was enormous, far larger than, for instance, Gray's *Anatomy,* which is the bane of modern medical students. The simple truth is that, from the thirteenth century to the Renaissance, medically trained university students appear to have learned little about birth control in their courses. The church regarded it as wrong, and the university was largely an institution of the church. The physicians' art was for disease and injury, not family planning.

As a result, much of the practical knowledge of birth control was left in the hands of "old women," some of whom became known midwives. Also pushed, shoved really, away from the central culture were women who knew the antifertility herbs and were thought to be witches. They were not suffered to live, as the King James translation of Exodus 22:18 reads: "Thou shalt not suffer a witch to live."

Women could advise one another about such matters as birth control. Some modern scholars believe that women accused of being witches did gather, in fact, in small groups and that the gatherings could reach as high as hundreds or even thousands on festival days. In these groups they may have engaged in "pagan religious worship" and in "trading herbal lore."[152] In fairness, assertions about how women may have exchanged information are speculative, not based on hard evidence. Not to be questioned, however, is that women were thought to know about herbal lore.[153] The magic associated with women was often connected to their use of herbs.[154] With the greater urbanization of Europe and the development of an industrial, commercialized society, people increasingly bought their bread from bakers, produce from greengrocers, and drugs from an apothecary. Herbal medicines for birth control were not simple—they had to be obtained from a midwife or from someone with special knowledge.

There are about 500,000 higher plant species. Medieval drug inventories and prescription literature have the names of more than 250 different species indigenous to Europe (plus some, such as pepper, cinnamon, and camphor, that were imported).[155] The average medieval person probably could identify more plants than the average modern person, even though there was no easy means, such as a field guide, to correct mistaken identifications in the Middle Ages.[156] Armed with picture books and a whole branch of science, taxonomy, the modern person finds it much easier to "look up" the name of a plant, but his or her medieval counterpart would have more "hands-on" experience. And both medieval and modern people know, no matter how they learned about them, that many plants are easily mistaken for others.

Information about natural products as antifertility agents is complex and not easily learned. One has to know how and when to harvest a plant. The chemistry of a plant containing active pharmaceuticals varies according to the season of the year. If taken at the wrong time—for example, spring rather than fall—a plant may provide extracts with negligible pharmaceutical qualities. Some herbalists say that the time of day can be important, mornings often being best. The correct part of the plant to be harvested must be known. For instance, only the seed or seed pulp of the pomegranate may be active as a contraceptive. With other plants the sap from stem, or roots, or flower, or bark, or seeds, or fruit may supply the active principle.

The method of extraction can be critical. Some compounds are not soluble with water extraction, others are. Alcohol extraction may be required. Some drug compounds are destroyed by heating, others are improved by it and are best prepared as a tea. Above all, one has to know the amount and concentration to use. Often the older recipes specified a concoction (cooking), others a decoction (boiling down to a concentrate). In addition, the route of administration must be known: orally, by cutaneous application, or as a vaginal pessary.

The complexity of drug administration does not end with the plant's proper identification, harvesting, extraction, and preparation. The amount and frequency of administration are critical, some herbs being potentially fatal. Take tansy and pennyroyal as examples. A small amount of tansy tea will not appreciably affect a pregnant woman. A certain number of cups of tea will cause an abortion in an early pregnancy, but too many will lead to disaster. Pennyroyal may be effective because it is fatally toxic to fetal tissue, but too much will damage the liver of the mother.

To prescribe the correct dose, one has to know the circumstances and duration of pregnancy. Some plants are contraceptive, even if administered post-coitally; Queen Anne's lace is effective, so the evidence suggests, only very early in a pregnancy. Judging from what the ancient medical literature says, some contraceptives are effective if taken for long periods, whereas others are active only for a short period. Most abortifacient plants, acting as hormonal stimulators or suppressants, are effective only in the early period of pregnancy. A few plants, such as birthwort or *Aristolochae* species and juniper, are effective late in term. Each plant has its own "secrets" concerning when it will have the desired effect and when its effect may be unsuccessful or even fatal. The secrets must be learned and transmitted to others in a chain of learning.[157]

A natural-product drug is truly a product of human knowledge. There is much more to birth control than knowing to take some of this or that herb. The ordinary people in the ancient and medieval worlds may have been common but they were not simple, as the line in Camelot reads. The use of natural products as antifertility agents is complex and not easily learned. A daughter had to be intelligent and give careful attention to learn exactly what to do.

We know that information about birth control primarily was orally transmitted. Ancient and medieval medical authorities were not re-searchers; they learned from their teachers. Somewhere in the ancient mists of time, someone discovered a medicinal usage for a substance. Trial-and-error experimentation was the next step, and then the per-son informed others about the experience. If a woman ate something and subsequently had a miscarriage, she made an association between the two events. Intelligent people can make such observations and, once armed with the knowledge, they know what not to eat to avoid a miscarriage or what to take to achieve one. Pliny noted the situa-tion.[158] So did Soranus, who gave a list of regimes to avoid miscar-riage. If one wants to miscarry, however, he advised simply to do the opposite.[159] Some animal science experts speculate that as many as 30 percent of all pregnancies end in miscarriages because of a plant diet.[160]

Another means by which contraceptives and abortifacients were dis-covered was the observation of animals that grazed on certain plants and failed to reproduce. Theophrastus spoke of learning about drugs through studying animal behavior.[161] This is the same method, after all, that modern science used to learn about the effect of plant sex hor-mones on mammalian reproduction.

Eventually, perhaps centuries or even millennia later, a person would write down the procedure and, if that work survived or, more likely, was incorporated in another written work that does, then the infor-mation was codified in a written authority. Information about birth control drugs usually was different in each writing; it was seldom that one author would copy precisely from another. Moreover, some of the writings in each time period introduced new drugs that had to be the product of the type of discovery just described.

From the evidence available to us, we learn that some drugs were discovered to be effective to control birth but that the chain of learn-ing was broken and the information, if not recorded, was lost. When that happened, future generations would not have the advantage of the product of human knowledge, once learned but then forgotten. Judg-ing by the medical records of the fourteenth and fifteenth centuries, many people in the late Middle Ages still knew about contraceptive and abortifacient drugs, but they may have used these drugs less fre-quently than their ancestors did.

5

Witches and Apothecaries in the Sixteenth and Seventeenth Centuries

Oyntment for flying here I have,
Of children's fat stoin from the grave,
The juice of smallage and nightshade,
Of poplar-leaves and aconite made . . .

> Mother Demdike in Shadwell's play, *The Lancaster Witches* (1692)

In 1484 Pope Innocent VIII issued *Summis desiderantes* against witchcraft. This papal bull is regarded as the official beginning of widespread persecutions. Particularly singled out by the Pope were the abominable crimes that witches commit to "ruin and cause to perish the offspring of women, the foal of animals . . . and hinder men from begetting and women from conceiving."[1] The new law, and others like it, demonstrated that the tolerance for abortion and birth control in Europe was waning. It decreased gradually, never dramatically, in the early modern period. A prime example of the change are the laws on abortion in the *Constitutio Criminalis Carolina* issued by Emperor Charles V of the Holy Roman Empire in the year 1532. The following provision originated in the ordinances of Bamberg and dated to the year 1507.

> Article 133: Penalty for anyone who aborts a woman pregnant with child. Item: anyone who through a blow to a pregnant woman, or

126

who gives to her a food or drink so to abort a living child, as well as anyone who makes a man unable to procreate or a woman to conceive, whether the deed is brought about deliberately or maliciously, the person should be given the punishment as for homicide, and a woman if she had done this to herself punishment to death by drowning or otherwise.[2]

A woman *(fraw)* who brings about an abortion on herself is guilty of a crime also severely punished. The law is not equating any abortion with homicide, just those that "abort a living fetus *(ein lebendig kindt abtreibt)*." The law adds that someone performing the same deed who terminates a "child, who still is not living *(kind, das noch nit lebendig wer)*," is guilty of a crime that is punished by a penance, punishment, or exile.[3] The law embraces the ancient and medieval distinction between the formed/unformed fetus *(foetus formatus/nonformatus)*. One whose actions in any way remove an unformed fetus from the womb is guilty of a crime, albeit not homicide. Here is where European law was extending itself in the protection of the unborn. The law does not recognize the fetus as a person. Just the same, the law was restricting acceptable behavior with respect to birth control more than had been done in the Middle Ages or antiquity.

Laws of Caroline

Another surprise lurks in the Laws of Caroline of 1532: anyone who causes a man or woman to be infertile is punished as a murderer would be.[4] The law does not clarify whether permanent sterility is at issue or temporary sterility (in other words, contraception).

The law was that of an empire, but it derived from a city law. As we saw in the previous chapter, particularly in respect to the town of Manosque, laws against abortion were locally enforced. The modern period saw local laws spread to larger governing units.

In the wording of the Caroline laws, once more, we must observe the means by which an abortion was expected to be delivered: through oral drugs. The German law used the words *essen oder drincken*, "food or drink," rather than *drogen*, "drugs." These words connote that the substances were common and that some were used as foods as well as abortifacients; also, there is a similarity with the expression used in the declaration in the Talmud that drugs that were eaten by healthy people could be taken on the Sabbath. While the actual drugs/foods were unnamed, probably they were the mints, rue, pennyroyal, spurge, sage, and other herbs that were foods as well as drugs.

Whether in Dante, Chaucer, church law, or state law, the means stated of administering contraception or abortion were always drugs (included in food and drink). The exception was an abortion caused by physical blows delivered by another party. In the Caroline laws, the substances were specified as oral. One wonders what a modern, clever lawyer would have done with pessary-administered birth control agents! One assumes that the lawmakers (men, to be sure) were acquainted with the normal or expected means but were not versed in birth control techniques.

English Law on Abortion

In 1460 John Baldwin wrote: "if a man strikes a pregnant woman, and then she is delivered of one who is dead; there it is not felony, for it cannot be known *(en notice)* whether it was not at such time *in rerum natura* etc., and so it cannot be tried."[5] Shortly before 1548 Sir William Staunford wrote the first systematic treatise on English criminal law. In discussing what we call abortion, he never referred to the principles stated by Bracton (although Bracton was often cited in other cases) and Fleta that made abortion of a quickened or formed fetus a felony, but he did discuss the Twinslayer Case (1327) and the Abortionist's Case (1348).[6] These actual cases, not pronouncements by jurists, he regarded as establishing the guiding principles. The tradition of law supported Sir William's position. If a person killed a fetus while in the womb, there was no felony. But if a person kills a child *in rerum natura*, that is, who exists in nature, or, in plain English, who has been born, he or she has committed homicide. In addition to the two cases concerned with the fetus in the womb, he cited a case of 1314–15, in which a woman gave birth to a child and immediately cut its throat (prior to baptism, it would appear). She was outlawed for homicide.[7] A similar situation arose in comment in the court of the Inner Temple (ca. 1490), when it was ruled that a sheriff could not arrest a person who killed a fetus "within its mother's belly" but should arrest one who killed a baby born but not yet baptized.[8] This case did not clarify whether the death was in connection with an abortion prior to delivery. Finally, an anonymous fifteenth-century commentary on a statute of Gloucester (1278) unambiguously stated that the dividing line that marks the commission of a felony in the case of an act that leads to an infant's death is birth *(in rerum natura);* if the act leads to the death of a fetus (abortion), there is no felony but the person who commits the act "shall be heavily fined, because the trespass is so heinous."[9]

The conflict between the jurists' position on abortion and actual case law was observed by William Lambarde (1536–1601). In the first edition of his *Eirenarcha, or of the Office of the Justices of Peace* (1581), Lambarde cited the 1314 case of the woman who killed her baby after birth as indicating that birth *(in rerum natura)* was the deciding factor in determining whether a felony had been committed. In the third edition of the same work, Lambarde discussed Bracton's opinion that the killing of a fetus in the womb after quickening was homicide. Here he cited the Twinslayer Case and the Abortionist's Case to conclude that Bracton was incorrect. By inference, of course, so would Fleta be incorrect. English common law differed from the German Caroline laws discussed above in that English law did not punish abortion as a felony at any period.[10] Abortion was an offense punished by ecclesiastical courts until about the 1540s or, if a case came before a secular court, it was treated as trespass or a misdemeanor. At least, secular courts in Norwich tended not to hear cases concerning abortion.[11] In contrast, up to the 1530s the Winchester consistory court presided over cases for concealed abortions, infanticide, and miscarriages brought about by herbs.[12]

No certain case have I found in English law where abortion prior to or after quickening resulted in a criminal conviction. A possible exception was the case of Maud, discussed previously. This is not to say that abortion was not punished, but the punishment was ecclesiastical, not civil. William Wodlake was indicted in 1530 in Middlesex for having given "with dissembling words . . . [to] Katharine to drink a certain drink in order to destroy the child then being in the same Katherine's body" and, as a result, she delivered a stillborn child.[13] Accused of other crimes as well, William died in the same year, apparently before his guilt or innocence was established, forever obscuring whether he was indicted for the murder of an unborn child.

It is possible that juries in William's time would have been more likely to convict than earlier juries were. When the details were recorded, the medieval common law cases on abortion specified only physical blows or manipulations and omitted chemical abortions. Because fifteenth- and sixteenth-century cases specified chemical abortions as well, it may well be that the law was extended to cover a subject neglected by medieval secular courts. This change in the perception of the law occurred because of Sir Edward Coke (1552–1634), the great jurist. Through some degree of deception, Coke altered English common law to punish more severely abortion before ensoulment by making the crime less than homicide—and he specifically stated that chemical abortion deserved the same consequences.

An abortion case whose details are uncertain came before the Queen's Bench in 1601. A man called Sims beat a woman, Cook, who was not his wife, and she aborted. He was found not guilty or liable because, in the same words from the Twinslayer Case, it could not be proven *(non constat)* that the beating caused a death. Among other things, we do not know whether the abortion was welcomed or solicited. The judges for the case expressed concern about abortions and how difficult they are to prove, but it is unclear whether they challenged common law precedent.[14] Edward Coke was Attorney General, but it is not certain whether he was aware of the Sims case. Some forty-one years after the case, Coke published his *Third Institutes*, destined to become an authority on law. In it he discussed the law on homicide as it applied to abortion. He wrote:

> If a woman be quick with childe, and by a potion or otherwise killeth it in her wombe; or if a man beat her, whereby this childe dieth in her body, and she is delivered of a dead childe, *this is a great misprision* [italics supplied], and no murder: but if the childe be born alive, and dieth of the potion, battery, or other cause, this is murder: for in the law it is accounted a reasonable creature, *in rerum natura*, when it is born alive.[15]

A misprision is a high misdemeanor. For his authority Coke quotes both Bracton and Fleta and cites them as well as other references. In the margins are citations to the cases of the Twinslayer and the Abortionist, but they are not otherwise the subject of comment. By citing these two cases in this context, Coke conveyed that they supported the principle argued by Bracton and Fleta when, to the contrary, they did not. In the opinion of Cyril Means, Coke has misrepresented the law in an "outrageous attempt," because there was no authority for saying that abortion before quickening was "a great misprision."[16] If so, according to Means, it was a deliberate misrepresentation of the law on abortion. Coke may have been disturbed by the 1601 case and felt that abortion, earlier punished in ecclesiastical courts, essentially went unpunished by law because civil courts did not assert jurisdiction.[17] The Puritan movement, which was strong in Coke's time, increased punishment for sexual crimes. Coke may have wanted to correct a wrong because of changed conditions, a sentiment with which modern American judges can identify. In the context of the seventeenth century, however, his change of course would probably amount to dishonesty.

A view more charitable to Coke is expressed by Robert Destro, who speculates that Coke was simply seeking to "bring the written common law into step with the times"—times that reflected the new science's concepts of fetal development.[18] Whatever is thought of Coke's writings, Coke gave more emphasis to abortion as a high misdemeanor rather than as a felony, and this position may not have been an affront to the trend in courts handling abortion cases. In Coke's writings, medieval common law was misrepresented but not totally misstated.

Coke's pronouncement was subsequently incorporated into common law and his position became law through the force of his authority. Coke took Bracton's *animatum fuerit*, or ensoulment at fetal formation, to mean "quickening" in English. Prior to the her perception of fetal movement a woman was "pre-quick with child," and thereafter she was "quick with child."[19] Ironically, Sir William Blackstone (1723–1780) cited Coke's view that abortion after quickening was only "a heinous misdemeanor," not homicide as Bracton had said, as an indication that Coke was more merciful than Bracton.[20] Matthew Hale in 1682 said homicide must involve a person killed who is *in rerum natura* but a woman "quick with child" who gave "a potion" to kill it has committed a "great misprision" but not murder. If the child is born alive, it is murder if the cause of death was attributed to "that potion." Interestingly, only chemical abortion was mentioned as a cause.[21] Gone were the medieval statements about physical manipulation, abuse, and assault. Hale complained, however, that the law was unfair: a person who attempted to help a pregnant woman by giving a potion would be punished for committing a felony if the woman was harmed, whereas physicians were safe from the law's justice.[22]

Midwives and Birth Control in the
Early Modern Period

Isabel Fernández was a practicing midwife in Málaga in 1492, the year that Christopher Columbus conveyed Spain's flag to the New World. Since the latter half of the fifteenth century, midwives in most areas of Europe had been pressured to submit to a licensing procedure that typically involved an oath. Midwives did not limit their services to pregnancies and births. Their employment included consultation on female maladies, including irregular menstrual cycles, breast-feeding, sterility, rape, and venereal disease.[23] In Málaga, Isabel provided such a wide range of services. She advertised that she produced some "medicines" herself, which she administered "if those who give birth with her suffer from any affliction of the womb or other distresses."[24] A half-century later in Cuenca province of Spain, María Luna, a Morisco or Moor, is described as "a woman well versed in medical matters and knowledge of herbs and a very good midwife."[25] In modern terms, Isabel and María offered "full-service midwifery."

In an exaggerated conclusion, Margaret Murray, a historian of witchcraft, wrote: "in the sixteenth and seventeenth centuries, the better the midwife the better the witch,"[26] a phrase said to come from the Middle Ages.[27] David Harley, a modern scholar, has entered a strong plea to reject the assertion that midwives were considered witches by advancing evidence that many midwives turned in witches, testified against them at trials, and enjoyed some degree of prestige.[28] Some, he admitted, fell victim to witchcraft persecutions, but often they were accused of magical and demonical practices unrelated to midwifery. He cited the case of Mrs. Pepper of Newcastle upon Tyne, a midwife, accused of administering magical remedies to a sick man who worsened after her treatment. Because Mrs. Pepper was accused of bewitchment, Harley exonerates her persecution as a midwife. Other innocent witches were the celebrated colonial New Englanders Anne Hutchinson and Jane Hawkins, who often are described as having been persecuted for their midwifery but were in fact accused of practicing magical medicine.[29] Midwives dealt with herbal medicines popularly known to be both curative and poisonous. Then, as now, the difference between a medicine and a poison is dosage and frequency. Many midwives were celebrated and respected because they did good; allegedly, some did harm and were persecuted as witches. The innocent burned in the same flames as destroyed those whose deeds *may* have kindled a cruel response.

Midwives used drugs to regulate fertility, to promote or suppress it. In addition to information from women like Isabel and María, there is ample information from people who believed that midwives engaged in the nefarious practice of abortion and infanticide, both associated with witchcraft and magic.[30] The number of cases multiplied during the sixteenth and seventeenth centuries in which women—almost always, women—who were tried for witchcraft were accused of infanticide.[31] In England 62 percent of the accusations against witches involved children.[32] This was a legacy of the thirteenth century, but by the sixteenth century the punishment was often death at the burning stake (except in England, where it was hanging).

In the Reformation it was believed that to burn witches and midwives was God's command—and the sixteenth century was a time when God's commands were heeded. Exodus 22:18: "You shall not allow a sorceress to live." The Greek Septuagint employed the word *pharmakis* (feminine gender), meaning "poisoner" or "sorceress," the base word also meaning "drugs." This was the same word employed by Paul (Galatians 5:20) and found in the Book of Revelation (9:21; 21:8; 22:15). The Latin Vulgate duly translated the term *maleficus* (masculine), the same term used in Roman law for one who performs abortions, through inference, by means of drugs or poisons.[33] The motif of the Protestant Reformation was that each person was his or her own priest, the Bible being a source of instruction directly to each person. For the passage from Exodus, Martin Luther translated the *pharmakis* as *Die Zauberinnen* (feminine gender), meaning "magicians," "sorceresses," or "witches" (2 Moses 22:17), whereas the 1560 English translation of the same passage, Exodus 22:18, reads: "Thou shalt not suffre a witche to live." The King James translation repeated the same words. In these cases, the sixteenth-century translations were more correct than the Latin or Greek. The Hebrew *měkaššēp* meant "sorcerer," but from other biblical contexts it was clear that the gender was feminine. In Deuteronomy 18:10 a male "sorcerer" was not punished by death, as was a female in Exodus 22:18.[34] A reasonable, literate person of the sixteenth or seventeenth century would know that God was denouncing female witches who were believed to be poisoners, especially when the poison was used against babies.

Midwives' oaths taken at the time of licensing were fairly explicit on the matter. A 1588 oath has the midwife promise that "ye shall not in any wise use or exercise any manner of witchcraft [or] charm." A Parisian oath of 1560: "I will not use any superstitious or illegal means, either in words or signs, nor any other way."[35] Embedded in the wording was the expectation that some of the devices employed were herbal drugs that were capable of working malicious deeds. Despite the oaths, in 1764 F. E. Cangiamila, an Italian prelate, said that midwives knew the medicines to take to cause an abortion ("medicamina, lunaria tributa moventia").[36] As late as 1795, according to the oath by the Barcelona College of Surgery for licensing in Cataluña, midwives swore "not to administer any medicament to women who are pregnant, parturient, or puerperal which has not been prescribed by a Latin surgeon or physician."[37] A similar English oath expressed the same prohibition but extended the pledge not to give counsel about "any herb, medicine, or poison, or any other thing, to any woman being with child whereby she should destroy or cast out that she goeth withal before her time."[38]

The midwives' oaths could be seen as primarily a means of preventing competition between midwives and surgeons and physicians and of raising royal revenue, were it not for the fact that those who gave out such "medicaments" were in danger of losing their lives. If in the modern world some people distrust medicine and turn to folklore and herbal medicine as an alternative, the same must have been true on at least an equal scale in the early modern period. In the late medieval and early modern periods, most women practitioners were not learned in the new academic culture of western Europe. Their herbal knowledge was learned from other women, not books. A church dictum stated, "If a woman dare to cure *without having studied* she is a witch and must die."[39]

A late-sixteenth-century ordinance in the city of Nürnberg stated: "Recently evil cases have taken place, that those women who live in sin and adultery have illegitimate children and, during birth or before, purposefully attempt to kill them by taking harmful, abortion-causing drugs or through other notorious means."[40] The very fact that this same ordinance prohibited midwives from burying the fetus or dead child without informing the city council is a probable sign that some midwives had been involved in such cases. When an infant was buried, a midwife was expected to have "three or four unsuspected female persons" to witness the procedure.[41] This may explain why Uge's mother took the aborted child away, presumably for secret burial, as the hapless, accused physician alluded in testimony in the trial in Manosque.

The laws of Caroline (1532), the same as those mentioned earlier that made abortion a crime, made witchcraft that harms people criminal.[42] (Harmless witchcraft was not punished.) Britain's law against witchcraft and sorcery in 1541 was more specific. It was a crime for anyone "to provoke any persone to unlawful love, or for any other unlawful intente or purpose."[43] When the law was repealed in 1547 under Edward, those convicted of such acts were pilloried. In revoking the criminal act these words were added: "unlaufull love or to hurte or destroye any person in his or her Body."[44]

Five years later the first law was reinstated, with some changes: it was unlawful to use any part of a dead body "in any manner Witchcrafte, Sorcerie, Charme or Enchantment."[45] Without providing details, the law was defining acts of witchcraft. When considered along with the other evidence cited, the wording suggests antifertility (and fertility) drugs and the manufacture of drugs from babies' bodies. Included in those midwives' oaths: one must not use or engage in any manner of witchcraft, or allow any woman's child to be murdered, and one must bury a stillborn child properly.[46] If any of these acts were considered unimaginable, there would have been no reason to include the words in the oaths. An English law in 1624 placed the burden on women to prove natural cause for an infant's death; otherwise they were accused of homicide, and often they were hanged. Increasingly, collaborative evidence from physicians, surgeons, apothecaries, and men midwives was required when women midwives testified about the viability of a live but premature baby.[47]

Women were the primary objects of witchcraft persecutions. About the year 1500 there was a shift and women were even more preponderantly its victims. Whereas men continued to be tried for heresy, women were those most often accused of witchcraft.[48] In 1602 a man proclaimed that 1,800,000 witches threatened Europe, a force stronger than any army that had ever descended on Europe.[49] In the French-speaking sections of Switzerland and in southwestern Germany, regions where data exist, approximately 80 percent of those burned were women.[50] In enumerating the reasons women are more inclined toward witchcraft, a male writer in 1576 asserted that Eve (not Adam) wanted to know everything, good and bad, and that women were more attracted to Satan.[51] In 1508 Abbot Trithemius explained, "It is a repulsive breed, that of the witches, especially the female among them, who, with the help of evil spirits or magic potions, bring to mankind endless harm."[52] In his century and the one that followed, twice as many witches were burned in Catholic areas as in Protestant. Thomas Gale, surgeon to Queen Elizabeth, visited two London hospitals in 1544 and reported 300 old and infirm, many suffering horribly. "All these [people] were brought to that mischief by witches, by women."[53] And he served a sovereign queen!

These data persuade some historians to surmise that the virulent witch hunts and the demonization of women, primarily by clergy, were caused by sexual frustration.[54] One modification of this theme is that in the sixteenth century people were reacting to "syphilitic shock," the fear of endemic syphilis and the fear of sexual relations that it engendered. Syphilis caused miscarriages and birth defects, and midwives were suspected of complicity in these events.[55] The syphilis idea has merit but the suppression of witchcraft has deeper roots, roots connected with the "root poisons" of biblical times.

Drugs were the means by which witches were supposed to enact their will: this much was asserted by contemporary accounts. Even before witchcraft was known or, at least, condemned, people in Anglo-Saxon England were warned to beware the woman who knew the herbs. Such knowledge carried an implication of magic.[56] One Yorkshire woman in 1590 attempted to clarify the matter: she cured cattle of diseases by medicine and drinks, not by charms and magic.[57] Pope Sixtus V's bull (*Effraenatam*, 1588) censured both contraception and abortion "by means of magical deeds *(maleficiis)* and by cursed medicines *(maleficiis medicamentis)*."[58] In speaking of how witches control people's thoughts, Scot (1584) said, "I grant there may be herbs and stones found and known to the physicians . . . but witches or magicians have power by words, herbs, or imprecations to thrust into the mind or conscience of man, what it shall please them, by virtue of their charms, herbs, stones, or familiars."[59] The charge is as ancient as the poetry of Virgil:

> she kept
> also the frute divine,
> With herbes and liquors sweete that still
> to sleepe did men incline.
> The minds of men (she saith) from love
> with charmes she can unbind,

> In whom she list: but others can
>   she cast to cares unkind.[60]

Johann Weyer (1583) disputed the claim by "some famous scholars" that "certain worthless objects or noxious drugs bring harm when they are hidden somewhere and later walked upon or passed by." The "old woman" worked her power "by virtue of witchcraft," not "the exhalations of a poison."[61] The herbs did not have the power, the witches did.[62] Frommann's treatise on wondrous things in 1575 said, "The Devil arranges through the midwives not only the abortive death of the fetuses lest they be brought to the holy font of baptism, but also by their [the midwives'] aid he causes newborn babies secretly to be consecrated to himself."[63] One woman confessed to preventing the baptism of twenty-three babies and another to killing babies in the womb.[64]

"Wise women," sorceresses, midwives, and witches were separate categories in the sixteenth and seventeenth centuries, but people, peasants and officials alike, often conflated them as all made of the same cloth.[65] Women who knew the herbs of healing were candidates for accusations of sorcery and witchcraft. Those who practiced midwifery were especially vulnerable because they knew the poisons that controlled fertility and could cause harm. An account from sixteenth-century Austria shows how a "wise woman" who practiced good magic with herbs came to be regarded as a witch:

> Such a woman cooked and mixed [certain herbs] and gave the soup or rather the water to women and men, so that when they washed themselves with it, no one could do them harm . . . Through this and other similar superstitions she developed a reputation as a witch *(Hexe)*; the peasants have such little faith that even when they have merely a pain in the finger, they run straight to such old women and have them do incantations, washings, and other such superstitious things, which they then tell to someone else, so that when he becomes sick or something else happens to him he should go to this or that [old woman] who can help him.[66]

And in the year of the plague, 1665, Daniel Defoe said that the common people

> ran to Conjurers and Witches and all Sorts of Deceivers to know what should become of them always alarm'd and awake, on purpose

to delude them and pick their Pockets. So they were as mad upon running after Quacks and Mountebanks and every practising Old Woman for Medicines and Remedies.[67]

Midwifery in the sixteenth and seventeenth centuries was connected with witchcraft, not as tightly as some modern scholars have suggested but more firmly than others say. Protestants associated the bad features of midwifery with Catholicism and *vice versa*.[68] One Danish minister referred to Catholic midwives as old "popish monks' women."[69] By organizing and by taking professional oaths, wittingly or unwittingly the midwives in each region of Europe conducted a public relations campaign to represent themselves as providers of care for childbirth and women's health. Their efforts were partially successful in the long run, but in the short run many died because they were accused of knowing and doing too much.

The Walwyn version of Aristotle's *Secrets* (1520) advised men "never to confide in the Works and Services of Women" and to "beware of deadly poison, for it is no new thing for Men to be poison'd."[70] In some instances, the abortifacient herbs could rightfully be called poisons. In 1505 a man from Nottinghamshire was named as an accessory to a crime whereby a woman "drank various bad and polluted potions in order to kill and destroy the child" in her womb and ended up killing both herself and the baby.[71] Men feared women who knew poisons. Women, especially old ones (or at least post-menopausal), were the practitioners of sorcery, and herbs were a principal means by which their powers were affected.[72] Little wonder, then, that physicians and learned people overlooked the utility of herbs and saw only their harmful uses. We need to know how much men—both physicians and laymen—knew about birth control herbs during the sixteenth century.

The Humanists

During the Renaissance humanists were devoted to the study of classical texts and the explication of the wisdom of the ancients. Through rigorous study and an energetic zeal for translating from the Greek, they brought out new editions and translations of the ancient texts, along with copious commentaries. When Galen's lessons on anatomy were replaced by new findings learned from the dissection of human cadavers, the change did not seriously alter the ancient notion that fetuses developed in stages, the male sooner than the female. The anatomists said nothing to challenge this idea, and some actually stated that at some point the *anima rationalis* (in an another word, the soul), having been sent by God, entered the fetus.[73] One would expect that explicating ancient pharmaceutical texts and actually identifying the plants mentioned in them would have revived traditional knowledge about birth control agents. Such was not the case, however.

To the contrary, the humanists appear to have known little about birth control, which was still associated with magic and witchcraft. The laws of Caroline and various city ordinances reflected increasing intolerance with abortion as it was then defined. Legal trends indicate that birth control information was being pushed underground, out of the public domain. The information continued to be published in herbals and in some medical works, but these were few in number.

Elsewhere I have shown how the translators of Dioscorides and, to a lesser extent, Galen and Hippocrates were fairly faithful in translating birth control terms; however, the translations do reveal some unfamiliarity.[74] A Hippocratic term for abortion in Greek was rendered into Latin as "embryo knocker" by Maurice de l'Corde (fl. 1570s),[75] and Hermolaus Barbarus (1480s) translated Dioscorides' text on squirting cucumber as "it makes an abortion *in pregnant women*"—a bit of redundancy atypical of philologists.[76] Even the great commentator on Dioscorides, a practicing physician in Venice, Petrus Andreas Matthiolus (first edition 1544), revealed that he knew surprisingly little about birth control agents. Despite the fact that his edition and commentary took three large volumes, by and large Matthiolus was content merely to repeat Dioscorides without comment.

One can presume two reasons for the humanists' paucity of data about birth control: either they knew little or they did not wish to reveal what they knew. I suspect the former reason was the more important. Those who published learned commentaries were usually philologists whose medical knowledge was limited, or they were physicians (and, as we have seen, physicians themselves were not well-schooled in birth control). Medical practitioners could have learned from their patients, of course, but the intellectual mood of the Renaissance caused them to distrust, even to scorn, folklore. And folklore is perhaps the category in which many Renaissance literati would have regarded the contention that plants could prevent conception or end pregnancy.

Herbals

While the humanists who dealt with the classical texts appear to have had scant knowledge of antifertility measures, the authors of herbals during the same time period were more aware and willing to disclose what they knew. One of the earliest printed herbals was the *Tractatus de virtutibus herbarum,* anonymously written and first published in Mainz in 1484. The edition I saw was printed in Venice by Simon Papiense in 1499 and contained woodcut drawings of the plants. Even though the author culled ancient and medieval sources, Arabic, Latin, and Greek, he digested his material and rewrote his findings. He employed some of the medieval circumlocutions, as when he said that celery, asarum (the fern), calamint, juniper, and parsley "stimulate menstruation" and when he related that artemisia and rue "stimulate menstruation *and* expel a *dead* fetus."[77] But birthwort and the round-leaved birthwort, administered either as a drink or a pessary, both stimulated menstruation and expelled a *dead or a live* fetus.[78] In a pessary, birthwort was combined with oil of myrrh and pepper for a dead or a live fetus, whereas a pessary made of just the century plant and sage expelled a fetus (without further ado).[79] Resorting to medical vagueness, the author said that mint, marjoram, peony, and pennyroyal were "wonderful for the womb." Marjoram, pennyroyal, and peony were said also to provoke menstruation. Each of the four was given with artemisia, and for the mint recipe birthwort was added.[80]

Given what we know from the ancients, there is no doubt as to what "wonderful for the womb" meant—or could have meant. We do not know who were the readers of the text, what their understanding was, or how they may have employed the information. It is unclear what was intended by the advice that cypress "comforts a cold womb" but, again wittingly or unwittingly, an abortion appears the likely outcome.[81] The description of savin, a type of juniper, is even more puzzling: it "provokes menstruation and the afterbirth," not mentioning a fetus at all, but the text then cited the *Pandecta* by Haly Abbas as saying it "provokes menstruation better than any other medicine . . . and it kills a living fetus and expels a dead one."[82] Finally, the author named three contraceptives: pennyroyal, willow, and poplar.[83]

Even though the inspiration may have come directly or indirectly from Dioscorides, the author omitted Dioscorides' magical references and gave the recipes without embellishment. Dioscorides, for instance, specified the poplar's bark,[84] whereas this unknown author said the contraceptive was a decoction made in water from its roots.

The herbals published in the early decades of printing sometimes would mention contraceptives and abortifacients. In comparison with the texts of previous centuries, the frequency of incidence was considerably less. For example, the herbal anonymously composed from older sources and printed in Vicenza in 1491 has only one contraceptive, an herbal amulet (saxifrages) to be hung around a woman's neck. Rue is stipulated as a menstrual stimulator.[85]

A number of the early herbals produced in Germany, and written in German (most anonymously), contained birth control information, although less openly than in the classical herbals. These often were called *Gart der Gesundheit*, or "Gardens of Health." Johann Wonnecke von Cube was named as author of an herbal published in Mainz in 1485, and a similar herbal was published anonymously in Strasbourg in 1515. Each contained beautiful woodcuts of the plants and began with artemisia *(Beyfüss)*, the "mother herb," the text explained. It was good for woman's sickness *(frauwen sucht)*. Soaked in wine, and taken orally, artemisia expelled all sickness that lurked in the womb, including those things that were swollen.[86]

The first four herbs listed in these massive works were menstrual stimulators, all being species of artemisia but none expressly abortifacients. Garlic, for example, *"bringen frawen menstruum* (brings menstruation to a woman)."[87] Birthwort, however, was described more explicitly: *"Holwurtz* [birthwort] mixed with pepper and myrrh is good for the woman so to have children. It also is used to abort."[88] The fern *filix* or *farenkrut* caused sterility.[89] That statement could not be seen as an advocacy; instead it was a warning. More antifertility drugs were named, as was rue: "soaked in wine and myrrh rue caused the flow."[90]

Gifted and eccentric are the words used to describe one of the Renaissance's greatest botanists, Hieronymus Bock or Herman Tragus (1498–1554). He broke with the practice of publishing herbals anonymously in German; he was the named author—as well he should be, because he was original and scholarly. The German edition appeared in Strasbourg in 1539. Generally Bock resorted to the indirect means of naming birth control agents as menstrual regulators. Birthwort *(weronmut, absinthium)* "disconnects a dead fetus and drives out the menses." Another birthwort *(wormkraut, abrotonum)* "expels a dead child."[91] No antifertility uses were alluded to in either the German or the Latin editions.[92] Under juniper (savin), the Lutheran Bock disclosed that a Catholic priest had attempted to lure "old witches and prostitutes" to mass and provided juniper to the young prostitutes so that they could abort.[93]

Otto Brunfels (1488–1534) produced one of the greatest herbals of the sixteenth century. This he did with the creative assistance of a great woodcut artist, Hans Weiditz. Unlike Bock, Brunfels did not avoid discussing birth control agents, but he did so circumspectly and through citation of old authorities. His knowledge of the subject was limited, it seems, to what he learned from texts.

The index of the 1554 edition lists fifty-nine stimulators of menstruation (including Queen Anne's lace, asafetida, birthwort, and the chaste plant), some of which were different species of the same genera. Under "*ducentia foetum* (cutting off of the fetus)" he named some thirty-five items. Many of those same items appear also under "*matrici convenientia* (comforts for the womb)" with nothing specifically stated about antifertility. Just the same, the agents named included juniper *(savina)*, birthwort, marjoram, and pennyroyal.[94] Birthwort "ejects the menses and a fetus *(partus)*" and a drink of aqua asarum (distilled) or decocted asarum "expels the fetus, whether alive or dead."[95] Celandine (*Chelidonium majus* L.) "stimulates the menstrua and comforts the womb."[96]

Periclumen (which by Brunfels's time meant honeysuckle) caused sterility if one drachma of it is taken with wine. Brunfels did not specify, as had Dioscorides, sterility *in males*.[97] Like his fellow herbalists of the time, Brunfels's knowledge of plants was greater in botany than in medicine. He gave no mention of the use of tansy as a menstrual regulator nor any hint of its use in birth control. Perhaps this was because tansy was not mentioned in the classical sources from which he derived most of his knowledge of medicine.[98]

One of the Fathers of Botany is Leonhart Fuchs (1501–1566), whose herbal, *De historia stirpium* (Basel 1542), is truly a masterpiece. Fuchs expressed irritation with physicians who did not know their medicinal plants. Fuchs was a practicing physician and knew the medicine as well as the plants. Writing on plants, supervising their illustration down to the finest detail, he conveyed precise medical knowledge about them. Most of medicine and perhaps all of the birth control information he wrote, however, was derived from classical sources, almost all being Dioscorides, Galen, and Pliny. For example, from Pliny Fuchs repeated that rue "as a food impedes generation."[99] From Dioscorides: "The menses, afterbirth, and fetus, all held in the uterus, are expelled by a drink of birthwort with myrrh and pepper in it."[100] And also from Dioscorides about the fern, *filix:* "It causes sterility [contraception] in women and, if they are already pregnant, it aborts."[101] He said it plainly, but he did not move from the ancient script with any new anecdotal experiences.

An herbal by Josse de Harchies, published in 1573, had less birth control information than most earlier herbals, but still the subject was not forbidden. It attributed no antifertility qualities to juniper but said that savin (a species of juniper), dittany, *panax* (a *Ferula*), and death carrot *(thlaspi)* expel the menstrua and the fetus.[102] Rue, colocynth, lupine, laurel, and myrrh were only said to stimulate the menses (without mentioning the fetus).[103] In a return to his classical sources, the herbalist listed *laser* or *silphium*, taken orally, for antifertility. Then he explained that the plant is now "asafetida."[104] In apparent and potentially dangerous confusion, he said that the fern, *filix*, "restored fertility in women."[105] His knowledge about the antifertility effects was bookish, impractical, and, in the case of *filix*, downright dangerous. Moreover, he referred to colocynth as a *secreta*, thus divulging his association of it with popular magic and, possibly, witchcraft.

The Renaissance herbalists should be applauded for their contributions to botany. On the other hand, either their knowledge of the uses of plants for birth control was limited primarily to their sources, or societal pressures required them to be circumspect. Even so, the herbalists continued the chain of knowledge about birth control agents indirectly. In a few instances, they actually contributed to the body of knowledge.

Pharmaceutical "Recipe Books"

It was during the sixteenth century that botany became a study in itself and lost its pharmaceutical trappings. People in the Middle Ages studied plants for medicinal purposes, for the most part, and the usual literary texts took two forms: herbals and receptaria or antidotaria (the latter two are compilations of recipes). The separation came about through lecturing on Dioscorides' texts in universities. In Italy the focus of lecturers remained on pharmacy, but in northern, German-speaking universities, the focus shifted to plants for the sake of plants; hence, "botany" was born.[106] Over time, herbals became concerned mainly with botany (and therefore drop out of the history of abortion and contraception); it is primarily in recipe books intended for use by apothecaries that we find information on antifertility qualities of plants in the early modern period.

One major exception to this rule was Valerius Cordus. Valerius's father was Euricus (1486–1535), a German who practiced and taught medicine at the University of Marburg and maintained a strong interest in botany *and* pharmacy. His son followed his father's interest and career. Valerius lectured on Dioscorides at Wittenberg between 1539 and 1543. While there he developed close ties of friendship with an apothecary. In 1542 Valerius submitted to the apothecary guild at Nürnberg a copy of recipes he wrote. So good was it that the guild adopted it as an official guide. As the decades went by, most German-speaking areas and many parts of the rest of Europe recognized Valerius's work, the *Dispensatorium*, as the standard. It influenced all parts for centuries to come.

So Valerius was in a good position to relate information about birth control and to influence the generations of the future. And he did have such an influence, but it was well disguised. Neither contraceptives nor abortifacients were among the recipes, but among the approximately 225 plants and minerals in his list were many substances that had those effects. One would have had to know how to read the guide before the information could be of use. Abortion was mentioned once, in a prescription containing opium and other narcotic alkaloids that prevented miscarriage *(abortum)*.[107] Valerius's practice was to list the title, the form (pill, syrup, powder, etc.) and the source of the recipe. Next he discussed problems with nomenclature and preparation, including adulteration (always a concern of apothecaries), and, in conclusion, the condition for which the recipe was given. Some recipes did not have any uses listed—the apothecary should know. The guide was, after all, for professionals who already knew their trade.

Valerius gave a number of recipes for menstrual stimulation. A typical one was a cordial tonic powder "according to Avicenna's description," that had sixteen ingredients, among them two species of birthwort (Aristolochiceae), pepper, and geraniums.[108] A Latin manuscript composed at the monastery of Lorsch around 800 listed geraniums as an abortive agent.[109] Geraniums were seldom found in earlier texts, but they did have abortifacient qualities. When my wife was pregnant, my mother told me to remove the geraniums from the living area because they would cause an abortion if eaten. I was amused and skeptical: how could a plant cause a miscarriage, and why should a pregnant woman eat a house plant? In the last chapter we shall speculate how my mother came to know this information. She did not get it directly from Valerius, nor the from Lorsch manuscript.

The powder formula containing birthwort and geraniums, Valerius said, "*menses ciet* (sets off menstruation)." Another powder, called a *diaprassium* "according to Nicholaus," was a complex mixture of sixty-seven ingredients and was employed for twenty-nine purposes, among them curing dizziness, purging arteries, and helping a sick liver; it also "*menses deducit* (leads out the menses)." Included among the ingredients were licorice, myrrh, birthwort, celery, dittany, and Queen Anne's lace.[110] Only one recipe was entirely for women: a powder molded into a cake (pill) called "Trochisca de myrrha D. Rasis," or "a pill of myrrh according to al-Rhasis." It was compounded of the following ingredients (note that 1 scruple = 20 grains = 1.2 grams):

3 scruple myrrh
5 scruple lupine
2 scruple opopanax (from *Ferula* species or closely related)
1 scruple *each* rue, wild mint, pennyroyal, cumin, blackberries, asafetida (*Ferula*), sagapeni (from *Ferula persica*), and artemisia

"It provokes menstruation and relieves passions that are a product of the retention of menses."[111]

Eight other recipes were for menstrual stimulation, and each contained the familiar abortifacient drugs.[112] Each recipe, however, had multiple uses (when they were enumerated at all). We have no way of knowing the reasons most clients bought these medicines. One compound almost startles us because of its ingredients. A "Syrup of Artemisia according to Matthaeus Gradibus" was made of forty-four substances, including artemisia, pennyroyal, a number of other mints, dittany, juniper, rue, betony, celery seeds, and cypress. "It calms the passions of the womb and retains things in their proper place, it resolves coldness, inflations (*ventositatem*), and sickness; it invigorates the nerves, opens pores, improves the blood, and commands and provokes menstruation."[113]

On the basis of what we know about the ingredients, it is difficult to imagine what the recipe would do except to cause an abortion. Even with modern phytochemistry at our disposal, it is difficult to assay single herbs and then to evaluate all the scores of a plant's chemical compounds and how they will act in synergistic relations with other compounds. Evaluating scores of herbs and other natural substances, mixed together, and the effect the mixture would have on the body is almost beyond the capacity of our science. Simply, we cannot know what the interactions of the drugs in the various ingredients would have been or the amount each client was instructed to take. Some herbs stimulate the production of estrogen, others of progesterone, while others countered hormonal production; some were gonadotrophic, others antigonadotrophic. It was as if Valerius or his source had gone through the manuals and listed in a single recipe most of the antifertility plants as they appeared in texts. Probably Valerius did not compose most of the recipes but merely compiled and refined customary practices, some of which might previously have been unwritten.

One wonders what may have been the purpose of two "simples" discussed in Valerius's guide. There is "oil of rue," which is a "warming and opening medicine, and warms the kidneys, intestines and womb,"[114] and an "oil of wormwood" (*absinthium*, a species of artemisia), which "warms and causes openings."[115] Other recipes are similarly vague, such as a powder that "is good for women, rectifies the disposition of the womb and airs it."[116] It contains a few abortifacient plants: celery seeds, pepper, and cinnamon, plus some sugar, presumably, to help it go down.

Modeled on the *Dispensatorium* of Valerius Cordus, another official guide to pharmacy recipes appeared in the so-called Augsberger pharmacopoeia, first published in 1564. The first edition had no contraceptives and no explicitly labeled abortifacients, but the recipes that caused an abortion were present. One recipe that came close to mentioning abortion was a "pill to provoke birth," but its ingredients—among them cinnamon (sometimes used as an abortifacient), crocus, and cassia—may not have worked.[117] Almost never did the work, in contrast to the *Dispensatorium*, list the application for which a recipe might be useful. In other words, the apothecary or physician would have to know.

Knowing, as we now do, which ingredients have abortive properties, we can look through the guide and find the abortifacients. For example, a "powder of opopanax from Mesue" consisted of opopanax (a *Ferula* or related species), colocynth, crocus, castoreum, myrrh, pepper, and other ingredients that would likely cause an abortion.[118] A similar recipe, this one an electuary (a paste or lozenge), was numbered as "4" and consisted of birthwort, pennyroyal, artemisia, parsley, juniper, rue, celery, and licorice, plus other ingredients.[119] Very similar to a recipe in Valerius's work was the "syrup of artemisia according to Matthaeus de Gradibus"; in other words, it was made from many of the known abortifacient plants.[120]

The Augsberger pharmacopoeia went through many revisions (in 1573, 1597, 1613, 1643, 1646, 1710, and, the last, 1734). Some of the revisions, contrary to my expectations, were more explicit than the first edition. The 1597 edition followed Valerius in noting that the "trochisk of myrrh according to Rhasis" would stimulate menstruation, if delayed, and was a good prescription for expelling a dead fetus, especially when delivery was overdue.[121] The same and subsequent editions said that oil of sweet marjoram together with myrtle leaves, abrotanum (a kind of birthwort), water mints, and cinnamon "expels the menses, afterbirth and birth [*partus*, or fetus]."[122] Even more explicit was an "oil of philosophers"(!), which was "injected into the vagina to provoke menstruation, discharging either a live or dead fetus."

Not only did the *Dispensatorium* become a standard pharmaceutical guide, it also inspired many imitators. A 1992 dissertation in German of these sixteenth- and seventeenth-century guides by Larissa Leibrock-Plehn established that, although the familiar recipes for abortions continued to be described, they seldom were labeled as having that action. A guide known as the Cologne Dispensatory, published in 1565 with subsequent revisions and printings, was written by three physicians in Cologne. It explicitly mentioned no abortifacients.[123] A pharmacopoeia by Thomas Guarinus (or Anuce Foès), first published in Basel in 1561, had one recipe explicitly labeled as an abortive agent, the "oil of sweet marjoram," and repeated the same wording as that in the Augsberger pharmacopoeia.[124] A guide published in Frankfurt in 1613 reprinted the same recipes and included only one explicit mention of abortion, an electuary that expelled the menses and "dead fetus."[125]

Just when our survey of pharmacopoeias of the early modern period would seem to allow us to make a generalization, the exceptions appear. The rule is that abortifacients were found in these guides (hence in real pharmacies) but that normally their use was disguised. The writings of an academic physician from Basel, Hans Jakob Wecker

(1528–1586), were an exception. Wecker named specific abortion drugs on a grand scale in his *Antidotarium speciale* in 1574 and his *Antidotarium generale* two years later. He designated forty-five plant and three animal products (castoreum, vulture feces, and a rabbit's stomach) as simples that caused an abortion. He cited numerous sources, but Dioscorides was his principal authority for birth control. He was explicit about what some of the drugs did: "*abortum facit* (it causes an abortion)"; "*abortum fieri* (to bring about an abortion)"; "*partus* [or *foetus*] evocat (it discharges a foetus)"; "*foetum enecat* (it kills a fetus)"; "*partus exanimat* (it draws off a birth)."[126] Various species of *Ferula*, asparagus seeds, anise, Queen Anne's lace, celery, fenugreek, and parsley, he said, only "move the menses."[127] He related one compound medicine, an electuary, consisting of fleabane (*Erigeron* sp.), myrrh, and cinnamon, that moved the menses and another similar one that added pennyroyal.[128] Wecker was among those scientists who applied chemistry (or spagyry) to apothecary skills to produce new distillates and prepared medicines.

Like Wecker but sixty-seven years later, Johann Schroeder updated the pharmaceutical arts with a book published in 1641 that received four later printings.[129] The new Paracelsian chemistry had its impact on the preparations he recommended. Numerous drugs chemically prepared through distillation and new extraction techniques made their appearance on the pharmacists' shelves.

Even so, Schroeder's work reflected a continuity with the past. Like Wecker, Schroeder knew Dioscorides' abortifacient drugs and, again like Wecker, he did not shrink from stating their uses. Among the new mineral salts and distillates, there were the familiar simple drugs artemisia, calamint, juniper, squirting cucumber (called *elaterium*), myrrh, and various *Ferula*-derived drugs. Despite the trends that pushed birth control away from formal medicine, despite the ecclesiastical and legal restrictions, the knowledge of the ancients could be found on the pharmacists' shelves throughout the sixteenth and seventeenth centuries.

Writings on Gynecology

The Germans were the pacesetters in sixteenth-century efforts to revive the ancient writings on gynecology, just as they were pioneers in developing botany and pharmacy as separate fields of learning. Such a pioneer was Eucharius Rösslin (ca. 1500–1526). Rösslin began his professional life, fittingly enough, as an apothecary in Breiburg, and he later became the city physician in Frankfurt and Worms. Before his untimely death, he wrote a title in German that translates "The Pregnant Woman's and Midwife's Rose Garden," which was published in Augsburg in 1529.[130] It received many subsequent printings as well as a Latin translation (*De partu hominis*, Frankfurt, 1532) and a popular English translation by Thomas Raynald in London (1552) entitled *The Byrth of Mankynd, Otherwise Named the Womans Boke*. The German edition and each of the translations received many printings, there being at least eleven issues of the Latin. Certainly, the work was widely circulated.

Rösslin did not hesitate to deal openly with abortion. When a woman's life was in peril, even if she just thought it was, it was necessary and justified for a physician to cause an abortion, he said. Signs of impending peril were trances (hallucinations), being weak and feeble, being unable to eat meat, and having a rapid pulse. If the medical evidence was present that she would not live long after the delivery, the physician should, in the English translation, "give all dylygence" to giving the proper recipes for expulsion.[131]

For an abortion the physician should first use recipes, but if they did not work surgery might be necessary. In the discussion that followed, Rösslin did not distinguish which abortifacients were good for administering at differing periods of the pregnancy. He did, however, begin his list of possibilities with fumigants (drugs administered by inhalation of fumes) and then graduate to oral drugs and, finally, pessaries. The first fumigant was created by placing on coals a dove's (?) stomach or an ass's dung, snake skin, myrrh, castoreum, and pigeon's dung. The second fumigant included opopanax *(Ferula)*, frankincense, and sulfur. The oral prescriptions consisted of familiar recipes, except that Rösslin did not include the complex polypharmaceutical prescriptions found in the apothecary literature of his time. Instead he prescribed simpler remedies: water soaked with figs and fenugreek, or dittany in warm water "to expel a dead fetus without any peril *(ausanschanden)* to the mother."[132] Other recipes included birthwort, juniper, rue, myrrh, castoreum, and two kinds of *Ferula*.[133]

If the physician judged, however, that the woman would die regardless of whether he administered an abortion, the physician should allow the delivery to proceed without interference. Although Rösslin discussed hindrances to fertility, he did not name any contraceptives.

Another gynecological text followed Rösslin's in subject matter, even in title. Walter Ryff's *Pregnant Woman's Rose Garden* was published first in Frankfurt in 1545 and subsequently in at least seven more editions. Those things that assisted births but could be taken as a drink for an abortion ("die todte Geburt") were named as galbanum (a *Ferula*), myrrh, laudanum (an opium preparation), "gummi elami" (unidentified), the rind of *Dannbaumen* (also unidentified), and savin *(Seuenbaum oder Seuenpalmen)*.[134] A similar catalog of abortifacients listed four or five drugs that included Cretan dittany and dill.[135] Pictured in the text were woodcuts of various instruments used to insert substances into the vagina.[136] Even though the subject of birth control was not taboo to Ryff, it was not central either. Other than the pictures of vaginal instruments, his work was derivative and not particularly useful to readers because he gave neither instructions nor recipes. Ryff also wrote a cookbook and household medicine guide (which contained little in the way of birth control information either).[137]

Closing the sixteenth century were two writers on gynecology, one Italian, the other Spanish. Scipione Mercurio (1538–1616) was a Roman physician who introduced changes in the caesarean section procedure. His knowledge of birth control, however, was limited, or so it would seem from his text. Under external causes of abortion, he named a few drugs (savin, squirting cucumber, colocynth), and, quoting older authorities, principally Avicenna, he conceded that sometimes "propria medicina" should be given to save the mother.[138] His knowledge was limited and his suggestions would have been of little practical, medical value.

Physician to the Emperor Philip II, Luis Mercado (1525?–1611) wrote a tract in four large books on the diseases of women. Surprisingly, he began with menstruation and, following a scholarly theoretical description, he discussed problems that accompany the retention of menses and how to relieve them. Future gynecology books would follow the example in Mercado's work by starting with menstruation. The list of drugs to relieve menstrual retention was fairly complete, divided into the weak (almonds, wild lettuce, lupine), the medium strong (celery, peony, iris, birthwort, artemisia, calamint, pennyroyal, hyssop, marjoram, and opopanax), and the extremely strong (distilled water of pimpernel, bryony, squirting cucumber, and spurge).[139] In all this great detail there was no advocacy for birth control. Indeed, some of the strong menstrual stimulators caused temporary sterility, he said.[140] A long section on sterility analyzed all aspects of the phenomenon except the sterility caused by sorcerers. That kind he said he would leave to priests and prayers.[141]

In the seventeenth century, two gynecology texts published in Holland and Britain had widespread influence. The first was by James Primerose (1598–1659), who studied at Paris, practiced medicine at Hull, and published his lengthy treatise on women's diseases in Latin in 1658. As was the convention in gynecology treatises, Primerose began with a general discussion of menstruation and next discussed menstruation suppression. He knew that the primary cause of menstrual delay was pregnancy. Sometimes even pregnant women would suffer menstrual retention, he explained, because it could be the third month before the fetus was of such size that it required all the menstrual blood for nourishment.

Dire consequences ensued when one allowed menstrual delay to go unchecked, even in pregnancy. He repeated the reasons given by Avicenna and Theodorus Priscianus to justify abortion (namely, a diseased womb, an opening too small, etc.).[142] In cases where justified, menstrual stimulation could be effected by means of diet, baths, exercises, and drugs. He detailed foods or additives to foods: thyme, hyssop, parsley, wild parsnip (carrot family), marjoram, mint, asparagus, saffron, pennyroyal, celery, and radishes.[143] Almost thirteen pages of text discussed the various drugs and preparations available for menstrual stimulation. He named a list of "gums": myrrh, asafetida and three other *Ferula* plants, storax, and frankincense. Under waters (distillations) he listed artemisia, pennyroyal, betony, parsley, hyssop, anise, and savin (juniper).[144]

Primerose wrote about sterility: "There are, in truth, also things by their occult properties are said to induce sterility, such as the roots of the female fern, a drink of powdered English ivy, a deer's heart, a mule's or a chicken's uterus, . . . [a number of semiprecious stones] . . . mint, fabian beans."[145] He was not advocating the use of contraceptives, merely relating the information from medical and occult sources. Interestingly, a means of treating the psychological disorder of a false conception was to give an abortion by drugs.[146] One ought not to move to abort a dead fetus until one knew the fetus was dead. The body naturally expelled a dead fetus, Primerose wrote.[147] Primerose's openness about birth control and his knowledge of it were comparable with Rösslin's expertise. These physicians' works reveal that, though midwifery knowledge was under attack, during the sixteenth and seventeenth centuries the "secrets" were still known.

The second seventeenth-century gynecological treatise originated in England, circulated widely, and was known as Aristotle's *Masterpiece*. This was a version of the "secrets literature" similar to the works attributed to Albertus Magnus. Little of the text came from Aristotle, but it became immensely popular because its contents appealed to the common people. Accompanying the *Masterpiece* was a similar, more detailed, work called *The Experienced Midwife*. The first edition of the *Masterpiece* was in 1684, the *Midwife* in 1700. Thereafter the two often were joined in publications with other pseudo-Aristotelian works under the title *The Complete Works of Aristotle*.

The *Masterpiece* and *Midwife* have been called sex manuals, because sexual organs and intercourse were described in a natural, if not erotic, manner.[148] Three or four times more information was given about females than males, probably indicating primarily a male readership. Young virgins were described as being girls about fourteen or fifteen when "their natural purgations begin to flow . . . , stir up their minds to venerate."[149] Freely and frankly advice was given to both genders with much detail to assist women in conceiving, bearing, and giving birth. What we would regard as common sense and sound medical advice was mixed with superstition and foolishness, from our perspective. The work was immensely popular and can be regarded as a gauge of popular knowledge.[150]

"Aristotle's Secrets" had much to do about sex but nothing on birth control. A long section on barrenness contained much practical advice, including changes in diet and behavior. Interestingly, one reason for barrenness was "want of love in the persons copulating." The medieval idea was repeated that "no conception following any forced copulation" was possible.[151] The *Experienced Midwife* added, "Love is that vital principle that ought to inspire each organ in the act of generation."[152] One test for infertility was to sprinkle a man's urine on a lettuce leaf and a woman's urine on another. The person whose leaf dried first was the infertile one.[153] Another cause of sterility is irregular or delayed menstruation. In order *to hasten the menses to promote conception*, the pseudo-Aristotelian author recommended "calac [calcium oxide], mint, pennyroyal, thyme, betony, dittany, feverfew [artemisia domestica], mugwort [artemisia], sage, peony roots, and juniper berries," all boiled together in beer and drunk.[154] Discussing the problem of delayed menstruation in general, many of the same drugs were repeated, plus others such as galbanum (a *Ferula*), and figs (in a pessary).[155] The pseudo-Aristotle's text never gave direct information about birth control, but, on the other hand, a savvy reader would discover some helpful hints.

Another great authority on gynecology in the seventeenth century was the French physician, Francis Mauriceau (1637–1709). His book, first published in 1668, went through many editions and translations into Latin, English, German, Dutch, and Italian. Among his achievements were the treatment of *placenta previa* and the condemnation of caesarean section (which he said was too dangerous to perform). He condemned Aristotle for disbelieving that women had seeds and challenged Hippocrates on the opinion that male fetuses have life earlier than females. Were this so, he said, males would come to full term sooner than the females, and experience shows that this does not occur. Moreover, he had seen fetuses in the fifth and sixth months of development and there was no difference between males and females, each "though small and very tender entirely formed and figured, at which time it is no longer than a finger."[156] An important cause of infertility in women was an inability to enjoy sexual intercourse; the reason, he said, is that those women who do have pleasure have a more open orifice.[157]

Mauriceau said there were two kinds of abortion, natural and unnatural, the latter usually deliberately attempted. An unnatural (that is, intentional) abortion was the same as homicide, he claimed. Mauriceau gave no information about drugs that caused abortion, not even to the extent of naming drugs and foods to avoid. Indeed, there was very little discussion of drug therapy in his work, showing the separation of pharmacy from gynecology and obstetrics. Ironically, in his condemnation of caesarean sections he ignored contraceptives and abortifacients that could have saved extremely young women whose lives were threatened by pregnancy.

Midwifery Guides

In 1671, a truly unusual event occurred: a Mrs. Jane Sharp published a guide for midwives because, in her words: "I have often sat down sad in the consideration of the many miseries women endure in the hands of unskillful midwives."[158] What was unusual was the fact that she was a woman. Sharp did not openly advocate either contraception or abortion, but she laid down those things to avoid that keep women from conceiving or, after conception, from carrying the child. To avoid contraception, a woman should not drink the wine from Holland known as "stum" nor eat ivy berries nor wear sapphire or emerald stones. To prevent a miscarriage, she supplied a longer list that included alpine snakeroot (*Eryngium alpinum* L.).[159] This is the first mention of the plant; modern studies have reported abortifacient activity in this plant.[160] By the fourth edition of the guide, this information was omitted.

Under menstrual stimulators, Mrs. Sharp gave some practical information. Weak women should rely on diet, exercise, and fumigants, she said. Drugs might be used by others. Artemisia, tansy, pennyroyal, and catnip (a mint), taken with cinnamon water, were useful to stimulate a delayed menstruation.[161] "To urge the terms [menstruation] in strong country people" she recommended that they take a number of compounds available at the apothecary, such as Syrup of Damask Roses, Oil of Aniseed, and "the pill" (without definition).[162] This is most interesting because why would country people, of all people, not be directed to use the simple drugs in their own gardens rather than to purchase compounded drugs at a store? In any case, Sharp knew what she was recommending: "But do none of these things to women with child for that will be murder."[163] Whether she wrote out of conviction or intimidation, we shall not know.

Interestingly, a situation in 1681 in Massachusetts may indicate how some guides were used. A defamation suit was lodged on behalf of Margaret Martin, a resident of Charlestown. In the trial, various women testified that Margaret was pregnant but had boiled up some pennyroyal, horehound, nip, and marigolds and that drinking this concoction had caused her to abort.[164]

Nicholas Culpeper (who will be discussed in greater detail in the next chapter) also wrote a "directory for midwives," published in London in 1651. His primary concern was to assist conception and childbirth, as he was motivated by having a sick wife who did not bear healthy children. Culpeper confessed, "Myself having buried many of my children young, caused me to fix my thoughts intently upon this business" of midwifery.[165]

Contrary to his personal feelings, Culpeper related birth control knowledge, albeit circumspectly. He discussed things that stimulate the menstrual flow: calamint, pennyroyal, thyme, mother of thyme [*Thymus serpyllum* L.], dittany, gentian roots, birthwort roots, betony, tansy, artemisia, sage, peony roots, and juniper berries.[166] He added a precaution: "Give not any of these to any that is with child, lest you turn murderers; wilful murder seldom goes unpunished in this world, never in that to come."[167] Thus, like Mrs. Sharp, Dr. Culpeper equated menstrual stimulators given to (and taken by?) pregnant women as a means of murder. Moreover, elsewhere he used the term *abortion* together with miscarriage, and said that abortions most frequently occurred within the first two months *"after conception."*[168] Culpeper was ahead of his time in defining conception as the moment when "twofold spermatical matter" mixed in a woman's womb and in calling the female sperm "tubae" or "eggs."[169]

What Happened to Contraceptives?

"What! the same thing to prevent a conception as to destroy the child after it is conceived?" exclaimed a cousin to a bride. The cousin recommended that the bride take a "physick," that is, a drug to kill unwanted children. The bride replied that she would not do that but would take a contraceptive, if they were available. In the play from which this scene came, *Matrimonial Whoredom* by Daniel Defoe (1727 edition), the bride explained, "I cannot understand your Niceties; I would not be with Child, that's all; there's no harm in that, I hope."[170]

As this scene may indicate, there were fewer contraceptive recipes in the herbal and gynecological literature of the early modern period than there were in previous centuries. Should we be surprised? Attention was given in Mauriceau's gynecology of 1668 to exercises and other things to do to *improve* fertility. The inclusion of this advice revealed that the admonition by the church against any form of interference in fertility was not heeded. Two late medieval Slavic Church manuscripts (the earliest being fourteenth century, the latest sixteenth century) stated that "those who make a potion to drink so that they cannot conceive a child" committed a greater sin than those who "by means of another potion . . . kill infants at each new moon." The reasoning was that a contraceptive drink caused sterility and one did "not know how many would have been born."[171] The obvious implication was that contraceptives caused permanent sterility, but no other testimonies were offered to that effect. It is interesting, however, that in this instance contraception was regarded as worse than abortion (by modern definitions). Also, the penalty for terminating a pregnancy was ineligibility to receive communion.

I can advance four reasons for the decline in the appearance of contraceptive drugs in written documents: (1) the drugs were never very effective; (2) their use was elementary, easy, and did not require a visit to an apothecary shop; (3) they were predominantly "simple" drugs free in nature and not effective in the complex compound medicines sold in druggists' shops; and (4) their use simply declined because of social factors not apparent in the documents, such as fear that they promoted promiscuity and the Reformation's aversion to infanticide and strong penalties for sexual misconduct.[172] Legal and religious requirements are not sufficient to explain the decline of contraceptives because the position of neither the church nor the various states was not that clearly defined. Defoe's bride thought that contraceptives existed but did not know what they were.

To be sure, knowledge of oral and pessary contraceptives continued among some people, as did their use. Of the reasons cited above, only the first one should be rejected straightaway, because we have good reason to believe that contraceptives were effective in reducing family size among the ancient peoples. Unless evidence is produced to the contrary, we should accept the proposition that the popular culture remained in possession of contraceptive knowledge but that this knowledge was less readily found in contemporary medical or pharmaceutical documents.

One reason to believe the knowledge was available, as we shall see in the last chapter, is that women alive today have the same knowledge as was recorded during the Middle Ages. The alternative is to claim that the old methods disappeared from common usage but were rediscovered only recently and made their way into folk medicine. But in fact we know that the information was there to be found in the medieval and classical works on which the Renaissance built. The texts were a part of the curriculum, although we have found no evidence that the information was stressed, highlighted, or emphasized in any way. Presumably, the religious, moral, and legal rules had some effect on people's behavior. Awareness of contraceptives was seldom found in sixteenth-century documents. Modern demographic studies show that women concealed contraceptive failures, thus leading to an underestimation of contraceptive use.[173] Whereas the modern phenomena may have been a factor in the historical records, the records still are unaccountably sparse about contraceptives but more abundant on abortifacients.

Still, a late-sixteenth-century apothecary shop would have had a number of ingredients on its shelves that caused an abortion. The apothecary's books would not be likely to have any listed as such. Just the same, a woman who came into a shop and properly described her needs could leave with a bottle or a package that served her reproductive needs. How explicit she needed to be we do not know.

We do not know either whether physicians helped women control their fertility; probably not. First, they were male; women were excluded from the profession by the requirement for university training and licensing procedures. Apothecaries escaped the accusation of witchcraft, probably because they were cleverly vague about birth control agents. They sold them, but nothing written in their shops said exactly what they did. In one sense, sixteenth-century drugstores resembled modern health food stores, where information and proof about usage are hard to come by.

Theology: No Cause to Change

On October 29, 1588, Pope Sixtus V issued a bull that was radically different from previous church positions on the use of birth control. The bull, known as *Effraenatuam*, began with a traditional embrace of Augustine but moved rapidly from Augustinian moderation to absolute condemnation of contraception and abortion:

> the most severe punishments [should go to those] who procure poisons to extinguish and destroy the conceived fetus within the womb . . . [and those] who by poisons, potions, and *maleficia* induce sterility in women, or impede by cursed medicines their conceiving or bearing . . . Moreover, we decree that they should by the same penalties be wholly bound who proffer potions and poisons of sterility to women and offer an impediment to the conception of a fetus, and who take pains to perform and execute such acts or in any way counsel them, and the women themselves who knowingly and voluntarily take the same potions.[174]

This is the strongest statement made heretofore by an official, to my knowledge. The severest of penalties went not only to those who succeeded in contraception or abortion but to those who even counseled the act. Women who did this on their own were equally guilty. What caused Sextus V to take such a drastic step? John Noonan speculates that the bull was the pope's personal expression and possibly a reaction to the prostitution in Rome. In 1527 there were, by a "conservative estimate," about 1,500 prostitutes in a city with about 55,000 people.[175]

The bull had a lifetime of about two-and-a-half years and was weak in influence. The succeeding pope countered it and returned to the traditional position that contraception was a sin and abortion a crime but that abortion could not occur until after the fortieth day, when the fetus was ensouled.[176] During the period of *Effraenatum*'s active status, it was unlikely that it had much impact on the consciousness or the conduct of Catholics. Once more, the only means specified by which contraception and abortion occurred were through "cursed medicines."

In 1679 Pope Innocent XI reacted to some tolerant theologians (discussed in Chapter 7) by condemning two propositions regarding abortion:

> 34. It is lawful to procure abortion before ensoulment of the fetus lest a girl, detected as pregnant, be killed or defamed.
> 35. It seems probable that the fetus (as long as it is in the uterus) lacks a rational soul and begins first to have one when it is born; and consequently it must be said that no abortion is homicide.[177]

The issues involved in therapeutic abortion were not explicitly addressed by the papal condemnation, but clearly this pronouncement was a reaffirmation of the medieval Roman Church's stance against abortion in principle.

The stern biblical injunctions by Calvin and Luther did not attack Catholic doctrine on birth control. In truth, little was spoken on the matter. Onan's sin of wasting seed on the ground was taken to mean that God's purpose was for men and women to propagate and that generation was the purpose of sexual intercourse. The misunderstanding from the Church Fathers remained that Onan's sin was wasteful ejaculation, not refusal to sire a child for his brother. Rightful sexual intercourse was vaginal penetration by a woman's husband. The new followers of Protestantism were not inclined to be open to accusations of permissiveness by allowing women to have sexual encounters without the possibility of pregnancy. Even within Catholic lands, the subject of contraception and abortion was not a focus of sermons.[178] Indeed, it may have been a subject to avoid.

High Culture and the Common Folk

Whether we are looking at the past or the present, we are never certain about the relationship between high and low culture. Did the ideas that were evolving in the learned works of science and theology, especially in relation to human reproduction, affect human behavior at the village and town level? In the medieval universities scholars were debating whether Aristotle was correct about only men having seed whereas women contributed nourishment or whether the Hippocratic-Galenic view was right that both men and women contributed seed to a fetus. Hippocrates and Galen won. Medieval scholastics decided in favor of the two-seed theory, that male and female alike contributed seed. In the victory women were more equal, but still not completely so. Female seed was not as strong, the experts declared.

Nevertheless, the troubadour and medieval Romances regarded women in an entirely different light. The Age of Chivalry was born: fair knights were in service to their ladies—no longer slaying the infidel, no longer raping seized women, no longer even seducing them. A look, perchance a handkerchief, or a raised eye was sufficient to motivate the bravest men. Some argued that, since a woman's seed was so important and was stimulated only by a pleasurable response in intercourse, it was more important for her than for her lover to have a climax. As wonderful and awe-inspiring as that sounds, it is an unconvincing version of reality, because one fails to find these ideas in operation in the general population in Europe. One might argue that the notions of chivalry were fashionable among a few and did not penetrate mass culture. The same may apply today: do the sentiments in modern musical lyrics affect our own behavior?

Attention to the egg came in the sixteenth and seventeenth centuries. In 1651 William Harvey wrote that "all living things come from an egg," but the realization was long in hatching. The great scholar on Dioscorides, Ulysses Aldrovandus (d. 1605), observed chicken eggs each day as they developed. Cracking one egg a day, he concluded that a fetus grows slowly, incrementally, a conclusion at variance with Pliny, Aristotle, and Albertus. Aldrovandus's research was based on the type of observation made by Leonardo da Vinci (c. 1490), who made two conclusions from the offspring of an Ethiopian man and an Italian mother: blackness is not environmental (caused by the sun) and a woman's seed is as potent as a man's.

Sixteenth-century science began the Scientific Revolution, the consequences of which eventually affected every man, woman, and child. In this era (1543–1687) the old ideas about reproduction gradually were swept away but never so dramatically as to capture the popular imagination. Millions of sperm in one drop, numerous eggs in a female—these ideas were too startling to alter most people's sexual habits. As best we can see, the old sexual practices prevailed, but women's sexuality was more recognized.

Jacob Ryff, Walter Ryff's father, claimed in 1554 that an egg-shaped mass developed out of a mixture of semen and menstrual blood or "of both seeds."[179] No important inferences that altered human behavior were drawn as a result of Ryff's assertion. Nor were inferences drawn seventy years later, when Thomas Fienus, a professor at Louvain, said the fetus was a product of a three-day mixing of a man's seed with menstrual blood. After the three-day mixing, the rational soul (not the vegetative or sensitive souls) entered the fetus. Thus from its beginning the fetus was ensouled. Fienus's ideas were not accepted. People of his age did not frame their experiences around what we in the modern era have come to regard as The Question: when does life begin?

On reproduction and the habits surrounding it, the cake of custom held fast despite the Scientific Revolution and, in particular, William Harvey. His emphasis on the egg in reproduction did shift central focus away from the male's semen and Aristotle's male-dominant theories. In De generatione, published posthumously, Harvey's observations of chicken eggs and dissections of deer led him to make a number of breaks with the past. The fetus develops so slowly that differentials between male and female fetuses were not observed, as said by Leviticus (12:1–5).[180] Harvey noted that the chicken could continue producing eggs after fertilization and concluded that the development of the egg was of primary importance. While the semen was critical to fertilization, there was a long period in which the egg could react to the semen and be fertilized. No particular event was observable during fertilization.

Harvey could find no menstrual blood, no regular blood, no semen, and no small fetus in the uterus in deer killed and dissected before and after coitus. Indeed, he could not find a conceptus or fetus in the uterus until after two months post-coitus. Harvey did not see an egg in a mammal or viviparous animal but thought that a female germ was present and that, after a period of time when it became fecund with male seed, it would form a fetus. The process of a gradual fetal emergence Harvey called "epigenesis."[181] There was no cause for the church or churches, fighting battles over much of Europe on many other issues, to reexamine their positions on birth control. Science discovered no event to determine when fertilization occurred and, therefore, fertilization could not be considered as the time of ensoulment.

Science in the seventeenth century only confused the issue for theologians. Harvey's epigenesis theory was countered from the beginning by the researches of Marcello Malpighi (1628–1694), who studied fetal development in chicken eggs through a microscope. Malpighi did not observe ovulation—which was not seen until the nineteenth century—but his ideas were built upon by others. Although he said that one could see nothing in an unfertilized egg, the care and exactitude of his drawings of fetal development led others to speculate that there existed in the body embryos prior to the fertilization process or prior to the epigenesis that begins with the egg.[182] Jan Swammerdam's study of frog eggs, published in 1669, built upon Malpighi (who did not actually say that germs of organisms pre-existed): the black spot in the egg is "the frog itself complete in all its parts."[183]

The controversy ensued, as we shall see in the next chapter, between the ovists (looking to Harvey) and the animalcultists (looking to Malpighi). The issue was not clear to theologians, certainly not to canonists, but philosophers rush in where others fear to tread. They were intrigued by the question of whether the germ of all animals existed in each animal. A group of scientists in Caen (1690s) argued that God created germs that float around in the air until absorbed by a male and made into a *animalcula*.[184] Descartes (*Traité de l'homme*, 1664) claimed that if one knew each of the parts that was in a single seed, "by reasons entirely mathematical and certain," one could then know exactly what the organism's individual details would look like after it was born.[185] Another Frenchman countered that generation is entirely different from the mechanics of a machine, as Descartes had implied. Put two watches side by side and they will never make little baby watches.

Through his newly invented microscope in 1677, Anton van Leeuwenhoek announced that each drop of a man's semen contains countless little animalcules. (Leeuwenhoek made the announcement even though one of his young students made the discovery—not a big surprise when you think about it.) Immediately, a reaction arose among scientists and, to a lesser degree, theologians: why would God (Nature) waste so many potential humans? The loss of seed by Onan on that fateful day was only a minuscule amount of his total lost seed.

Harvey's book was published in 1651, but it was not until the 1690s that the egg began to be recognized as important by French scientists. Did life come from eggs, from *animaculae*, from both? And when did it come? The slow acceptance of the new science was partly due to the fact that so many questions were unanswered.[186] The new embryology provided a weak, unclear case as to the relation between an egg (if that is what they saw), *animalicules* (so many in a single drop!), fetal development, the anatomy of ovulation, fertilization, and implantation (really not seen until the late nineteenth century), and whether the form for the new individual existed prior to fetal formation or developed incrementally. It is easy to replace the female "semen," seen in Hippocratic theory as a fluid that appears at climax, with an egg and to associate male sperm with those "worms" seen under the microscope. After that, the old theories continued in use to explain fetal development.

The Scientific Revolution was not a reason to regard birth control any differently from the traditional interpretation of the Church Fathers and canon law. The Catholic theologian Paul Laymann (1574–1635) said that one who took or gave something "maliciously" to prevent conception or ensoulment (what we would call early-term abortifacients) "commits not a true but a quasi homicide and sins mortally."[187] He raised a practical question: "Can a woman take a drug to prevent conception, if a doctor says or her own previous experience indicates that the birth of a child may cause her death?"[188] Contrary to the answer provided by physicians who raised the question (such as Theodorus and Avicenna), Laymann's solution was a sad but firm no. If such a blanket permission were to be given, it would be "wonderfully abused."[189] When sexual pleasure was involved, people just could not be trusted to make correct judgments. It was better for the church to stand steadfast in facing the issue. Just say no, Catholics and Protestants alike enunciated.

The Married Woman, an Herb, and Demographics

The sixteenth century witnessed one of Europe's most revolutionary changes in the history of population.[190] The average age at marriage rose from approximately 16 to 23 for women and then to approximately 27 and for men to approximately 30.[191] The altered marriage pattern was confined to western Europe, roughly west of a line from Trieste to Leningrad.[192] In earlier European society, most women who could marry did, but with the changed marriage customs as many as 20 percent of the women never married. Add to that a very low level of illegitimacy, which means that population increased statistically within the matrimonial bonds.[193] Add to that the approximately 10 to 20 percent of the women who were widows (as seen on tax rolls) and we have a picture of a radically changed society.[194] Add also to this change a modest increase in population.[195]

From the experiences of medieval towns, people began to see a connection between population size and economic-political power.[196] Mercantilism, the economic philosophy of early modern Europe, was town policy applied at a national level. Public policy promoted population growth through encouraging fecundity, punishing illegitimacy, and rearing poor and abandoned children through public support.[197] Little wonder, then, that the crime of the sixteenth century was bastard infanticide. Infanticide was often masked: exposure of children through withheld care; giving them away to nurses, in whose care they died after a few weeks; and withdrawal of timely breast-feeding. These actions are not easily regulated or measured, but they have been interpreted by Heinsohn and Steiger as a form of resistance against "enforced procreation."[198]

The French law (1556) that followed the Caroline laws on witchcraft also condemned as a criminal any woman who concealed her pregnancy and allowed a fetus to be killed or a child to die prior to baptism.[199] English law (1623) said that in the case of a bastard child born and subsequently claimed to have been stillborn or dead, the mother would be held liable if she attempted to conceal it. In other words, the presumption was guilt unless the mother could prove otherwise.[200] These examples indicate how much secular authorities were concerned about births. As in the Middle Ages, governments continued the protection of the right-standing (or, in our term, the public morals) of their communities, but there also may have been an underlying economic factor. This point will be explored more in the next chapter. The question here is whether there is a connection between the demographic changes of the sixteenth century, the suppression of witchcraft, and the loss of practical knowledge about birth control?

In the sixteenth and seventeenth centuries about as many women were executed for infanticide as for witchcraft, although, to be sure, the two were connected.[201] One reason may have been that lawyers who were responsible for witchcraft trials were reluctant increasingly to prosecute witches because the burden of proof was so heavy. On the other hand, infanticide was more easily proved when it was blatant and not disguised as poor care giving. Reginald Scot (1584) spoke of the law in connection with witchcraft:

> If anie womans child chance to die at her hand, so as no bodie knoweth how; it may not be thought or presumed that the mother killed it, except she be supposed a witch; and in that case it is otherwise, for she must upon that presumption be executed except she can prove the negative or contraries.[202]

In England, because of the law to which Scot referred, the prosecutions for infanticide increased to such a degree that some jurists asserted that the common law principle of "innocent until proven guilty" was being violated. Scot was in favor of these measures because it was the best way to get the witches. A defender of the draconian infanticide law, however, countered its critics by asserting that in "secret murders . . . half proofs are to be allowed."[203] Far from abandoning the law because of its affront to common law principles, the act of King James I (mentioned above) reaffirmed the provision that a woman who disposed of a delivered child was guilty of murder unless she could prove it had been stillborn or had died of natural causes.[204]

Elsewhere in Europe secular authorities tightened laws on infanticide. In Nürnberg, for example, between 1513 and 1777 eighty-seven women were executed for infanticide. All but four were single. In the same period six were executed as witches.[205] Fifty-one women in the county of Essex in England were tried for infanticide between 1575 and 1650, and two-thirds were found guilty and executed. Two hundred sixty-seven women were tried for witchcraft during the same period, with only one-fourth paying the extreme penalty.[206] Seldom was a man accused of infanticide.

Large numbers of single women, spinsters and widows, the increased intolerance for *maleficia* (harmful magic), an intense unprecedented misogyny, and the conflict between the Protestant and Catholic churches (which raised standards for behavior all) contributed to making birth control information dangerous. The question arises as to what societal changes were the result of the suppression of birth control information. The age of women at first marriage, concern about illegitimacy, the proportion of women who never married, the age of women at the birth of their last child, and altered life styles (for example, changing occupations and wet-nursing)—were these in fact new methods of birth control that arose because of declining use of drugs for the same purpose? The answer (probably not) will be examined in the next chapter. Neither the medical-pharmaceutical sources nor the demographic evidence indicate that birth control knowledge declined sufficiently to explain these larger societal changes. Just the same, the cumulative effect of the churches' and states' positions on abortion and birth control, together with the association of sexual and procreative habits with magic and witchcraft, must have been factors to some degree.

An ancillary change was the rise of prostitution and, in some cases, approval of it as a means of postponing marriage. Town councils saw organized prostitution as a means of keeping young men, especially unattached immigrants, away from the town's daughters.[207] As noted earlier, the prostitutes knew birth control procedures, but possession of that knowledge by other women was considered dangerous.

Little wonder, then, that physicians knew less and less, that midwives were cowed into restricting their activities to assisting births, that women were reluctant to tell their daughters what their mothers had taught them, and that apothecaries sold birth control drugs under the cloak of false labels. Physicians censured and incriminated charlatans who sold unknown substances as abortifacients.[208] An example is a widow in Goosnargh, England, who died after eating some "berries" given as an abortifacient by a flax-dresser. The man was unable to find pennyroyal and white mercury and so he gave her a substitute that turned out to be poisonous, according to the physician who performed the autopsy.[209]

If a woman sought not to become pregnant (in the age's definition of the term), she might have had little difficulty preventing motherhood if she consulted early, before the fetus was "quick," the right woman, physician, or apothecary. She would be advised (perhaps not by a physician, however) to take any number of menstrual regulators, or emmenagogues, as they would be called a century later. What she lacked that her counterpart a couple centuries earlier had had was access to the wise women who could give her precise, careful, and expert directions. The wares sold in the apothecary shops appear to have been complicated and (if I may judge without the benefit of scientific proof) less effective than the simple drugs of antiquity and the Middle Ages. Even if mixed properly, these commercially sold drugs very well might have been dangerous if carelessly or inexpertly taken. If her life were in danger because of a pregnancy that had quickened, there were physicians who would assist her just as there were those who would not. What happened is that fewer physicians and fewer women themselves knew what once was known by many. The sixteenth and seventeenth centuries seem to have "deleted from the record" a great deal of knowledge from millennia past.

6

The Broken Chain of Knowledge

[The College of Physicians has kept] the people in such
ignorance that they should not be able to know what the
herbs in their gardens are good for.

    Nicholas Culpeper, 1649

Modernization was built on the bodies of slain women and witches, so
claims a recent theory. In 1985, Gunnar Heinsohn, a sociologist, and
Otto Steiger, an economist, both at the University of Bremen, came
to a startling conclusion: The Scientific Revolution, the economic incentives for procreation, and the contemporaneous suppression of
witchcraft marked the destruction of the *weisen Frauen,* or "wise
women." As Christina Larner expressed it, "witch-hunting *is* woman-
hunting."[1] The hunts were not for just any women but for special
women, those who had special knowledge that to others was considered suspicious, magical, and, above all, not scientific as defined by the
new age.

When "huge numbers of women were burnt to death," the surviving women became dependent on physicians (rational men of science)
for help with matters that their ancestors had usually handled among
themselves, so argues the thesis.[2] Heinsohn and Steiger figure the number of women persecuted as witches as around one million women
charged, half a million killed.[3] Furthermore, they regard as an effect
of the suppression of the "wise women" the upswing in population beginning at the end of the fifteenth century and dramatically increasing

in the eighteenth century.[4] They reject Claudia Honegger's view that the suppression of witchcraft was a means of reducing the status of women and focus instead on the demographic consequences of the measures taken.[5] King James I of England expressed his view succinctly: "The more women, the more witches."[6] Heinsohn and Steiger attribute the reason for the suppression to economic needs. The mercantile philosophy adopted by business and political leaders led states to undertake a policy of pro-natalism, to encourage population growth. Standing in the way of such growth were those who helped women to limit the number of children they bore, the "wise women."

Heinsohn and Steiger's theory assumes that the reason for the relative stability in population during antiquity and the Middle Ages was that women had the means to control reproduction. The usual explanation for stable population levels in the pre-scientific age—extremely high fertility rates accompanied by extremely high mortality rates—in this theory is rejected in favor of deliberate decisions and conscious choices made by millions of women. In the modern period, at the same time that women lost reproductive control, they lost the knowledge of nature that enabled them to function with some measure of independence in respect to reproduction. If women's increased autonomy in the nineteenth and twentieth century is connected to access to accurate information and various options regarding fertility, then the reverse is true: if women lose the knowledge, they lose autonomy.[7] It is on this crucial point that Heinsohn and Steiger build. The suppression of witchcraft was a deliberate, conscious decision by political and religious leaders to halt the decline in population, they say. Witches, with their wares for birth control and infanticide, were a genuine threat to the economic prosperity of the Christian community, and so they must be destroyed.[8]

Direct connections between the extermination of witches, women's dependence on men for knowledge of reproduction, and the modern increase in population are not as closely tied as Heinsohn and Steiger allege, however. Their theory has been criticized, for example, by the historian of witchcraft Wolfgang Behringer.[9] Noting that Heinsohn and Steiger implied that the medicines and *maleficia* mentioned in the documents, and the spells, ligatures, and the evil eye, must have had some effect in reducing the population, Behringer pointed out that they proposed no scientific arguments that the wise women in the Middle Ages actually possessed the means to control population. By and large, Heinsohn and Steiger argued that women were victims of modernization and the rationality of science. Before deciding which argument to believe, we need to examine four topics: the population changes during the period of witch hunts and thereafter; whether the information about birth control was suppressed so much that it was largely lost to women following the suppression; whether the position of women in European society changed from relative freedom to dependence; and how influential the new theories of science and theology were in altering birth rates through behavioral changes.[10]

Demography

Many demographers believe that Europe, before the Scientific Revolution, was unaffected by birth control.[11] This is, of course, the reverse of Heinsohn and Steiger's thesis. The impact of birth control on gross population size can be measured, demographers surmise, beginning with the late eighteenth century and culminating in the nineteenth century. Modern demographic techniques using family reconstitution data fail to detect whether European populations prior to the late eighteenth century used birth control to the extent of being statistically detectable.[12] (Roger Mols said that "birth control . . . crept in in some restricted circles at the end of the 17th century.")[13] In most demographic models, reproduction prior to about 1770 was independent of birth control (not believed to be practiced) and largely dependent on external factors: wars, celibacy, famine, plagues, land use, and nutrition, plus infanticide.[14] For most of the people, most of the time, the available means of birth control was timing and incidence of marriage and restraint within marriage, according to some modern demographers.[15] Nursing for as long as possible after childbirth can be a partial factor in prolonging intervals between children, but only by a matter of around five months.[16] One demographer, Michael Flinn, raised the question of whether early modern population control could be explained by "the mechanical and pharmaceutical contraceptive devices" and concluded emphatically that these measures "can be ruled out" as having any influence.[17] The thesis of this book is just the opposite. The devices in use were drugs, both contraceptive and abortive, and they may have influenced meaningfully the results that I shall summarize next.

After the large population increase from the tenth through the thirteenth centuries, European population underwent periods of decline (notably in the fourteenth) and rapid recovery in the early fifteenth century (except in England and southern France). There followed slow growth and relatively steady growth through the seventeenth century. Between approximately 1000 and 1300, European population rose from 36 million to an unprecendented 80 million.[18] By the eve of the Black Death (1347), Europe's population was approximately 90 million, but it declined for the rest of the century (−3 per thousand) and was followed by a slow recovery in the fifteenth and sixteenth centuries and stagnation in the seventeenth.[19] Chief among the causes for the problems of the seventeenth century were Thirty Years War, other conflicts, plagues, and a general economic instability brought about partly by monetary problems caused by New World discoveries. In the late eighteenth century there was, in the words of H. J. Habakkuk, "a sustained cumulative increase."[20] The gross population data, that cited by Heinsohn and Steiger, indicate a dramatic population increase after 1800, a period when birth control became an issue of public policy, as seen in Table 5.

The table's data were prepared by different people, each using various techniques, and the results should be regarded only as approximations, because not all Europeans lived in states that collected census data.[21] The estimates by Josiah Russell (cited in Chapter 1) for the population in Europe were 32.8 million in 1 C.E. and 38.5 million in the year 1000, compared with 37 and 42 million, respectively, in this table.

A graph prepared by John D. Durand (1977) displays the estimates prepared by various demographers.[22] Although they differ especially in the early modern period, the figures are reasonably close to one another, and there is universal agreement about trends (see Figure 2). Of course, the more recent in time the more accurate the data.[23] The overall trends appear certain, according to the scholars' reports. The dramatic increase in population *(die europäische Bevölkerungsexplosion)* began in the last half of the eighteenth century.

The European population rarely increased at an estimated rate of over 38 per 1,000 people annually in the pre-modern period prior to the late eighteenth century.[24] England's lowest birth rate, for example, was 22.9 (in 1659) and the highest 44.3 (1815).[25] Thomas Pierre Chaunu, the French historian, called late marriages "the real contraceptive weapon *(la véritable arme contraceptive)*" of classical Europe.[26] The pre-modern European rate compares with birth rates in modern

Table 5. European population estimates, 400 B.C.E.–1970 A.C.E.

Year	People (millions)	Year	People (millions)
400 B.C.E.	23	1400	45
1 A.C.E.	37	1450	60
200	67	1500	69
700	27	1550	78
1000	42	1600	90
1050	46	1650	103
1100	48	1700	115
1150	50	1750	125
1200	61	1800	187
1250	69	1850	274
1300	73	1900	423
1350	51	1950	594
		1970	636

Sources: Shepard Clough and Richard T. Rapp, *European Economic History: The Economic Development of Western Civilization*, 3d ed. (New York, 1975), p. 52; reproduced from Gunnar Heinsohn and Otto Steiger, *Die Vernichtung der weisen Frauen: Beiträge zur Theorie und Geschichte von Bevölkerung und Kindheit* (Herbstein, 1985), p. 95, with addition of 1970 data.

underdeveloped countries (where little birth control is practiced, it is assumed); rates were usually over 40 and often over 45 per 1,000. For example, the birth rate for the French village of Crulai[27] in comparison with the death rate was as follows:

	Births per thousand	*Deaths per thousand*
1675–1749	36	31
1750–1789	31	28

Although delayed marriage had an influence on population size, another important factor was that women after marriage were increasing the intervals between children. Some demographers dispute this point by holding that up until the nineteenth century (slightly earlier in

**Europe, Including European Russia
or European Part of the USSR:
Population Estimates since A.D. 1600**

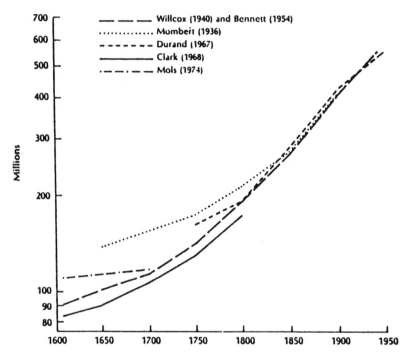

Figure 2. Estimations of Europe's population (including European Russia) since 1600. Citations are to the following references:

Willcox, Walter F. 1940. *Studies in American Demography*, Appendix 2. Ithaca, N.Y.: Cornell University Press.

Bennett, M. K. 1954. *The World's Food*. New York: Harper and Bros.

Mombert, Paul. 1936. "Die Entwicklung der Bevölkerung Europas seit der Mitte des 17. Jahrhunderts." *Zeitschrift für Nationalökonomie*, 7: 533–545.

Durand, John D. 1967. "The Modern Expansion of World Population." *Proceedings of the American Philosophical Society*, 111, no. 3: 136–159.

Clark, Colin. 1968. *Population Growth and Land Use*. New York: St. Martin's.

Mols, Roger. 1974. "Population in Europe, 1500–1700." In *The Fontana Economic History of Europe*, ed. Carolo M. Cipolla, 2: 15–82. Glasgow: Collins.

(*Source:* From Shepard Bancroft Clough and Richard T. Rapp, *European Economic History*, 3d ed. [New York: McGraw-Hill, 1975].)

France) a deliberate birth spacing did not inevitably lead to smaller families.[28] In Geneva between 1650 and 1674, only 10 percent of families had children within an interval less than eighteen months. Fifty-two percent had children within eighteen to thirty months, and 39 percent with an interval greater than thirty months. Indeed, 14 percent produced a child after a forty-nine month interval. The intervals between the first, second, and third child fell slightly in seventeenth-century Geneva, but the mother's age at the birth of the last child fell sharply from 38.5 to 34.3 and, with it, the average family size shrank.[29] By the period 1625–1772, the interval was less than eighteen months for only 6 percent of families, whereas in the same period a majority of 54 percent of families had children at an interval of thirty-one months or greater (and in 25 percent the interval was greater than forty-nine months).[30] Heinsohn and Steiger maintain that from the late fifteen century to the late eighteenth century each married woman had, on average, between 5 and 6.5 children. Without the revolutionary change in European marriage patterns, the figures would be much higher, say between 9.8 and 11.6 children per married woman.[31]

Unless one hypothesizes that unknown biological factors were decreasing fertility, the conclusion from the data is that a cause for the low birth rates was deliberate family planning *after marriage*.[32] The means was usually nothing more complicated that the event described in the diary of Martha Ballard, a midwife, on September 27, 1789: "She is suffering from obstructions and I prescribed the use of particular herbs."[33] It was the same as in 1427, when Bernardino accused Tuscan wives of arranging "that they cannot conceive; and if they have conceived, they destroy them in the body."[34]

Population data for the early modern period are spotty and come from a variety of sources, none definitive for large areas.[35] When the data are considered as a whole, however, the patterns I see support the idea of continuous use of contraceptive and abortifacient medicines among some, but limited, populations over a long period of time. Occasionally there are a few references in contemporaneous documents to manipulative or surgical abortions. Mostly, however, when a birth control procedure is found in the sources, the means prescribed were herbs to be taken orally.[36]

The case for continuous use of birth control herbs in the early modern period is not apparent in the larger picture. A few examples of extremely rapid growth demonstrate that economic and social factors sometimes allowed, or even encouraged, large family size. In 1300 England's population was 3.75 million, the same as in 1500, but it recovered slightly to 4.25 million in 1600.[37] The Irish population moved from approximately 3,042,000 in 1725 to 4,753,000 in 1791, but it jumped from 6,802,000 in the twenty-year period of 1821 to 1841 to 8,175,000 (data based on actual census collection).[38] The explanation for Ireland's case is the potato. The new food source enabled Irish farmers to subdivide their land and support more families on smaller acreage, and the fertility rate increased; of course, it decreased when the food source disappeared because of the infamous potato blight.[39]

Between 1550 and 1680 the population of England moved from an estimated 3.0 million to an estimated 4.9, but between 1651 and 1680 there was a decrease from 5.23 to 4.9.[40] However, during what E. A. Wrigley calls the "long" eighteenth century (from 1680 to 1820) England's population increased from 4.9 million to 11.5, a rate of increase much higher than that in France, Germany, or the rest of Western Europe.[41] Thus, from a relative balance between the fertility and mortality rates in the third quarter of the seventeenth century, the population began to grow, and this rise is explained mostly by economic forces at work in England. The life expectancy at birth increased from about 32.4 years in 1680 to 38.7 around 1820.[42] The mortality rate did not cause the dramatic results so much as the fertility rate, which rose from a low of 30.7 to 39.6 in the same period. In another view, the rise of the fertility rate was two-and-a-half times greater than that of all the mortality rates.[43] (However, some demographers believe the nineteenth century's increase is better understood by postulating a decrease in the mortality rate in part because of improvements in hygiene and public health.)[44]

In contrast, the marriage rate varied, with some decrease in women's age at first marriage. Even if people were confident that they could have children when they planned on it, they might have other reasons to delay marriage. Children are only one important economic factor in the decision to establish a new marriage and, in England's customs, likely a new household. Whereas the illegitimacy rate increased during the "long" century from 2 percent of all births in 1680 to 6 percent in 1820, the births within marriage account for the bulk of the fertility increase. (This is a strange phenomenon, because normally one expects illegitimacy rates to increase when marriages are being delayed and to decrease when people marry young.) As a rule, an increase in population brings about increased competition for wages, which causes a decrease in wages and an increase in food prices that in turn cause a population decrease. England escaped the cycle because its economy produced increased goods and services that sustained an increased growth rate and improved living standards.[45] Neither England's nor Ireland's gross demographics in the early modern period supply evidence about the use of birth control medicines.

In contrast to Europe, the population of North America in the seventeenth and eighteenth centuries increased at an unprecedented rate, one that caused Thomas Malthus to marvel.[46] After about 1810, however, it had one of the lowest fertility rates.[47] From 1800 to 1860, the fertility of the white population in the United States fell precipitously (although with immigration the population increased).[48] Fertility among the provinces of Italy were more variable with higher mortality rates during nineteenth century, but with generally reduced rates between 1866 and 1875 as compared with the 1814–1816 rate. After 1862 there were constant population increases, varying from 6.0 to 7.5 percent per decade until 1900.[49] In contrast, during the eighteenth century and first half of the nineteenth century, pre-industrialized Japan's population was relatively stable, supposedly through a combination of methods, such as infanticide, abortion, and late marriages.[50] Whether the Japanese, like the Chinese, practiced herbal birth control awaits study.

While some regions of Europe decreased in population in the sixteenth and seventeenth centuries (such as the Scottish Highlands), other regions increased but none dramatically. Spain's total population is estimated to have declined from 8.5 million in 1591–1594 to 7.5 million in 1717 and then increased to 9.3 million in 1768, the date of its first census.[51] Economic and political factors associated with Spain's political decline and attendant monetary problems help explain the decline. These regional patterns are sufficiently varied so that one cannot explain the data on the basis of the availability of birth control measures. Complex local conditions produced different population sizes and rates of growth. Nevertheless, we do see patterns that can be better understood by postulating continuous use of contraceptive and abortifacient medicine among those populations that saw the need to limit family size or individual reproduction. For example, when Spanish families were enduring economic hardships, what means did they have to limit fertility?

France was at variance with most of Europe. Between 1660 and 1750 France's population held steady but then it grew until 1790.[52] The gross reproductive rate declined from about 2.4 per thousand in 1770 until reaching 1.0 per thousand in 1935.[53] Swedish birth rates for the general population were approximately 34.2 per thousand in 1691 and 33.7 per thousand in 1750, with an average for the intervening years of 32.9 per thousand.[54] The estimated French birth rate was 38.6 per thousand in 1771, but it steadily dropped to 32 per thousand in 1800. The usual explanation is the discovery of coitus interruptus by the French peasantry.[55] That was only the beginning of a decline that lasted more than a hundred years. In 1801 the crude birth rate was only 21.7 per thousand in Calvados (Normandy), and it steadily declined to 17.9 per thousand in 1851–1855.[56] After 1800 French population statistics are based on census data. By 1850, the nation's population rate was definitely declining.[57] Whatever the cause of France's low birth rates, the trend began in the seventeenth century and continued in the next.[58] Mortality rates, although high during the Revolution and the first half of the nineteenth century, do not adequately explain the data. Illegitimacy was declining during most of the seventeenth century. In France it was below 2 percent prior to the mid-eighteenth century.[59]

The conclusion reached by demographers, as we have seen, is that the masses discovered contraception and various other forms of birth control prior to the French Revolution.[60] Louis Henry's study of the eighteenth-century French data indicates tentatively that some form of birth control within marriage was practiced at the end of the seventeenth century. But, Henry wrote, "there is scarcely any evidence enabling us to verify the assertions of authors" who claim that birth control had spread to the peasants in the late eighteenth century.[61] Henry raised doubts about the "discovery" of birth control by the masses in the late eighteenth century. So too did Alan Macfarlane when he concluded that an assumption of some form of birth control is necessary "to bridge the huge gap" between the number of children in English families and the number that would be expected if fertility were unrestrained.[62] By and large, demographers contend that birth control was used often enough to affect population size in the decades prior to 1800. A treatise written in 1778 allegedly by Baron de Montyon about the population in France denounced the "pernicious secrets, unknown to all animals save man," that women used to avoid children. Fearing harm to France, the author proclaimed in alarm that "it is time to halt this secret and terrible cause of the depopulation."[63] Earlier, in 1764, a similar denouncement of *medicamina* used to prevent children was heard in Italy.[64] Without knowing the techniques used by pre- modern people, Henry based his doubts on the evidence presented, as Baron de Montyon said. Not only did pre-modern women know as well as their eighteenth- and nineteenth-century counterparts what to do to prevent or end a pregnancy, but probably more of them knew it better.

Numerous factors played a part in the demographic changes of the sixteenth and seventeenth centuries: late marriage ages; time intervals for bearing children; wars; immigration and migration; economic opportunities to establish work and living space; infanticide; famines; diseases (especially in the sixteenth century); plagues;[65] illegitimacy (although it appears insignificant); and altered life styles (the rise of factory-workshops; wet-nursing; prostitution *inter alterum*). All in all, the human will to reproduce or not to reproduce was the crucial component that determined population size, that in conjunction with the mortality rate.[66]

A contrasting picture comes from a study of the fertility rates of Venetian nobles that evidences birth control. From 1563 to 1790, the rate of decline of the Venetian nobility was precipitous but steady, while the total population's rate was up and down (see Table 6). These data come from a long period during which Venice declined in economic importance.

Judging from the data alone, one would be remiss in concluding that Venetian nobles knew how to control their reproductive rates and French peasants did not. Demographer Massimo Livi-Bacci found evidence that aristocracies and Jews engaged in fertility control prior to the modern era, but his findings are confined by other demographers to a restricted few.[67] Emmanuel Le Roy Ladurie and Philippe Ariès assumed that the means employed by the elites was coitus interruptus.[68] Were this so, the aristocrats and elites were remarkable in their self-restraint, enough so to deserve their position. To withdraw before a climax is a torturous act for a male, and a male's cooperation is necessary for the effectiveness of the technique. Not suffering the dangers of pregnancy and childbirth or the difficulties of raising small children, males as a rule are less concerned about family size.

The sources inform us that the primary means to limit population was drugs, although other things (manipulative abortion, interruptus,

Table 6.   Fertility rates in Venice, 1563–1790 (births per 1,000)

	1563	1586	1642	1766	1790
Nobility	38.8	34.3	27.6	20.6	20.0
Total population	34.1	31.8	37.2	32.2	31.7

Source: Roger Mols, *Introduction a la démographie historique des villes d'europe du XIVe au XVIIIe siècle*, 2 vols. (Louvain, 1955), 2: 328.

infanticide, celibacy) played their roles. Birth control was employed by many if not most women, I believe, who wanted to limit their reproductive rates. In order for fertility control to take place, three things conditions must be met: (1) people must perceive that they have a choice; (2) couples must desire to limit the number of children; and (3) the means must be available.[69] Evidence seems adequate to postulate that conditions (1) and (3) existed; condition (2) is a matter of the deepest recesses of human motivation—albeit these feelings are affected by economical, social, and religious influences—and in the end it escapes historical analysis.[70] Sometimes, it is obvious, fertility *was* controlled. Still some scholars have argued that, prior to the modern era, parents wanted large families and that therefore there was no family limitation.[71]

One reason that pre-industrial Europe's population history is complex is that it represents the collective effect of millions of reproductive decisions that varied according to time, class, region, and economic prosperity. Indeed, any individual woman, even in the most pronatalistic and prosperous of societies, might believe herself to need birth control in a special circumstance. A study of attitudes toward menstruation in seventeenth-century England found that women who did not menstruate on time expected the reason to be pregnancy. The absence of menstruation, if a woman did not wish to have a child, was a symptom requiring treatment.[72]

The data do not conclusively support the thesis that birth control was a modern (that is, late eighteenth or early nineteenth century) discovery. On the other hand, those data do not prove that a characteristic of modernity was the loss of birth control means once known to wise women and witches. In fairness, Heinsohn and Steiger believe that people's resistance against enforced parenthood did not become exhausted and that the means to prevent or end unwanted pregnancies continued, albeit at a reduced level.[73] Complex factors were altering former, more stable patterns of change. The question is whether, despite legal and religious sanctions against birth control and despite the suppression of witchcraft, the same herbs were available and known to the general population to a sufficient extent to affect gross population numbers.

Menstrual Regulators and Abortion

To prevent women from killing infants, an English law in 1624 placed the burden on an accused woman to prove that an infant that died in her care died of natural causes. In Essex between 1620 and 1680 the rate of conviction and execution by hanging for women accused of suspicious infant deaths was over 40 percent, much higher than the conviction rate for those accused of other homicides.[74] By the eighteenth century, the number of cases was decreasing, which shows the degree to which English society was stressing legitimacy and child raising. Faced with the prospect of prosecution for infanticide, some women sought refuge in old remedies that prevented things from getting to that point.

A unique set of statistics from County Lancashire in the seventeenth century gives us an indication of the prevalence of abortion. By some chance, the burial records between 1581 and 1710 here list the deaths of newborn and aborted babies. The aborted babies varied from 10 per 1,000 live births in 1601–1610 to 30 in 1631–1640.[75] These figures certainly are low, but we must remember that an abortion was recorded only when the act was declared, and undoubtedly those cases were fairly late-term abortions. Midwives would give baptism to stillborn infants, and this custom served as a reason to register their deaths in this shire. The miscarriage or stillbirth rate ranged from 29 per thousand live births (in 1641–1650) to 96 per thousand (in 1691–1700); this compares with miscarriage rates from 10 to 20 per thousand live births in the twentieth century.[76] Also compare these figures with an average number of stillbirths in fourteen German villages in the eighteenth and nineteenth centuries of only 10.8 per thousand live births.[77] Thus, compared with the modern data and the historic German data, the Lancashire data probably indicate a high number of miscarriage-abortions in the later part of seventeenth century.

Evidently, most of these miscarriages were induced by women deliberately taking menstrual stimulators in order to avoid pregnancy (in the definition of the time). "Making themselves regular" was the phrase of the age.[78] This judgment I make without absolute proof because in most of these cases no one but the woman would have known, let alone recorded, that an abortion had taken place. A historian (or even an anthropologist) could have lived in the woman's home and still not have known—and this in a time when houses afforded little privacy (it was only with the use of the hallway in the eighteenth century that bedroom doors came into fashion). In order for a miscarriage to be recorded, the pregnancy (as measured, by our reckoning, since implantation) would be somewhat advanced, at least well in the second trimester. King Henry II of France in 1556 sought to check women who concealed their pregnancy by asking them to declare their condition so that, should a child be born dead or prematurely, the proper rites could be given.[79] The edict was unenforceable, but its presence demonstrates a perceived problem and the willingness of the secular state to provide solutions.

It is questionable that a woman would inform anyone, or even know herself, if by taking a drug a week or so after a delayed menstrual period she had ended a potential pregnancy. In addition, as we have noted earlier, there are hints in the sources that women regularly took some herbs, namely rue, with food as a prophylactic to prevent pregnancy, and these women obviously would make no declarations. The fact remains that pre-modern women had a period of time after every delayed menses to decide whether or not to have children during which they were largely unchecked in their decisions. An eighteenth-century physician in Eisenach expressed it this way, "Menses can be said to be the principal cause of abortion . . . Abnormal menses, however, either are a hinderance to conception or cause an abortion through a minimal flux."[80]

There are cases of individual choices, of course, coming before the public. A criminal case of abortion was tried by a municipal court in the German city of Cologne in 1629. A young woman described as having an "unchaste life style" secured some "fresh savin [juniper] and other things" and aborted her pregnancy. Certain details were brought out that enlighten us, although they incriminated her. She had difficulty finding the herbs, which apparently were not readily sold in the city. This is strange in light of the official apothecary guide for this same city, which was discussed in Chapter 5. Acting on advice received from a female friend ("Kollegin"), the woman went to a vineyard worker, but he had nothing to give her. She had better luck when she was sent to a gravedigger at the Church of St. Johann the Baptist. She was told that the herbs secured from him "would not allow her to become pregnant or, if she already were, that they would abort her fruit."[81] Confirming the information from her colleague was the same advice she received from her sister, she was found guilty.

Twelve years later in the same city, another case came before the court that confirms our suspicion that apothecaries were selling birth control drugs, just as the pharmacy sources inform us. A young woman in 1641 who was pregnant, on the advice of a woman friend, was dispatched to an apothecary for a drug to alter her condition. Her friend warned her that she could not come right out and say what she wanted because not all druggists would sell it to her. She had to be indirect.[82] According to the diary of a physician in Eisenach who practiced in the 1720s, local women received menstrual promoters, which he knew could end pregnancy, both from other neighborhood women and from "lower" healers who traveled from village to village, town to town.[83]

In seventeenth-century England a married man seduced a maid and, when he discovered her pregnancy, went to the maid's aunt to "buy something at the apothecaries and give it to her kinswoman to destroy her conception."[84] Another young man was faced with a slightly different situation: he wanted to do the right thing and marry his pregnant lover but his father objected. His father's advice was to let some blood (blood-letting being a common practice and commonly performed on pregnant women) and "to take some herbs as may be convenient to destroy the child that was conceived." The lover objected by pointing out that it was "a thing" that destroyed his own sister.[85] Another pregnant woman was given a box of powder within a fortnight of delivery, but apparently she did not take it.

The two Cologne cases were, after all, tried in criminal court, which considered abortion a crime. The historian G. R. Quaife, who studied the "wanton wenches and wayward wives" of England during the seventeenth century, believed that abortions were widespread and successful but that women resorted to them only reluctantly and cautiously. He remarked that their wariness stemmed not so much from religious reasons as from fear of what might be a threat to their physical safety.[86] A study of sex in seventeenth-century Middlesex, Massachusetts, pun unavoidable, uncovered testimony that the knowledge of abortifacient herbs was widely known. Despite this, there were only four cases where the use of herbs, savin among them, resulted in trials in the county courts between 1649 and 1699. There was only one case of infanticide, and the accused was a married couple.[87]

According to the anecdotal information, local women were the source about which herbs to take. For example, a pregnant woman in Kilton, England, was approached by a village woman who "did offer to make her a medicine for to destroy the child."[88] Another case in Kingsdon reveals that the local apothecary was the source for such medicines as the local "whores" knew. In this same case one woman reproved another because she had a "base child," as she was not "acquainted with it [the medicine] in time," and consequently her reputation suffered.[89] Not all herbal lore came from women. A young woman in Eisenach in the 1720s feared that she had taken the Holy Eucharist while being unworthy and for months thereafter her normal menstrual flow did occur. Her worried parents took her to a university-trained physician, whose remedies did not work. Believing that witchcraft was involved, they obtained a remedy from an executioner that apparently did work.[90]

As noted in Chapter 5, birth control information was not as readily available in the seventeenth and eighteenth centuries as it had been before, but it was available. In 1653, one person said that there were "creatures [who] will give a dram ... [to] make an abort if need be, keep downe their paps, hinder conception [and] procure lust."[91] An Italian canon, F. E. Cangiamila, complained in 1762 that women were procuring miscarriages by dancing and, if that did not work, by purchasing drugs from midwives, "debauched women," and even from surgeons and apothecaries.[92] Advertisements for medicines proclaimed drugs for a variety of sexually related controls, which indicates that people were not estranged from the idea of gaining control from a bottle.[93] To learn just how well known the birth control drugs were, we need to look at the herbal, medical (including midwifery), and pharmaceutical sources.

Herbal Lore through a Veil

"Then little by little [I will] conduct thee through most pleasant gardens, and other delightfull places where any herbe or plant may be found, fit for meate or medicine." Thus did John Gerard begin his immensely popular herbal in 1597. He was a surgeon-barber, the curator of the "physic garden" of the College of Physicians of London, and owner of a tremendous garden of his own at Holborn in London. Gerard knew plants well and was competent to speak of their medicinal usages. Speak he did, to the extent of 1,392 pages and nearly 2,200 woodcut illustrations.

On birth control he spoke as well, but neither loudly nor clearly. He employed the common circumlocutions and evasions. Those plants that "bringeth downe the menses" he named as: parsley, mountain parsley, chervil, love-in-a-mist (*Nigella* sp.), wild horehound (*Stachys* sp.?), sea madder (*Rumex aquaticus* L.?), *carlina* (?), larch (*Larix decidua* Miller), *tamariscus* or myrrh, spurge laurel, laurel, almond, and cinnamon.[94] Under the rubric of plants that "bring down [or provoke] the termes," which is the equivalent of the above, he named: southernwood (*Artemisia abrotanum* L.), galingale (*Cyperus longus* L.), camel's hair (of *Juncus* or *Eriophorum* genera?), iris, asphodill (*Asphodelus* sp.), "sorcerers garlick" (*Allium* sp.?), mustard (*Sinapis alba* L.), anemone (*Anemone* sp.), and "butter burre" (*Petasites officinalis* L.).[95] The authority named was most often Dioscorides.

Gerard saw an association between menstrual stimulators and birth. Wild horehound, artemisia, and marigolds, he said, not only provoke menstruation but also expel the afterbirth.[96] Interestingly, he said that angelica (*Angelica* sp.) was similar to *silphium*, and it "draweth downe the tearmes [menses], driveth out or expelleth the secondine [afterbirth]."[97] Of course, angelica little resembles *Ferula* physically or botanically, and so he may have thought of it as similar to *silphium* in its actions. Angelica is a member of the carrot family, just as Queen Anne's lace is, and there are reports in modern literature that it has abortifacient qualities.[98] Also he said that horse tongue, a kind of laurel, stimulates menstruation and hastens a speedy delivery.[99]

Gerard perhaps knew more than he told. Chaste tree seeds are taken with pennyroyal to "bringeth downe the menses," he wrote, but under pennyroyal he expressed it in these words: "provoketh the monthly termes, bringeth foorth the secondine [afterbirth], the dead child and unnatural birth."[100] By unnatural birth he meant, I presume, an abortion rather than a miscarriage, both being the same thing except that the latter was not intended and the former was. Under savin, a type of juniper, he was even more precise: it "bringeth downe the menses *with force*, it draweth away the afterbirth, expelleth the dead child, and killeth the quicke."[101] This description definitely indicates that he knew

it meant abortion, because by the use of "quicke" he meant a quick fetus. In the vernacular this meant a fetus that was fully formed and kick-
ing, so to speak.

Gerard used the word *abortion* only once: Xyris (*Iris foetidissima* L.)
"profiteth being used in a pessarie to provoke the termes and to cause
abortion."[102] The information was not a caution against its use, because he said it "profited being used" as an abortifacient. Gerard related no birth control information about various species of *Ferula*, but
he said that these plants were good for cramps and for women in childbirth.[103] Clearly he knew about the "herbe Grace" or rue: "the juice
of rue drunke with wine purgeth women after their deliverance, driving foorth the secondine, the dead childe, and the unnatural birth."[104]

Given Gerard's background, he was in a position to know the uses
of these plants, but he was obscure about their effects in most instances.
He prevaricated more often than he explained. Just the same, he was
definite about some of the plants' birth control qualities. He saw that
some of the plants that could bring on an abortion were the same as
could be used to assist in difficult deliveries. Nowhere, however, does
he say that abortion was wrong or that a menstrual stimulator was a
form of abortion.

About the same time that Gerard wrote in English, a very elaborate
herbal was produced in German by Jacobus Theodorus (Tabernae-
montanus, d. 1590), which had many editions. The work was intended,
he said, for physicians, apothecaries, gardeners, cooks, and house fathers and mothers. When discussing dill, he said that he wanted to
thank all the women who had given him information about the
plants.[105] In relating what he learned, far from excluding birth control
information, Theodorus included it but indirectly. Rue's qualities to
interfere with birth received great detail; however, most plants did
not.[106] He said only that cypress was an emmenagogue and that birthwort caused an abortion.[107] Artemisia expelled a live or a dead fetus.[108]
Nonetheless, he listed three abortifacient recipes, prepared from
asarum, pennyroyal, artemisia, and rue, as distillates in the new pharmacy.[109] As detailed as Theodorus's herbal was, clearly the issue of
birth control was handled gingerly, much more so than the *Gart der
Gesundheit* herbals of a century earlier. Just the same, the use of distillates indicates that Gerard was knowledgeable and current for his
time, a standard that the anonymous authors of the earlier herbals did
not meet.

Almost a century later, yet another herbal was published that veiled the identity of birth control drugs. As a practicing physician in London, graduate of Oxford, John Peachey knew the medical aspects of plants when he wrote his innovative herbal (1694). Eschewing scholasticism and citations of earlier works, Peachey's work is the product of personally experienced knowledge. He divided the work into two parts: plants growing in England and those imported. Never did he explicitly recommend a birth control drug; seldom did he miss the opportunity to inform those who were savvy about the terminology what effect a plant would have. Native plants that "provoke the Courses" were calamint, cypress, agrimony, horehound, juniper, parsley, pennyroyal, rue, sage; imported plants included the chaste tree and sassafras.[110] Those plants said to "cure women's Obstructions" were bryony, Queen Anne's lace, and catnip from England, and tansy and walnut from abroad.[111] Artemisia and laurel stimulate menstruation and remove the afterbirth, whereas wild basil removes the "birth" as well and lovage expels a dead child.[112]

Savin ("Sabina" or juniper) provokes the "Courses," "causes Miscarriage," and expels a "dead Child." For this reason, Peachey wrote, savin is "too well known and too much used by Wenches."[113] Nowhere could he be said to advocate abortion. Snakeweed, fennel, and sea holly *(Eringium)* prevent or hinder abortion.[114] Just the same, he conveyed the information; for example, the fern, *filix,* "is reckon'd injurious to Women, and occasions Barrenness, hinders Conception, and causes Abortion."[115] The wild cucumber is listed as growing in England, and he tells us that it "moves the Courses and kills the Child; wherefore it is seldom used."[116] I assume that this was the wild or squirting cucumber of the *Ecballium* species that under close cultivation can be grown in England. Aloe stimulates menstruation but "Women with Child must not take it."[117] Mustard (*Thaslpi* or giant carrot?) is "injurious to women with Child."[118] Finally, he gave the recipe for syrup of artemisia, much the same formula as that provided by Valerius Cordus and sold in drug stores, and he said of it: " 'Tis frequently used by Women, inwardly and outwardly, in all the Diseases peculiar to them."[119] Syrup of myrtle, whose recipe he also gave, is seldom used "now-a-days."[120] So some contraceptives and abortifacients he said ought not to be taken and others were seldom taken. Nowhere did he say to take them. Never did he advocate usage except for the menstrual stimulators, which he did not connect with birth control.

Culpeper's Revelation of Secrets

In contrast to most other herbals published in the sixteenth and seventeenth centuries, which were intended for apothecaries and physicians, one work appeared that presented current knowledge for the public. Its author, Nicholas Culpeper, was a revolutionary on two fronts: he supported Parliament against the king, who was beheaded in 1649, and in that same year he challenged the English medical establishment. Culpeper published a translation of and corrections to the London Dispensatory, an official guide to drugs written in Latin. He said that he wanted people to know the secrets about the herbs in their gardens that the physicians and apothecaries kept from them. The College of Physicians, reacting indignantly to the challenge, pronounced through a royalist paper that the translation was a product of "two yeeres of drunken labour."[121]

Culpeper revealed secrets about birth control, but he did so cautiously and soberly. As we saw in the previous chapter, Culpeper was personally biased toward having children, perhaps because of his wife's childbearing problems. The fern called *filix* and laurel, he said, were dangerous for "women with child." Dittany "hastens travail in women and provokes the terms," whereas iris "provokes the terms," though he did not specify that it induces labor.[122] These four herbs were listed near the beginning of his *Physical Directory*, as he named his translation/ correction. For later entries he changed his vocabulary, even though seemingly describing the same thing. Lily and tamarisk, he said, stimulated menstruation (without any reference to birth control); cinnamon bark speeds menstruation and delivery; artemisia, juniper (savin), carrot seeds (Queen Anne's lace?), *Ferula (galbanum)*, and myrrh stimulated menstruation, the birth, and afterbirth, whereas pennyroyal provoked menstruation and removed the afterbirth (without mention of assisting in childbirth).[123]

Two contraceptives are listed, wild mint and rue: "Rue or herb of grace: hot and dry to the third degree [meaning very strong, not extremely strong], consumes the seed and is an enemy to generation."[124] Strangely, no abortifacient qualities are cited for rue. Asafetida and birthwort's qualities in respect to birth control he omitted entirely[125] and, more bizarre, "the very smel of it [tansy] staies [halts] abortion or miscarriage *in women*" (italics added).[126]

While Culpeper did not explicitly advocate birth control, neverthe-less he provided the information so that a savvy reader of English could know what those "herbs in their gardens are good for." By the mid-seventeenth century people were accustomed to taking their medicines in compounds—that is, pills, liquids, and so forth, in complex mixtures. In revealing the secrets of compounds, Culpeper gave careful instruc-tions. There was an "Aqua hysterica" for women, which was composed of bryony, rue, artemisia ("mugwort"), mint, pennyroyal, dittany, and myrrh: it "is a most excellent remedy to bring away dead children and the after-birth, a spoonful or two of it being given; therefore let mid-wives make much of it."[127] Concerning syrup of artemisia, attributed to Matthaeus de Gradibus, with much the same ingredients listed by Va-lerius Cordus (above), Culpeper said only that it provoked the "termes" or menstruation.[128] A powder for the womb with (in its entirety) asafetida, *Ferula*, myrrh, birthwort, juniper, dittany, mint, rue, cas-toreum, and asarum ("asarabacca") helps "fits of the mother, expel both the birth and the after-birth, and expel the relics of a careless Midwife."[129]

There were several prescriptions that stimulated menstruation, each with familiar ingredients, but nowhere did Culpeper say that they caused an abortion.[130] In exasperation he listed one compound men-strual regulator attributed to Conrad Gesner (1516–1565), the Swiss medical writer, that was composed of about twenty-seven ingredients, with elaborate instructions. "It is such a mess . . . ," Culpeper lamented, "I verily think the labour and cost of it put in an equal ballance would outweigh the benefit."[131]

Culpeper knew whereof he wrote. Born in London, a student at Cambridge, he became an apprentice to an apothecary, but about 1640 he crossed the line and became a physician. In the previous chapter I mentioned his expertise and interest in midwifery. After his revolu-tionary revelation of the physicians' secrets, he wrote an even more detailed herbal (first published in 1652 as *The Physitian*). More men-strual stimulators were named in the herbal than in the guides to drugs and midwifery. He named, for instance, allheal (probably opopanax, a *Ferula*), angelica, and betony as stimulating menstruation and expelling a dead child.[132] He wrote of bryony that it "clenseth the Mother, . . . expelleth the Child, and Afterbirth, but is not to be used by Women with Child, for fear of abortion.; a dram of the Root in Pouder taken in white Wine bringeth down their Courses."[133] Administered either orally or in a pessary, stinking iris (*Iris foetidissima* L.) stimulated the onset of menstruation "but causeth abortion with women with child," for which reason it ought to be "utterly forbidden to women with child."[134] Much the same was said about ground pine ("chamepitys").[135] Thereby Culpeper disclosed that he knew what the menstrual stimulators did. In Chapter 5, where Culpeper's guide to midwives was discussed, we saw that he called one who gave a menstrual stimulator to a pregnant woman a "murderer."

Why would he be more open and less inhibited in his herbal and medical works than in his treatise on midwifery? Perhaps it was because midwives should not administer the drugs he described. Obviously, he was reluctant to be too specific about birth control in whatever he wrote; for example, even in his *English Physitian* he said that sweet basil expelled the birth and afterbirth and "helps the deficiency of Venus in one kind, so that it spoils all her actions in another." And he concluded with these remarks: "I dare write no more." But, he added a curious observation: "Something is the matter with this herb and rue will not grow together, no, nor near one another; and we know rue is as great an enemy to poison as any that grows."[136]

As Culpeper said in the *Physical Directory*, he occasionally noted when drugs should *not* be taken, as when, under ferns, he said: "They are dangerous for women with child to meddle with, by reason they cause abortions." He added that they "causeth barrenness" as well, that is to say, contraception.[137] Calamint "hindreth conception in women," but he warned that it could do violence to women.[138] A more typical example, however, was pennyroyal, about which he said only that it provoked menstruation, expelled the "dead" and "afterbirth."[139] For rue he entered a precaution that is very interesting: he said that people put rue on their meat or in drinks as a food, but long-term use of it "destroys the ability to get children."[140]

Culpeper regarded tansy in an eccentric way, to say the least:

The Dame Venus was minded to pleasure women with child by this herb, for there grows not an herb fitter for their use than this is; it is just as though it were ordained for the purpose . . . Let those women that desire children love this herb, it is their best companion, their husband excepted . . . [It] procures women's course [stimulates menstruation] . . . It is also very profitable for such women as are given to miscarry in child-bearing, to cause them to go out their ful time.[141]

In his drug guide, Culpeper was similarly inconsistent. Tansy, the plant that Hildegard of Bingen first disclosed as an abortifacient, was touted by Culpeper as an aid to pregnancy *and at the same time as a menstrual stimulator*. It may be that those plants that are estrogenic or that stimulate progesterone could be both helpful and harmful to a pregnancy, depending on the dosage. Possibly, he may have been confused by what women told him, but we are in the dark on this matter.

We are not in the dark about most of what Culpeper knew and told his readers. He showed that he knew the birth control plants very well indeed, but he was not advocating their use for that purpose. It was not only what he said but what he left out that raises questions. In relation to birth control, nothing, explicitly or implicitly, was said about celery seed, pomegranate, or wormwood (artemisia).[142] Savin (juniper) was recommended for external medicines but "inwardly it cannot be taken, without manifest danger."[143] He had many readers, as is known by the number of printings and editions. To no one did he recommend birth control.

Culpeper was involved in another project that was ostensibly published to give guidance to the poor, but again he obscured information about birth control even as he presented it. The project was a medicinal guide prepared by Jean Prevost (1585–1631) in Latin (published in 1641), and it was translated by Nicholas Culpeper. Earlier, Prevost had published a guide listing drugs under various categories. For example, under drugs that extinguish a man's semen "to impede generation" were such things as the chaste tree, rue, juniper, ginger, and willow.[144] Under drugs that stimulate menstruation there was a long, exhaustive list of simple drugs and the names for compound medicines, but nothing explicitly for abortion.[145]

This earlier volume was merely list making. Prevost wanted to call to "common people's" attention those drugs that grew in their garden, so that they did not have to rely on physicians and apothecaries for their wares. The work he produced would have been helpful to a woman seeking birth control information, provided she could read and provided she knew the code, namely that "remedies that move the courses" are abortifacient as well. If she did not read and already possessed the information, Prevost's herbal would not be helpful at all. It could only be of use in extending the range of herbs she used.

Prevost listed three classes of abortifacients, depending on the severity of the case. In mild cases of menstrual retention, he gave three recipes that used a fern *(capillis vel polytrich)*, chick-bean flowers, walnuts, saffron, and cinnamon.[146] Significantly, Nicholas Culpeper's translation was imprecise—or, maybe, vague. Culpeper translated the fern as "maidenhair," an English name for the fern but also a name for a plant, *Galium verum*. The chick-bean flower he translated as "red chiches," which could be the plant *or* chicken because it was to be made into a broth. Whereas Prevost's Latin had three separate recipes, each with measurements carefully given, Culpeper's translation omitted the details.[147] Culpeper had been stung by criticisms of having done more harm than good in publishing the London Pharmacopoeia and causing many people to poison themselves.[148]

The medium-strength remedies were birthwort, artemisia, cinnamon, saffron, calamint, dittany, tansy, marjoram, pennyroyal, mercury, basil, horehound, and savin (juniper).[149] Again, Prevost gave precise recipes whose detail is obscured by Culpeper. The strongest were so forceful that they should be used only when others fail and then only in pessaries, fumigants, or infusions.

The statement that pessaries were the most extreme procedure paralleled an ancient warning: Soranus had said in the second century that pessaries were more dangerous and had greater side effects than did oral-route drugs. Those drugs used for pessaries or fumigants were laurel, juniper, marjoram, myrrh, lesser calamint, gagate stone, thyme, rue, and gums (such as asafetida and sagapenum or *Ferula*).[150] These herbs (and one mineral) were mixed in various recipes according to precise directions. One wonders, however, how a poor person in England would find myrrh growing in her yard or garden. One wonders, too, whether some recipes, such as those advertised to "root out the cause that is offensive" (poisons, internal corruptions, and worms), were in fact abortifacients in disguise.[151]

Culpeper's English translation would have been virtually useless if all the reader knew was what she found in the text. Even Prevost's Latin, much more detailed than the translation, was inadequate. The poor woman who read Prevost's guide needed knowledge more than money if the work was to be of any use. What a contrast between Prevost's guide to the poor and Peter of Spain's four hundred years earlier! The medieval guide, written by a pope, was much more detailed and explicit about birth control than was the guide written by a physician in the seventeenth century. What a difference time made!

De Tournefort, France's Foremost Botanist

No one knew plants better than Joseph Piton De Tournefort (1656–1708), who studied at Montpellier and whose love for plants led him to journey to Spain to find species unavailable in France. He eventually became director of the botanical gardens in Paris and instructed physicians in herbal lore. For this reason, the herbal he published was much more clinical than other botanical works, and in this respect it was relatively open about birth control. A decoction of horehound *(stachys)*, De Tournefort said, brought on menstruation and caused an abortion and, strangely, he added, "in women."[152] Along the same line, he was more cautious about ground pine *(chamaepitys):* "It expels a dead foetus and the afterbirth and operates so powerfully that the use of it is forbid wholly to such as are with child because it causes miscarriage."[153] He repeated Dioscorides on the contraceptive use of cabbage flowers, and he added preparation instructions not found in Dioscorides.[154] Stock *(leucoium;* earlier this word may have referred also to wallflower) expels "a dead child, nay, and the living one too, says Galen, if it be drunk after the child is quick."[155] Although Galen was cited as his authority, Galen did not say that this plant was a late-stage abortifacient.[156] De Tournefort's discussion of rue is interesting. Rue has been "discarded from tables and is of no use in the kitchen" because of its disagreeable taste and smell. He cited the School of Salerno *(Schola Salernitana*—by which I assume he meant one of the Regimen treatises attributed to the Salernitan school) for the saying that "Ruta facit castum" (Rue makes one chaste). Why, he asked, should rue make men chaste and make women lustful, as was claimed by Jacobus Theodorus and Regimen Salernitana? He rejected the reason that since men were of a hot nature and women cold, the same herb could have opposite effects on each the two sexes. He said, "There is sufficient reason to doubt [this]."[157]

De Tournefort also offered insights into what we would call anthropological speculation. Like many humanists, he explored nomenclature for what it might tell us about plants. He cited Cicero as saying that birthwort *(aristolochie)* received its name from its "inventor," a man called Aristolochus.[158] It was "hardly credible that Cicero fram'd this story out of his own brain," and so he concluded that it came from even more ancient accounts. De Tournefort embraced a comment by a scholiast of Nicander and said he believed that some woman must have discovered that the plant brought away the afterbirth and gave birthwort its name. He also cited a case of a woman who had struggled in childbirth for four-and-one-half days and was near death. When she drank a decoction of birthwort, she delivered straightaway a healthy child with no more complications. The plant also, he added, provoked menstruation (in other words, implicitly, it was an abortifacient).[159]

Iris, De Tournefort wrote, provoked menstruation, "but in women with child, it caused abortion, and therefore must in any such case, be very carefully avoided."[160] Thus, the herbalist was not advocating its use as an abortifacient. He gave neither contraceptive properties to willow nor abortifacient qualities to black hellebore.[161] There were, however, some baffling passages: tansy provoked menstruation *and is given in a syrup with its juice to prevent miscarriage!*[162] This claim is similar to the one made about tansy by Culpeper. Much later, in 1865, tansy was listed as one of the powerful emmenagogues, and nothing was implied about its powers to help a pregnancy, only to terminate one.[163] Queen Anne's lace "provokes menstruation," De Tournefort claimed, and he gave this formula: "Two drams [approximately 9 grams] of the seed infused in white wine and drunk cures hysterical fits or fits of the mother."[164]

De Tournefort cannot be seen as an advocate of birth control. Asparagus stimulated lust in both sexes but, he warned, there were contrary reports that it hindered conception and caused sterility.[165] Calamint provoked menstruation "but at the same time killed the birth, and therefore [was] to be refused to women with child."[166] Under giant fennel (*Ferula* sp.) he listed the following plants: *Ferula foemina, F. galbanifere, F. fingitane, F. lucida hispanica, F. flauces, F. orientalia, sagapenum,* and *serpinum.* They provoked the menses, he said, without adding a warning about pregnancy.[167]

Doubtless learning this information on one of his botanizing trips, he said that "an old woman doctoress in Salamanca in Spain used the root of [death carrot] particularly to bring down the terms and to purge the body, which it doth with so much violence both upwards and downwards, that it frequently put those who take it in great hazard of their lives."[168] The death carrot was *Thapsia garganica* L., a member of the same family as *Ferula.* De Tournefort may have uncovered (for the Europeans) some interesting folk usage. The death carrot was known as an abortifacient in antiquity. Pliny, for instance, said that it stimulated menstruation "but it kills the fetus."[169] But the plant had strong effects and could lead to death in sufficient dosage, as its English name implies. This effect may have been what persuaded Dioscorides to exclude it from the list of emmenagogues/abortifacients. An Italian scholar, Vann Beltrami, who in 1989 compared descriptions of the death carrot with various species of *Ferula*, believes that the plant may have substituted for *silphium*.[170] As recently as 1983, the death carrot is reported to be used as a female contraceptive ("sterilità femminile") in North African folk usage.[171]

De Tournefort continued the herbal tradition, but clearly he was not advocating birth control; indeed, he specifically warned against it in many instances. Just the same, he made the information available in much the same way that Pliny had related similar data in the first century A.C.E.

Gynecology and Midwifery in the Eighteenth Century

Although the texts of the eighteenth century were a bit more varied in their approaches to gynecology, they followed much the same strategy in presenting birth control information as the writers of the sixteenth and seventeenth centuries had—they disguised it. John Freind prefaced his work, the *Emmenologia* (1703), with the remark that "Misera profecto videtur et iniqua foeminarum conditio," translated as "Wretched surely and unequal seems the condition of the Female Sex."[172] Freind devoted his attention entirely to menstruation and developed a unique theory that attributed its inception within the uterus according to a mathematical model. He called Galen's assertion that menstrual blood nourished the fetus as "utterly absurd" *(perriducula)*.[173] "Plante Emmenagogae" or "menstrual-stimulating plants" did not actually provoke the menstrual flow, but they had the quality of accelerating the rate of the flow.[174] Suppressed menses caused such severe symptoms that the condition ought to be treated; such therapy was inappropriate, however, when a woman was pregnant or nursing.[175] The use of drugs to assist menstruation was good, and did no harm even in weak women (provided the drugs were taken under the correct conditions), especially if a paregoric (opium) draught was taken afterward.

Freind named some acceptable "stimulating" agents, such as aloe, jalapa, scammony (a purgative), elaterium (prepared from squirting cucumber), but he assumed that his readers would know what the others were, because he ended the short list with "et cetera."[176] Some of the agents he named were merely laxatives without known hormonal actions. Some of the remedies that restored the blood also acted to stimulate menstruation. They were found in the kitchen *(culina)* as frequently as they were in apothecary shops *(ex officia)*.[177]

Freing distinguished between emmenagogues and astringents. Emmenagogues altered the *crasis*, that is to say the "mixture," because their "attenuating *(attenuatrice)*" quality produced "sensible effects *(effectus sensibles)*." Many of these drugs could be identified by their taste, acrid and bitter. Examples included "opium, gentian, myrrh, asarum, birthwort, savin juniper, rue, pennyroyal, century plant, etc., all being hot and aromatic, to which could be added quinine [*cortex Peruvianus*]."[178] The attenuating qualities of emmenagogic drugs could be proven by the following experiment: when an emmenagogue was mixed with warm blood, the blood would not coagulate.[179] Freind delivered to his readers a number of recipes for manufacturing and compounding emmenagogues.[180] His ideas, while they did not survive long, inform us that people continued to experiment, even after the period of witchcraft persecution, with birth control agents, although never did Freing call them by that name nor even hint at their purpose.

Nearly seventy-five years after Jane Sharp published her book, another treatise on midwifery appeared that omitted altogether such sparse information as she had included on birth control.[181] William Smellie wrote a popular treatise on midwifery, published in 1752, in which he ridiculed Freind's menstruation theory and returned to the traditional explanations. He also provided some definitions for the termination of a pregnancy: a "miscarriage" happened before the tenth day of pregnancy and was nothing more than a "liquid conception"; from the tenth day to the third month, anything that ended a pregnancy was known as an "expulsion"; "betwixt that period and the seventh month, she was said to suffer an abortion."[182] Smellie mentioned neither contraceptives nor abortifacients, but he did say that there were "prescriptions" that could be taken for delayed menstruation (although he did not name them).[183] Unlike Sharp, Smellie did not even say what to avoid.

Exactly one hundred years following Sharp's book, Henry Manning published a work on female diseases that adopted some of the same format as in Primerose's larger volume. Manning started with a discussion of the theoretical causes of menstruation and then described treatments for its malfunction. Because of the problems it caused, menstrual retention ought to be treated with the best emmenagogues (the term used in the new pharmacy) because "those [are the] medicines which strengthen digestion, such as the bark, bitters, and steel."[184] The purpose of administration was to strengthen digestion, Manning claimed, but his classification of medicines was also interesting.[185] Under medicines from barks were willow and cinnamon, but under bitters he listed most of the other birth control medicines. This reminds us of the warning in the Gospel of the Egyptians that said "eat not of that which has bitterness in it."[186]

The term *steel* presumably was an alchemical product, iron chloride, called also "vitriol of Mars."[187] As early as Dioscorides, iron filings or rust were given as contraceptives.[188] When a woman took these medicines, she should sit for some minutes over steaming water, the vapor being induced into the vagina by means of a funnel, to relax the uterine vessels. Manning's favorite medicine for menstrual retention was *tinctura sacra* ("Sacred Tincture"), whose formula was not given but which presumably was sold at the local apothecary shop.[189] Manning rejected the advice to give drastic purgatives because they "excited hysterical symptoms."[190] Concerning the expulsion of the afterbirth, in earlier works an indirect reference to abortifacients, Manning said to employ "emollient and emmenagogic materials" rather than "purgative" materials.[191] Thereby he disclosed that the same drugs given for an abortion were given for the elimination of the afterbirth. Manning gave no recipes or formulas for the medicines but left those details to the woman and her druggist.

In works written for physicians, too, many details concerning birth control were left out. In 1761 Jean Astruc, professor of medicine at Paris, began publishing a series of volumes on gynecology. In general, his work is regarded as the best written on the subject for the century. Astruc rejected Freind's theory on menstrual discharge or, at least, he observed that it mattered not, because the therapy was not altered by the causation.[192] For relief from suppression of the menses, Astruc recorded the familiar recipes, including Aqua Artemisia et Melissa—calamint *(Melissa calaminta)* or balm *(Melissa officinalis* L.)—with some of the same ingredients described by Valerius Cordus more than two hundred years before. The compound medicine had a long shelf life in European pharmacies.

Astruc's discussion of other emmenagogues was thorough. He recommended those that could be taken *"sans danger."*[193] Birthwort, artemisia, and myrrh were frequently given in various recipes. He spoke highly of iron ("le Fer ou l'Acier"), said to be very effective when mixed with other simples.[194] One recipe called the Syrup of Savin (omitting the amounts) was "un secret admirable": pennyroyal, artemisia, betony, calamine, savin juniper, calamint, birthwort, century plant, anise and fenugreek seeds, celery, asparagus, and asarum roots, polypodum (a fern), spikenard,[195] zedoary, and dittany.[196] All in all, Astruc's knowledge of emmenagogues in the late eighteenth century was as detailed as that commanded by writers before the suppression of witchcraft. Did he know that emmenagogues could cause an abortion? Yes, of course; one did not write six detailed volumes on gynecology, even in the eighteenth century, without knowing this fact. Among the external factors causing an abortion, he wrote in the fifth volume, was the taking of emmenagogues.[197] He knew.

Our survey of early modern herbals and books on gynecology and midwifery sampled only some of the large number that were produced. It is possible that a more thorough study will find a pattern different from what this study has uncovered. On the basis of what I have seen, early modern medical and botanical books either showed restraint in divulging birth control information or omitted it altogether, even when some of the information they used was from classical sources.

New World, New Drugs, Old Applications

Having looked at the literature dealing with botany, gynecology, pharmaceuticals and midwifery, one might be inclined to conclude that knowledge of birth control was in decline in the early modern period and what remained was static. The decline appears to be a correct conclusion; but it is not true that what was known about birth control remained static. Anyone who has lived through the second part of the twentieth century knows the enthusiasm that greets the discovery of a new drug. After the modern state began classifying drugs as unrestricted and restricted, legal and illegal, and made even the possession of some a criminal offense, people became imaginative and resourceful in discovering new hallucinatory, narcotic, and stimulative drugs. These discoveries are made in the popular culture and have so far kept legislators busy attempting to catch the law up with the newest designer drug. One noteworthy example comes from the seventeenth century: a new ingredient was added to the ointment that witches smeared on their bodies before going to the Sabbath. The new drug was tobacco.[198] This is interesting for two reasons: first, it shows that, despite the persecutions, witchcraft pharmacy was adaptive and experimental and, therefore, alive. Second, tobacco is a member of the Solonaceae family, the same as most of the other alkaloid-producing herbs in medieval recipes.

The early modern state did not attempt to regulate drugs, but, as we have seen, it did attempt to regulate practices—for example, by making abortion criminal in defined circumstances. While the practices remained essentially the same as they had been for millennia, new drugs were being discovered.

The discovery of the New World made new drugs available. The mendicant orders in Spain and Portugal were nearly as diligent in looking for new drugs among the "occidentall Indians" as they were in converting them to Christianity. Souls and bodies were to be saved.[199] Antonio Brassavola (1500–1555) attacked the authority of Dioscorides because he scarcely knew one plant out of a hundred on the planet. Nicolås Monardes (1493–1588) researched the new medicinal plants by talking with travelers on the docks at Seville. Monardes practiced medicine, and his books made him the most widely read Spanish medical writer in Europe. Appropriately, an English translation by John Frampton (who was a merchant!) in 1596 was entitled: "Joyful News Out of the New-found World!" The friars and monks who searched for medicinal plants were not interested in sending back to Europe birth control plants.[200] They did so anyway, but, as we know to expect, their deeds were disguised.

A widely acclaimed drug was *mechoacan*, named after the Mexican province, that was a species of bindweed (*Convolvulus mechoacana* or *Ipomaea* sp.). Later it was commonly called jalapa (now classified as *I. purga* Hayne). Monardes said that it cured "*pasiones de mujeres en especial males de madra*," which his translator, Frampton, rendered "paynes of women and especially the mother."[201] The description makes it clear that its purpose was to stimulate menstruation, without saying so directly. Careful attention, he warned, should be given to the amount, which should be varied according to age, size, and constitution, but, in the single exception of women, it was better to give too much than too little (as it was, for instance, with children).[202]

Similarly, tobacco was good for "*dolor de muelas*," or "griefs of women," when administered with oils into the navel.[203] He was more direct about sassafras, prescribed for *"retencion de menstruos"* or, in Frampton's less direct translation, "griefs of women."[204] One plant baffled modern botanists. He called it *carlo sancto* and it acted as a purgative when taken with water soaked in cinnamon and coriander.[205] Now we believe that the plant from Mexico was a species of birthwort *(Aristolochia)*![206]

The Peruvian bark or quinine mentioned by Freind is an example of a new birth control agent being added to the list of ancient herbs known to Europeans. A physician in Virginia described its abortifacient qualities in 1734.[207] An inappropriate synonym for it was "Jesuit's bark."

The use of cotton root *(Gossypium arboreum* L.) for abortions appears to have been discovered in Africa and was brought to America by slaves.[208] The active substance is identified as gossypol. Other species of *Gossypium* are native to India and China, each of which was used for birth control.[209] Negro slaves drank a preparation made from its root for an abortion, which became widespread in the southern United States.

Ergot, a fungal infection of grain (especially rye), has already been discussed in Chapter 3 as an abortifacient. The ancient Mesopotamians may have referred to it in connection with miscarriages during certain periods. Throughout the Middle Ages and the early modern period, epidemics of ergotism (known as St. Antony's fire) were prevalent. In order to grow, ergot needs the correct conditions, notably, cold weather in winter and spring and warm summers. Researchers have found a statistically significant relation between the occurrence, from 1660 to 1739, of the optimum temperature for ergot growth and low birth and high mortality rates.[210] The intentional use of ergot as a drug was dangerous because of the problem in controlling dosage. Ergot appears to cause an abortion only in the later stages of pregnancy, which is not when most women attempt to end a pregnancy. Late-term abortions are most hazardous. The earliest gestation that can be terminated by ergot is probably four months.[211]

The use of ergot-infested rye was first reported by Lonicer in 1582, for the purpose of terminating pregnancies and assisting in childbirth. By the eighteenth century there are reports that ergot was employed as a drug in folk medicine, as, for example, by Rathlaw, a Dutch abortionist, in 1747.[212] The German name for ergot, *Mutterkorn* or "Mother corn," testifies to its folk usage in the same way that a common English name for artemisia is "mother wort." An English source in 1832 reports that regular use was made of it by quacks and midwives in Germany. The medicinal use of ergot in the United States was reported in 1807 (for abortion), and in 1824 it was recommended for the control of postpartum hemorrhage.[213] Some physicians, so it is claimed, employed ergot when they tired of awaiting a long, inconvenient delivery.[214]

The description of the behavior of the women accused of being witches in Salem in 1692 matches the symptoms of ergot poisoning. This leads one scholar to conclude that witches were possessed not by the devil but by a devilish drug.[215] Because it was considered useful in bringing on childbirth, ergot was admitted to the London Pharmacopoeia in 1836.[216]

A pharmaceutical prescription for ergot, primarily a custom of the nineteenth century, would call for a dosage of 2–8 grams administered through an extract or a tincture of 5–30 drops. In folk usage, however, there was no dosage control; a person would simply eat contaminated rye grains. A woman told me that she had seen ergot rye sold in the herb market in Cairo in the 1960s, where she was told it was "for women who did not want a child." There can be no doubt but that ergot was employed first in folk medicine and that it worked its way into official medicine by the nineteenth century. When it was first deliberately used as a drug, however, is not known. Certainly by the sixteenth century it was so used.

Birth Control Information in Everyday Life

An old Swedish folksong, the musical text dating around 1600, preserves a bit of herbal folk wisdom:

Uti vår hage

Out in our meadow the blueberries grow
If you want me for anything we'll meet there.

[Refrain:] *Kom, rosor och salivia, kom, luva krusmynta, kom, hjärtan fröjd.* [Come roses or sage, come lovely mint, come, balm.]

Pretty little flowers there invite one to dance
If you want to, I'll make a wreath for you.

Kom, rosor och salivia, kom, luva krusmynta, kom, hjärtan fröjd.

> The wreath I'll then put in your hair
> The sun goes down, but the hope rises.

Kom, rosor och salivia, kom, luva krusmynta, kom, hjärtan fröjd.[217]

Excepting the roses, all the plants mentioned in the refrain are abortifacients: sage, mint, and calamint (*Melissa officinalis* L., or balm). The exception, rose, was named by an American medical writer in 1832, who recorded that he put red rose petals in a vaginal infusion.[218] When the "sun goes down but the hope rises," these plants were there. The memory of their use is preserved in a song with a lovely melody. How many Swedes who sing the song today know its meaning?

Snippets of details from everyday life in the seventeenth and eighteenth centuries reveal the continuous knowledge and use of birth control plants. French provincial journals were filled with advertisements for "restoratives," drugs that restored order and regularity to the menstrual cycle.[219] A seventeenth-century single woman was told by her lover to drink bearsfoot (*Helleborus viridis* L.) and "savon" (savin) boiled down, or to drink "madder chopt" (probably birthwort)[220] boiled in beer.[221] These statements came from England, where abortion was tolerated more than on the continent.[222] The rabbi who headed the Talmudic Academy in Poland in the seventeenth century noted that other rabbis permitted the "cup of roots" (contraceptive) to be given to a woman with childbearing problems.[223] In eighteenth-century France a "would-be surgeon" was unable to attract a practice in his home village and moved to another area. He proclaimed that he "healed motherhood, treated the spleen, [and] restored the disordered womb." His house was soon filled with patients.[224]

Physicians and apothecaries were not the sole sources for drugs in this period. Midwives and barbers knew what people needed. Toward the end of the eighteen century a traveler from Göttingen reported:

> When I traveled through the countryside in Swabia and saw a savin bush in a farmer's garden, it confirmed what I had in many cases already suspected, that the garden belonged to the barber or the midwife of the village. And to what purpose had they so carefully planted the savin bush? If you look at these bushes and shrubs you'll see them deformed and without tops, because they have been raided so often, and even at times stolen.[225]

Similar sources indicated that it was ordinary women in households who planted and used the savin juniper in the countryside, and those in urban areas raided public gardens.[226]

In pre-modern Europe abortion-inducing drugs were more often than not camouflaged as menstrual regulators, but how much awareness was there that they also functioned to control births? Storch, a physician of the early eighteenth century, expressed it this way: "when the fluxus mensium stayed away owing to an external and patent cause [such as 'fright,' or as we would say today, stress], women rarely want to hear anything about being pregnant until halfway through the term they are convinced by quickening in the womb."[227] The tricky part was that physicians and women believed that on some occasions "expulsives" or menstrual regulators promoted, not ended, pregnancy. Bad blood and "filth" and other "useless stuff" not expelled in a normal menstruation could stagnate inside the body, thereby thwarting pregnancy. Storch, for instance, did not regard stagnation as an indication of pregnancy. He knew, however, to be especially cautious in prescribing expulsives for single women and widows.[228]

An advice pamphlet called *Every Man His Own Doctor, or The Poor Planter's Physician*, published in America, said that a common complaint "by unmarry'd women" was the "suppression of the Courses." One should take "Belly-ache root" (angelica, *Angelica archangelica* L.) for "a week before you expect to be out of Order; repeat the same 2 Days after; the next Morning drink a Quarter of a Pint of Pennyroyal Water." Drops of the spirits of hartshorn (century plant, *Centaurea scabiosa* L.?) worked as well.[229] A description of Indians in North Carolina (published in 1714) described "trading girls" who trafficked in nightly sexual liaison with boys prior to marriage. They seldom had children "for they have an Art to destroy the Conception."[230] The Indians were not taught by the Europeans about such ways. They drew on their own experiences. (Historical study needs to be made of Native American birth control agents.)

The Late-Eighteenth-Century Druggist Shop

At the same time that the herbals maintained some continuity in presenting the birth control information known to the ancients, the apothecary shops were hiding from their past. This is the conclusion one reaches from the pharmacopoeias of the era, the guides to drugs that apothecaries were supposed to have and to know. In English the greatest guide was the Edinburgh New Dispensatory, with editions published in the United States. Through the editions of the 1790s, the following were listed as drugs, without being named as either birth control agents or menstrual stimulators: asafetida, asarum, artemisia, birthwort, Peruvian bark or quinine, Queen Anne's lace, dittany, squirting cucumber, *filix*, hyssop, juniper, lupine, myrrh, parsley, and sage.[231] The subject of birth control was not censored entirely. The guide called distilled oil of savin and a watery extract one of "most powerful emmenagogues . . . as well as rue." Savin also was compounded with powder of myrrh.[232] Common artemisia was "formerly used in the *suppression* [italics added] of menstrual evacuations [but] it is now, however, very little employed."[233] Asafetida "promotes the fluid secretions in either sex" and the "ancients" attributed "other virtues, which are at present not expected from it."[234] Southernwood (a kind of artemisia) is "at present very little employed in practice" and an extract made from another kind of artemisia was "rejected by Edinburgh pharmacy."[235]

Even though the pharmacy guides failed to mention the purpose of the birth control plants, there was some continuation of the historical recipes. Pennyroyal "has long been held in great esteem" for "suppressions of the uterine purgations." After giving simple preparation instructions, the 1791 guide adds that "any form of it is now less frequently employed than formerly." Distilled pennyroyal (*Spiritus pulegii*, as it once stood on the pharmacy shelves) "has no place in the Edinburgh pharmacopoeia," but it is "frequently employed as a carminative and antihysteric."[236] Hysteria was then considered a problem with or in the uterus. A carminative was a drug that expelled gas from the stomach; an antihysteric was any treatment of female uro-genital problems. The recipe for powdered aloe with iron was listed for "obstructed menstruation" without any other usages listed.[237] Myrrh powder's manufacturing formula was delivered, with other ingredients being savin, rue, and Russian castor for the same purpose.[238]

By the late eighteenth century, anything explicitly causing an abortion was dropped from the official publications. The mention of menstrual stimulators, which had the same effect, was sharply reduced in pharmaceutical discussions. These trends notwithstanding, the fact remains that there was a faint hint, an echo, of the ancient remedies in the official pharmacy guides. Reading between the lines, for that is what must be done, one surmises that the same drugs were on the druggists' shelves as were there for centuries before.

One way to know what apothecaries sold is to judge from the references in practical guides to pharmacy practice. One study of premodern European pharmacy showed that among those drugs most frequently mentioned were camomile, century plant, figs, ginger, hyssop, licorice, mint, myrrh, parsley, pennyroyal, pepper, pimpernel, pomegranate, rue, and wormwood.[239] Some of these, of course, had multiple uses, but menstrual regulation and birth control were perhaps the primary or only usages for others. For example, it is difficult to find a use for pennyroyal except as an insect repellant and an abortifacient.

Another way we know what was on the pharmacy shelves is the survival of the drug jars. Many apothecary jars, in beautiful porcelain with labels artistically drawn, testify that these drugs once stood on the shelves in shops. For example, there is a beautiful English jar from the late seventeenth or early eighteenth century with the label: "O. SABIN" (oil of savin).[240] Another double-handled jar from the early eighteenth century contained "Aqua rutae" (distilled rue).[241] Inventories exist from each century beginning with the fourteenth that show not only what drugs were on the shelves but also what their prices were.[242] Thus, when herbals or the guidebooks for the poor prescribed rue, pennyroyal, and myrrh, we know that they were available.

Dr. Olivier's Great Discovery

The divorce of information about birth control agents and modern "professional" medicine is illustrated by a small article in a French medical journal in 1760. Dr. Olivier wrote about an interesting case in his medical practice at Saint-Tropez. A woman six months pregnant came to him and explained that she no longer felt any movement. After an examination, he concluded that her fetus was dead. Not knowing what to do, he read in Aëtius (of Amida) about expulsives or abortifacients *(Foetus vivos interficit, mortuos extrudit)* and so, on this authority, he prepared a decoction of *fougère*, which she drank. The same day she aborted and soon was well.[243] *Fougère* is the fern that we have encountered in the classical sources as *filix*. In his time, it was almost certainly *Aspidium filix mas*. The implications are that Dr. Olivier did not learn about abortions from his regular medical training and that he had to turn to the classical medical authorities. On the face of it, the case was considered important enough to merit a journal article entry, a contribution to knowledge. Here in the mid-eighteenth century, we have a physician who is close enough to what we call "the cutting edge" of research to contribute to a medical journal, but who knew nothing of an important abortion drug that had been used for millennia.

A postscript: the use of *filix*, which Dr. Olivier thought he rediscovered, remained in German folk medicine until the twentieth century, when in 1908 a Dr. Aigremont wrote that the fern was a contraceptive and an abortifacient. Interestingly, he said that this fern was a witch's drug *(Hexenkraut)* and a prostitute's drug *(Hurenkraut)*![244] Aigremont's association of this abortion drug with witchcraft and prostitution informs us that the legacy of events that began this chapter—the suppression of witchcraft—survived until the twentieth century. This story demonstrates how much the knowledge of birth control drugs had faded by the advent of the modern period, when momentous changes in birth control took place.

After the Witch Hunts

As I explained at the beginning of this chapter, Heinsohn and Steiger's theory asserts that the extermination of the wise woman and the repression of witchcraft were a deliberate result of secular and ecclesiastical authorities' alarm over a low birth rate. The demographical data for the period of the sixteenth and seventeenth centuries simply do not support their theory conclusively. Indeed, Behringer asserts the contrary: where witch hunts were most extensive, the population was growing.[245] The period of the suppression of witches was from approximately 1450 through 1700, and large population increases began in Europe in the late eighteenth century. If the former led to the latter, as Heinsohn and Steiger claim, cause and effect are separated by a very long lag time. The data do not prove the hypothesis conclusively, but they also do not reject it.

Jütte is correct in saying that information about birth control remained among some women and in some apothecary shops, a fact not disputed by Heinsohn and Steiger.[246] Such information held by the popular and high culture was slow to be erased. In support of Heinsohn and Steiger's theory, practically all of the anecdotal data concerned single women in distress. Most of the information came from court cases of persons indicted for using or providing birth control medicines. Quite possibly the witch hunts, by suppressing the practice of midwifery, altered conventional family planning. A married woman would measure the risk of taking an abortive, especially if she waited a month or so past her missed menstrual cycle. If family planning was a victim, I am still puzzled about what happened to contraception. All the more do I suspect that married women employed both contraceptive and abortifacient drugs throughout the early modern period. A study of abortion in the eighteenth-century village of Pomfret in New England concluded that the restriction on abortion seemed to apply to single women who were sexually promiscuous.[247] As we shall see in the last chapters, married women were the primary users of birth control drugs in the nineteenth century. It is foolish to believe that, when single women knew what to take, they somehow forgot what they had learned upon marriage.

Notwithstanding these qualifications, we should not regard Heinsohn and Steiger's thesis as "absurd," as Jütte called it.[248] As they say, the modern population rise is partly attributable to pro-natalist views and suppression of birth control measures. A trend that began in late antiquity to restrict abortion certainly was accelerated by the witch scares in pre-modern times, with the effect that birth control information became a subject to be dealt with cautiously, or not at all.

7

The Womb as Public Territory

> I have reason to believe that there exist among us the Science and the Art of Abortion. The worship of the goddess Aphrodite finds its father-confessor in the foeticide.
>
> Ely Van de Warker, M.D. (1872)

In 1803 Lord Ellenborough introduced an omnibus crime bill that was intended to apply only to Ireland. So pleased was he with his commission's work that his Lordship said it ought to apply to both Ireland and Britain. Thus modestly came the advent of statutory criminal abortion in the English-speaking world. Ellenborough wanted to close loopholes, such as the law that made it only a misdemeanor for one to administer a poison with the intent to murder. While the commission was on the subject of poisons, it sought to rewrite the law of James I that declared a woman who delivered a bastard child and subsequently was suspected of burying, drowning, or disposing of it to be considered a murderer unless she could prove otherwise. In erasing James's law, the Ellenborough Act said the court was obliged to determine whether the child was born dead or alive and whether it would have been a bastard.

Lord Ellenborough's act did not stop there:

[It is a crime of murder for anyone to] unlawfully administer to, or cause to be administered to or taken by any of his Majesty's subjects any deadly poison, or other noxious and destructive substance or thing, with intent [for] . . . his Majesty's subject or subjects thereby to murder, or thereby to cause and procure the miscarriage of any woman, then being quick with child.[1]

As we have seen (Chapter 5), common law did not hold the same principles as Roman law.[2] Mindful of the difficulties facing courts in proving whether quickening had occurred, the authors of the act extended the state's concern to the pre-quickening period: anyone who administers such poisons or employs other means to "cause or procure the miscarriage of any woman not being, or not being proved to be, quick with child at the time of administering such things or using such means, that then and in every such case the person or persons so offending . . . are hereby declared to be guilty of felony."[3] The punishment for a felony was specified as fine, imprisonment, pillory, public whipping, or transportation to a penal colony for a term not to exceed fourteen years.

The debate on the bill raised few concerns. The mission of Lord Ellenborough's commission was to tidy up the laws and to make it easier for courts to convict the guilty. Lord Auckland confessed that the laws governing murder were numerous but the crimes "enumerated by the Noble and Learned Lord were such as to call for severe and exemplary punishment."[4] In the debate, Lord Ellenborough spoke of the need to provide fairness and justice to the woman who had a "bastard" child and wished to rid herself of it. Whatever his and Parliament's intent, the act made abortion after quickening murder by statutory law and abortion (or, willful "miscarriage") prior to quickening a felony. Nothing in the law made it applicable only to out-of-wedlock pregnancies. As written, it could have been interpreted as applying equally to married women, but it was not so interpreted. In practice, abortion was defined as an act taken by a single woman late in pregnancy that led to a termination of that pregnancy, the assumption being that she wanted to avoid the consequences of an illicit affair.[5]

Let us not overlook the fact that the Ellenborough Act stated explicitly that the expected means of performing abortions were chemical. The habits of the British were not suddenly altered because the law was made. The law had little initial impact, but through the course of the century its significance grew. English juries were not stampeded into changing what had been the long-standing custom, namely, to consider abortion before quickening no crime. Only gradually did juries regard abortion after quickening as criminal. In 1811, Phillips, a young man from the county of Monmouth, was charged with administering savin to his unmarried girlfriend, Hannah Mary Goldsmith, who was alleged to be quick with child. In the first trial, she claimed that she had not felt fetal movement prior to taking the medicine. She was careful not to call it "a noxious and destructive substance," as the law said. Various medical experts were brought in, but they differed as to when a fetus could be said to be quick. All agreed that there were individual variations. Most said that it *usually* was about the sixteenth or eighteenth week after conception. On one point they all agreed: by tradition, quickening occurred after the woman felt the movement. On the basis of testimony, a mistrial was declared.[6]

Subsequently Phillips was charged with having "wilfully, maliciously, unlawfully and feloniously" delivered a noxious and destructive substance that caused Goldsmith to lose her fetus not yet quickened. The indictment alleged that six ounces of savin (juniper) leaves were prepared in a decoction, the amount being "divers large." Phillips's solicitor was clever. Phillips testified that he prepared the medicine by pouring boiling water over the leaves. Expert apothecary witnesses testified that type of preparation he described was an infusion (tea, to us), not a decoction (a boiling down), as the indictment read. The defense raised doubts about whether the leaves were actually from a savin scrub, some testifying that they were not. The Crown's prosecution countered that in any case the preparation was "noxious and destructive" and intended to cause a miscarriage. The defense easily checked that argument by saying that if it could not be proven what the substance was, it could not be declared noxious and destructive. As for Phillips, he testified that he gave her an innocent brew to amuse her because she was distraught enough, he implied, to commit suicide. The jury's verdict: not guilty. In this case, at least, the jurors were not prepared to apply the spirit of Lord Ellenborough's Act.[7]

Criminalization of Abortion in Other Countries

France made abortion criminal in 1791, some twelve years before Britain.[8] The national law was based on the same principles that local courts had enforced since the Middle Ages. Later, in 1810, Napoleon's Penal Code, generally guided by Roman law, set aside the older laws and took new directions on abortion. Article 317 reads in part: "Anyone who by food, beverage, medicines, violence, or any other means procures an abortion on a pregnant female, regardless whether it was with her consent or not, shall be punished by incarceration." The article added more: any other person who attempts the same shall be guilty, whether or not the abortion succeeds. And, adding even more, any "physician, surgeon, or other health-care official, and that includes apothecaries," who administer an abortive agent will be transported to a penal colony.[9] A second article said that anyone who attempted a crime, whether or not it was manifested and independent of the wishes of the other parties, would be guilty of a crime as if it had taken place.[10] The Napoleonic law omitted the pregnant woman from punishment if the drugs were self-administered. Anyone who assisted or advised her on what to take—regardless of medical status, from physician to midwife—was criminally guilty. Seven years later the French law was amended to apply to women who secured their own abortions.[11]

In colonial America abortion was treated on the basis of common law, but few cases are known. In colonial Maryland there were only four cases, which raises the question why prosecution was so rare. In 1651 or 1652 a Captain Mitchell was charged with giving an abortifacient to a widow, Susan Warren (age 21), with whom he had had an illicit affair. She was probably about three to four months into her pregnancy and subsequently gave birth to a stillborn child. In Warren's deposition she said that "he prepared a potion of Phisick over night unknown."[12] Mitchell was brought to trail on other charges and, waiving a jury trail, elected to pay a fine.[13] A somewhat similar case in the 1650s concerned a medical practitioner who gave a "fisick" or drug to a servant whom he had impregnated, allegedly by force. Following the delivery of a dead fetus, he had the charges dropped by marrying her.[14] No cases are found in which a woman was charged with administering an abortion to herself.

No American state had a statutory law against abortion prior to 1821, when the state of Connecticut passed one that would be the model for other states over the next twenty years. Certain phrases of this law appear to have been borrowed from the Ellenborough Act, but others were avoided. Any person was guilty and subject to jail who administered or caused to be administered, regardless of whether the motive was malicious or benevolent, "any deadly poison, or other noxious and destructive substance" with the intent to cause a miscarriage of any woman "then being quick with child."[15] Some of the other states that followed Connecticut's precedent omitted the clause about quickening, but, whether the deletion was deliberate or not, the result would be the same as in the Connecticut law. Proof could be obtained only if the person who performed the act was aware beyond doubt of the woman's pregnancy.[16]

Missouri and Illinois followed Connecticut's law closely, but the State of New York passed in 1828 and enacted in 1830 a law that made abortion after quickening second-degree manslaughter for the person who performed it. The woman who had the abortion was not liable. The New York law's wording followed Lord Ellenborough's act: "Every person who shall wilfully administer to any pregnant woman, any medicine, drug, substance or thing whatever, or shall use or employ any instrument or other means whatever . . ."[17] But the law permitted a physician to administer a therapeutic abortion to "preserve the life of such woman," provided two physicians made a judgment that her condition merited the procedure.[18]

The effect of these early American laws was to make statutory law reflect the same principles embodied in English common law. By 1850, seventeen American states had criminal abortion laws that were similar to the New York law: abortion after quickening was a felony by whatever means unless administered by a physician to save the mother's life. Wisconsin led the first change in intent of the law in 1858 by making the self-administered abortion or abortion attempt a felonious crime.[19]

Other states in Europe and the Americas did not adopt new criminal laws against abortion in the first half of the century. This is not to say that abortion was not punished, only that the old laws were derived from medieval precedent, canon law, and Roman law. The law in England did not continue to refer to historical practices very long either, once it was written as statutory law. In 1828 the Ellenborough Act was amended to include the phrase "or shall use any instrument or other means."[20] Surgical or manipulative abortion had been omitted from the original act, and now this procedure was covered. The very fact of its omission for twenty-five years indicates that it was not in widespread use. The most common practice was what all the laws specified—chemical abortion.

In 1837, the first year of Queen Victoria's reign, the law on abortion was modified significantly. The capital crime of abortion was eliminated, and abortion at any period, before or after quickening, was made a felony, punishable by transportation to a penal colony for not less than fifteen years or imprisonment not to exceed three years.[21] Juries indicated reluctance to assign the death penalty, so the punishment was lessened. Significantly, however, for the first time since Sixtus V's Bull of *Effraenatum* in 1588 (in effect for only two years), abortion was defined as the elimination of a pregnancy regardless of its stage. Gone was the distinction between formed or quickened fetus and unformed fetus in Victoria's new law.

Pharmaceutical Guides and the Availability of Drugs

Two years after the Ellenborough Act made abortion criminal, the London *Dispensatory* was published. This guide to drugs was based on the official London Pharmacopoeia, and the items it names suggest that most of the drugs used for abortion and contraception were sold in drug stores. The list of official materia medica begins with aloe, angelica, asafetida, and asarum.[22] Under prepared drugs there were the familiar formulas, many with recipes and names going back to Cordus, though usually with fewer ingredients. An example is powder of myrrh, made with asafetida, sagapenum *(Ferula)*, Russian castor, and opopanax *(Ferula)*.[23] Under essential oils made from leaves there is this list: marjoram (sweet and wild), peppermint, spearmint, pennyroyal, rosemary, rue, savin (juniper), wormwood (artemisia).[24] All are abortifacients, although the text omits any indications of usage. A reader could be instructed about preparations but not be informed that the guide contained birth control data.

By 1818 there were some references in the London *Dispensatory* to birth control, however indistinct. Pennyroyal was "formerly regarded as an emmenagogue . . . but it is now justly considered of no value, and seldom used in regular practice."[25] But, without qualifications the guide said that juniper (savin) was a "powerful stimulant . . . [and an] emmenagogue."[26] Tansy is "formerly regarded as a powerful remedy in . . . obstructed menstruation."[27]

The Edinburgh *Dispensatory*, published in New York in 1818, was more straightforward, but even so it lacked information that issues of the same work had contained twenty-five years earlier. Garlic was "by some supposed to be an emmenagogue," though the guide did not endorse the drug. Aloes and asarum were listed to stimulate menstruation, but artemisia was "rarely used in any way."[28] No birth control usages, even disguised, were mentioned for Queen Anne's lace, juniper, laurel, pomegranate, and quinine.[29] Pennyroyal was not listed at all, although we know from inventories it was in most drug stores. Savin (juniper) was called a "warm stimulating medicine" that "excites haemorrhagy [bleeding] especially from the uterus."[30] Myrrh was "supposed to act especially upon the uterine system," and the fern, *filix*, was "formerly used in secret remedies," although this dispensatory does not say for what.[31] "Some physicians have a great opinion of [tansy] in hysteric disorders, particularly those proceeding from a deficiency or suppression of the uterine purgations."[32] Finally, under compounds is found the formula for pills of myrrh, but their effects were not specified. The work was published at a time when there were no laws in the United States making abortion a criminal offense, except for the common law protecting only a formed or quickened fetus. Just the same, information about birth control was well-nigh gone from official medicine.

A guide to drugs published by physicians in the United States of America in 1836, when there *were* laws against abortion, had less information about birth control. No birth control uses were named for a number of traditional contraceptive and abortifacient drugs, despite their inclusion in the list of approved drugs. The following drugs were listed without being accompanied by any birth control information, overtly or covertly: garlic, wormwood (artemisia), asafetida, asarum, colocynth, squirting cucumber, male fern, pomegranate, jalapa, juniper, and Virginia snakeroot (birthwort).[33] Some mention was made of "women's problems": "It [savin] has been much used in amenorrhea . . . At present, however, it is not generally employed . . . In pregnancy it should always be avoided."[34] *Amenorrhea*, the suppression or absence of menstruation, was a new word used to describe the familiar effect.

Using language to avoid the appearance of advocacy, the American guide said that ergot was "popularly used in parts of Germany, France and Italy . . . empirically by midwives" to induce contractions of the uterus. It could be dangerous, the guide warned. Next the dosage was given: fifteen to twenty grains (of fungi-contaminated seeds) were given to women in labor.[35] A few menstrual regulators were named: pennyroyal was "much used as an emmenagogue in popular practice, and frequently with success."[36] Myrrh, tansy, and rue also were named, but rue was "particularly [used for] amenorrhoea."[37] Aloe was a different case: the guide seemingly recommended the drug, although not specifically for an abortion. Aloe was used as an emmenagogue "perhaps more frequently than any other remedy, entering into almost all the numerous empirical preparations which are habitually reported to by females in this complaint."[38]

With the exception of aloe, all other entries were carefully discussed without advocacy or approval. Just the same, the drugs were listed and, as such, generally were available in drug stores. In some descriptions the reader is aware of glaring omissions by the writers. Elaterium, the drug made from squirting cucumber, was not identified for its menstrual or antifertility uses, but the guide says that it was in "disfavor" because some people had died as a consequence of taking it, without stating the reason for the fatal action.[39] Nevertheless, the guides published in the early nineteenth century all indicate that in the very years that abortion was criminalized the means of performing an abortion were commonly available.

Changing Attitudes toward Sex and Birth Control

The nineteenth century marked a perceptible change in people's attitudes toward birth control. Once the principle was breached that fetal development was not marked by dramatic changes in different stages, the focus of discussion became the gravity of the offense of killing a fetus, whatever its developmental period. The tendency was for states' laws to protect an "unformed" or pre-quickened fetus. This change first occurred only in small areas of Europe and the Americas, but it was steadily extended to most regions by the end of the century. In seeking to find some answers to what may have brought on the change, one finds several factors: altered attitudes and habits in sexuality and the role of the church; the development of embryology and the dissemination of debates about fetal development; the awareness of and, in some cases, alarm over the relationship between population size and political and economic power. Each of these topics is extensive but will be discussed here only briefly.

To understand what was new in the nineteenth century about sexual mores and ideals, one must have some idea of sexuality in European culture in previous centuries. Anyone who has read works by Giovanni Boccaccio, Pietro Aretino, Hans Sachs, or François Rabelais is aware of the striking contrast between the bawdiness and eroticism of the society they portrayed and the stern religious character, inspired by Calvin, Luther, and the Counter-Reformation, that became predominant in Catholic lands. Bawdiness and piety were contemporary features of early modern society, but the sexually explicit aspects of art and literature revealed more than flesh. They revealed attitudes. English seventeenth-century works of pornography—and they were numerous—portrayed women, even those eager for sexual contact, as being passive. When the sexual act was described in all particulars, it was the male who jumped on the female and threw her around.[40] With the breakdown of the Puritan ethic, from the mid-eighteenth century, premarital conception as a reason for marriage was increasingly prevalent in English society.[41] Roughly one-fifth of the brides between 1540 and 1700 were pregnant at marriage, and this proportion rose to two-fifths in the later centuries.[42] In England and Germany, the increasing percentage of pregnant brides leads us to conclude that there was an overall increase in premarital sexual activity not restricted to brothel visits.[43]

In the early modern period the Catholic Church's position on sexuality saw some liberalization. Martin Le Maistre (1432–1487) abandoned the Augustinian-Tomistic doctrine of intercourse only for procreation. He fashioned a "golden mean" assertion that pleasure in sexual relations was not itself bad.[44] Could not a married couple have sexual relations even when one was sterile? In the course of the sixteenth and seventeenth centuries, other theologians built on Le Maistre's ideas to the degree that one Scottish theologian likened copulation for pleasure to eating an apple for pleasure.[45] That was too radical for subsequent theologians and, of course, was never adopted by church as doctrine.

A Jesuit theologian, Thomas Sanchez (1550–1610), modified the reaction against Aquinas on procreation—sex engaged in for pleasure alone was sinful, but it was not a sin if its purpose was to foster mutual love.[46] A woman could dispose of a man's seed deposited during rape just as she was allowed to strike a thief.[47] Similarly, a woman could remove her fetus should the fetus clearly be a threat to her life. What if the threat to her life, however, was her parents, husband, or someone who would be angered by a pregnancy? Yes, said Sanchez, abortion was acceptable because here too her life was at risk. He drew the line at the point where an abortion to protect a woman's reputation was unjustified. A fetus that had already received its soul was not to be killed. A fetus whose existence threatened the mother and had not been ensouled could be removed by wounds, beating or poisonous drugs.[48]

Sanchez gave an analogy based on Thomas of Aquinas' theory of a just war. Christians may engage in a just war even when it is known that war involves killing and, when war is directed against a city, the killing of babies. "Just war is waged against lethal humors by applying medicine," Sanchez said.[49] A pregnant woman may run from a charging bull even though she knows that in saving herself from the animal she would lose her potential child.[50]

On abortion Sanchez was relatively munificent, but contraception brought up difficult issues. He raised a moral question: could a person engage in contraception (defined as a "potion by which conception of offspring is obstructed") in order to protect an estate from being divided among heirs?[51] No, he asserted, and clearly he was referring to contraception by drugs within the marital bonds.[52] This was a practical question of a kind seldom raised by church writers, at least not since the early medieval penitentials that said contraception was less offensive if its purpose was to restrict children in a poor household. The church was not unmoved by the plight of women, although, in truth, it was not moved to action either. By and large, neither Protestant nor Catholic churches were directly concerned with sexuality until the issue was forced upon their prelates by science.

During the late eighteenth and early nineteenth centuries there was a change in attitudes about sexuality not necessarily favorable to women.[53] The loss of traditional knowledge formerly held by female healers and midwives resulted in a new dependence on male physicians and midwives and led to new epistemological views that lowered women's status.[54] According to Thomas Laquer, the impulse for change arose with the new industrial social order and was quite independent of changes occurring about reproductive theory in the natural sciences. The new sexuality was epitomized by the new expression "the opposite sex"[55]—women were opposite, separate, unequal, just not men, in other words. No help did the medical profession give. Physicians, male all, viewed menstruation as a manifestation of women's special weakness, whereas women thought themselves normal for having the "monthlies."[56]

On one hand the Enlightenment should have liberated sexual feelings: the theme of the age was that sex was natural and that which is natural is good, provided reason prevailed. There is the image of André Morellet, who wrote of two sets of parents watching while their boy and girl explored one another's body until they discovered, through trial and error, penis-vaginal intercourse. The parents rejoiced at their children's newfound happiness.[57] This theme was not limited to Morellet's simple lesson.

The study of anatomy changed attitudes on sexuality in the late eighteenth century in a way that decidedly did not liberalize sexual expressions. The Greeks proposed that the female reproductive organs were the equivalent of the male, but in reverse. The vagina was the penis, the ovaries the testicles, the labia the foreskin, the uterus the scrotum.[58] In the fourth century the Christian Bishop of Emesa wrote: "Theirs are inside the body and not outside of it."[59] The ancient observations were given new meaning in the eighteenth century.

The eighteenth-century Enlightenment's study of nature led to a reversal of the medieval notion that a woman must climax during intercourse in order to become pregnant. First, scientists observed that female sexual climax was not necessary for conception, since women who were raped could become pregnant. (Always the maxim: nature provides the clues to rightful human conduct.) Second, by a simple syllogism, since women were the opposite of men and since men had pleasure in intercourse, women should not enjoy sexual activity. In 1803 Jacques-Louis Moreau expressed the relationship between men and women as "a series of oppositions and contrasts."[60] What a reversal historically from the thirteenth-century notion that female climax was as important as if not more important than that of the male![61] The new proposition held that women were naturally (hence, rightfully) passive and should receive the generative seed without a scintilla of pleasure.[62]

The Problem of Population

Around 1780, language and public discourse made childbirth a matter of public concern. Court testimonies were increasingly concerned with intimate details, and courts became a means for pornographic indulgence.[63] In 1735 Prussia required the registration of post-menopausal unmarried women.[64] An article on miscarriage in Diderot's *Encyclopédie* in 1770 asserted that women were using herbs with harmful side effects (fever, inflammation, derangement) and, increasingly, surgery (with its own dangers) to induce miscarriages.[65] Married women did it to prevent property from being divided and unmarried women to protect their reputations.[66] In 1778 Hanover outlawed the use of ergot by midwives.[67] Police uprooted cypress trees in public parks so that women could not use them to induce abortion.[68] Doubtless, juniper trees were included, just as today's police raid marijuana patches. Although cypress and juniper trees were not protected from the law, the police of the nineteenth century did not inspect the herb garden.

After 1800, French population statistics were census-based and gradually policy makers became aware of an alarming, unexplained fact. The expected increase did not occur. By 1850, the nation's population was feared to be in a decline (even though there was a slow rate of increase).[69] In 1800 the French were 15.7 percent of Europe's total population, but by 1900 the percent was 9.7, low enough to strike fear in any political or military leader or businessman and most church prelates.[70] In contrast, England went from a population of approximately three million in 1550 (4.9 percent of Europe's total population) to 30.5 million in 1900 (15.1 percent of Europe). Between 1820 and 1900 English and German growth rates were 166 percent and 142 percent, respectively, compared with 26 percent for France.[71] By 1870, the year that Bismarck won a war against France, there were more Germans than French; fifty years before, France was two-thirds larger in population.[72] No wonder the French were concerned about their reproductive rates. "Cowardly in the face of duty" is the way a journal editorial described females who practice birth control.[73]

In 1798 Thomas Malthus published anonymously his first essay on population. He developed the law, as it came to be regarded, that humankind is doomed because increased prosperity is accompanied by an even greater rise in population. Two propositions captured the bleak laws governing humankind just as mechanics govern matter: (1) "The power of population is indefinitely greater than the power in the earth to produce subsistence for man"; (2) "Population, when unchecked, increases in a geometrical ratio. Subsistence increases only in an arithmetical ratio."[74] Malthus recognized that the "arts," such as agriculture and technology, could alter these laws, but the picture he portrayed was bleak. Practically, these dismal axioms allow three choices: self-restraint from sexual intercourse, misery, and vice. Included under vice's rubric is contraception. Neither Malthus nor the Malthusians who followed him considered women central to the issue. A commentator on Malthus, S. Chandrasekhar, observed that one can read

Malthus's *Essay* without "ever [having the] thought women had anything to do with population."[75]

Inasmuch as the care of the community was in the hands of government officials, the strong connection felt to exist between population size and economic and political power could not be subject to individual decisions, especially if women made the choices. Councils and various municipal and government entities no longer considered reproductive matters private. In the words of Ivan Illich, "The womb was declared public territory."[76] Michel Foucault's history of sexuality stresses the complex array of social factors and emotions revealed by sexuality, and one of those components is "power."[77] It was an exercise of power, on the part of government, business, and institutions, that made reproduction a matter of public concern. A woman's duty was to bear children, declared Henry Wright in 1858, stating what many regarded as a rule of human conduct.[78] The Marquis de Condorcet (1743–1794) said that the law of nature regarding procreation was set aside by humans alone among the animals; recognizing just this, Malthus saw a danger with "unnatural passions and improper arts to prevent the consequencies of irregular connection."[79] The fear of too small a population was greater than the fear of too many people.

Let us postpone until later the justification for invoking public concern for the welfare of all. First, let us look to the consequences.

The Public Womb

By the nineteenth century, a woman's body was literally revealed to the public, through the physical examination for the determination of pregnancy. To find out if she was pregnant, a woman would go (or be sent) to a physician, whose eyes would observe the darkening of the areola and examine her vagina and whose hands would feel her breasts and whose fingers, inserted in the vagina, would feel the cervix.[80] The vaginal examination was for the so-called Hegar's sign, enlargement and softening of the uterus and cervix. Medieval physicians would not or could not have made such intimate inspections. (An exception existed in English common law, which allowed a sheriff to examine a woman, suspected of being pregnant, by "feeling her breasts and abdomen" and other unspecified ways[81] in cases where the husband died before pregnancy was apparent.) There was no medical reason for a physician to conduct a pregnancy examination, because pregnancy was announced when a woman, not a physician, said it was so (unless her body, through layers of cloth, made the announcement unnecessary).

Midwives were in a better position to assist, but prior to the mid-nineteenth century they could not definitively determine a pregnancy before quickening, even though some claimed they could. In the eighteenth century an increasing number of males were becoming midwives, to the point that in France the male *accoucheurs* were driving female midwives from the birth chamber.[82] In England, male midwives were said to believe that female anatomy was designed to fit the male midwives' fingers.[83] Physicians would be expected to give testimony in alleged abortion cases, especially in a dispute over whether quickening had occurred. More routinely, however, a woman going to a physician for a prescription for a drug to induce menstruation probably would be subjected to full examination, as was illustrated in some landmark court cases. The physician was risking not only his practice but his personal freedom by giving a menstrual regulator to a woman simply on her word that she was not pregnant. He could not rely on the case-history approach (asking about the last menstrual cycle and timing of sexual intercourse) because his independent judgment was expected.

In the late seventeenth century a French physician, Philippe Le Goust, first reported hearing a fetal heart by placing his ear directly on the woman's abdomen.[84] In 1818 Théophile-René-Hyacinthe Laennec announced the invention of the stethoscope, which could amplify heart sounds.[85] As the use of this important diagnostic tool spread, physicians were more able to hear a fetal heart beat. The early stethoscopes were fairly effective (the instrument remained essentially unchanged until the early 1940s). There was no absolute date at which physicians could be sure the heart could be heard, because of individual variations. By the 1840s and 1850s, patients expected physicians to have a binaural stethoscope around their necks[86] and physicians expected to hear a fetal heart by the fourth month.[87] The fetal heart is not synchronous with the mother's pulse, and so it is easily identifiable when heard. For the first time, the technology gave a physician a certain means to determine pregnancy even when a woman declared no perception of fetal movement. A woman experienced with pregnancies can perceive movement between the sixteenth and twentieth week, but a primigravida (first-time pregnancy) may not be perceptible until about twenty-two weeks. Prior to the nineteenth century, the declaration of a pregnancy was the responsibility of the woman. After about 1850, this responsibility belonged to physicians or, in some cases, licensed midwives.

The Beginning of Life: The Haller-Wolff Debate

Diderot's *Encyclopédie* (1757) prefaced its remarks about reproduction with these words: "La génération des corps en général est un mystère dont la nature s'est réservé le secret."[88] Already the secrets were being exposed. In the late eighteenth century a controversy arose between Albrecht von Haller (1708–77) and Caspar Friedrich Wolff (1734–94) over organic generation. The debate sharpened issues, formed and divided opinion, and focused attention on what conception is and when life begins. Haller's first position was that of his teacher, Boerhaave, who asserted that the rudiments of the embryo existed in each male animalcule or sperm. The female was essential for completing the process of generation. In the mid-1840s Haller converted to the theory of epigenesis, the position of William Harvey that life developed incrementally in the fertilized egg. In other words, all the parts were not there in the beginning; they developed. By the 1850s Haller recanted his conversion because of recent studies on reproduction. Trembley reported the artificial division in the freshwater polyp, which reproduced by budding without sexual union with another polyp. Other studies reported the regeneration of a lizard's tail, the division of a worm with two organisms resulting, and parthenogenesis in the aphid.

Back to the preformation theory went Haller, this time with forceful arguments. First he rejected the existence of female semen. He disavowed the claim that a female seed was necessary to explain the similarities in appearance between mother (as well as father) and child. Haller said that children were not similar to their parents; moreover, were it so that an organism or person had components of both parents' parts in each seed, a deformed person would pass on the deformity, but this did not happen. Finally he asserted that every detail of each of two bodies being in each seed was too much. "There is missing a building master," Haller wrote, for how could it be decided where all the particularizations go, in what order, and which parent's quality is selected?[89] Such reliance on chance was not in keeping with the belief in God as the Director of all things. In 1757 he concluded, "It appears very probable to me that the essential parts of the fetus exist formed at all times."[90] The tiny embryo of a female was stimulated by male semen that contained the form, beginning with the heart, and from that developed the fetus.

Working in St. Petersburg, Caspar Wolff corresponded with a number of people, including Haller, his rival. Wolff's major work, *De formatione intestinorum* (1768), gave a careful account of the formation of a chick's alimentary canal on the basis of microscopic examinations, and it included splendidly detailed drawings. The early embryo developed from "leaf-like" layers that formed different tissues. He saw a heart being born, one developed where none had been before. It was not there, hidden, only to appear later; it never was there prior to being formed.[91] In Wolff's words, "The beating heart, making its appearance while other parts are still largely so inconspicuous as to escape the untrained observer, is perhaps the most striking, indeed, the most dramatic feature of the early embryo."[92] The new organism formed in the egg according to patterns of development, not according to pre-formed parts.

Haller and other supporters of animalculism regarded Wolff's ovist or egg theory as dangerous to belief in God's part in the creation of a new organism. If things developed gradually, mechanically, God had no part. Wolff and his followers conceded that point but raised the question whether God would create millions of forms in each drop of semen, only for them to be lost. Wolff was too much of a biologist to raise the question, but others did: did the form have a soul within it? Too many souls would perish in each man each day.[93] Reacting to the specter of such images, churches in the early nineteenth century decried all the more the sins of masturbation and onanism.[94] Those condemnations did not relieve the frightening question about wet dreams that loomed in their conscience-stricken minds.

Wolff argued that an "essential force" caused the development of an egg into the form of a new organism. This did not challenge the role of God in creating the essential force, only his direct involvement with the details. Like an egg, the science of embryology developed slowly but, unlike the egg, it had no predetermined form. Over the decades Wolff's position emerged victorious, but significant contributions were made by his antagonists, Haller and the animalculists. The debate narrowed the issues for research, and the results of the debate changed the popular concept of life's beginnings. Chemical means of staining tissue, new techniques of slicing tissue for examination, and better microscopic instruments allowed the avid scientist to see the vivid details of embryological development. By the 1830s spermatozoa had been found in almost all invertebrates, but it would not be until 1876 that Oskar Hertwig actually could see and demonstrate a sperm penetrating an egg, thus causing fertilization.[95]

By the 1830s, however, educated people had developed an awareness that the notion of quickening was untenable. There was no event to record, no happening with which a soul could enter a fetus. Physicians and lawmakers alike knew the old principle of quickening was invalid in light of what was known about nature.[96] As we saw, in 1837 English law abolished the distinction made between the unformed/ formed fetus. The soul entered the body at some point, but when? Especially through the sketches of Wolff, the science of embryology showed the gradual development of a fertilized ovum as it became an embryo and then a fetus—and showed also the absence of any landmark points. In light of science, the Christian churches no longer could hold the position they had held for over a millennium and a half.

"From the Moment of Conception"

A committee of the American Medical Association was appointed in 1857 to "investigate the subject of criminal abortion, *with a view to its general suppression.*" Declaring the physician's responsibility to save lives, the unanimous resolution challenged the "wide-spread ignorance" that the fetus was not alive before the period of quickening.[97] In 1866 a Dr. Dana reported to the Maine Medical Association what he claimed was conventional wisdom: "It is now an established and universally admitted fact of physiology that life in the embryo commences with the very moment of conception."[98] Chief Justice John S. Tenney of the Maine Supreme Court (1859–1862) said that the old legal mark of quickening "had been abandoned by jurists in all countries where an enlightened jurisprudence exists in practice."[99] Never mind that he was exaggerating, the quickening concept no longer held among the elites. Regard for the fetus as something more than pre-life was growing. To call the fetus human was becoming more common, although *feticide* was the word of currency for abortion. There are "*no* circumstances" that justify the procuring of an abortion, declared a Massachusetts physician in 1870.[100] A southern medical practitioner said that abortion was clearly prohibited by the Bible in the

Ten Commandments: "Thou shalt not kill."[101] A northern counterpart expressed it, "foeticide is [a] murder."[102]

In 1869 Hugh L. Hodge, M.D., told physicians in Philadelphia that the fetus before birth was no different than after birth because at both times it was dependent on the mother for nourishment.[103] In the same year E. Frank Howe delivered a sermon to his parishioners in Terre Haute, Indiana: "Taking the life of the unborn child is a crime, and that crime is none other than murder."[104] And the following year, 1870, Dr. Andrew Nebinger said before his colleagues in Philadelphia that he had learned from physiologists, physicians, Christian priests, and rabbis that "the embryo is a living being from the moment of its conception."[105] With emphasis, the New York Medico-Legal Society declared in 1872: "The foetus is alive from conception, and all intentional killing of it is murder."[106]

In 1851, Pius IX declared "scandalous" and "erroneous" Catholic writers who accepted onanism (the code word for contraception) in marriage provided the reasons were good.[107] In 1869, the First Vatican Council met in Rome to attend to many matters of faith. Pope Pius IX, whose pronouncements were deemed by this Council as infallible, dropped references to ensoulment. In retrospect, Pius's statement on abortion was mild, but it had the effect of abandoning the Aristotelian position of graduated or staged development.[108] The exact words were, "Excommunicationei latae sententiae . . . declaramus . . . procurantes abortum, effectu sequuto" (We declare an automatic excommunication [on one] procuring a successful abortion).[109] Contrary to the way these words usually are interpreted, the pope did not say that life began at conception. By using the term abortion without qualification (except "successful"), he removed the unformed/formed, animal soul/human soul terminology as an event.[110] Many people interpreted him as agreeing with what science was saying about the development of the human embryo. Pius's motivation could have been just the opposite of bringing the Church into compliance with science. Angus McLaren notes that the pope was alarmed over the English neo-Malthusians and what was happening with birth control in France. He may have seen a strong Church stance against birth control as a way of stemming the medicalization and the artificial regulation of pregnancy.[111]

The 1869 pronouncement cannot be seen as revolutionary; indeed, the surprise is that the Catholic Church waited as long as it did before abandoning the position of ensoulment at quickening, long after medicine, science, and the law had come to new understandings. Without saying so explicitly, the Catholic Church moved to believe that life began at the beginning, that is to say at conception. Its increasing militancy against contraception was more evolutionary and represented a greater change. Even so, as with abortion, the anti-contraception stance was not without a long historical development.[112] The issues in Pope Sixtus V's bull (*Effraenatum* of 1588) were revived.[113]

A New York physician summed the changed view: "quickening is absurd and false; that there is no time for the moment of conception to the moment of birth when the foetus is not a human being; and that its life is as sacred at one period as at another."[114] One by one the nation-states of Europe and the Americas passed criminal abortion laws without reference to the formed/unformed fetus or quickening: Austria, 1852; Denmark, 1866; Belgium, 1867; Spain, 1870; Zürich Canton of Switzerland, 1871; Mexico, 1871; Netherlands, 1881; Bosnia/Herzegovina, 1881; Norway, 1885; Italy, 1889; Japan, 1907; and, interestingly, Turkey, 1911 (a first in a Moslem society).[115] A marginal note beside a Responsum in a Warsaw synagogue in 1849 stated: "In these times in Europe it is forbidden to give one the [contraceptive or abortifacient] 'cup of roots' to drink, without permission of the medical authorities appointed by the government."[116] Some laws (as alluded to here) pointed to drugs as being the expected means of effecting an abortion. The wording was usually comprehensive enough so that all forms of abortion were outlawed, except in some cases for the so-called therapeutic abortion to save the mother.[117] For example, the Belgian law of 1867 specified "by food, drink, medicine, violence or any other means" to procure an abortion and, like most of the laws, it applied to physicians, surgeons, apothecaries, or anyone else and to the woman who contrives in her own abortion.[118]

The Queen Versus Dr. Pascoe

The medical profession did not react adversely to the newly expressed Catholic position. Under the laws holding medicine's practitioners criminally liable for administering or assisting in abortion, doctors were under great peril even when pregnancy was a woman's declaration. If pregnancy was defined to be at or near conception, physicians not women were more in command. The profession's role in decision making increased.[119]

By the mid-nineteenth century, a physician who knowingly administered an abortion (such as by administering an abortifacient drug) when he knew a woman to be pregnant was guilty of a crime in England, France, the United States, and in many other countries. One case in England demonstrated the physician's peril. In 1852 in the Assize of Cornwall, Dr. Pascoe was indicted for a criminal abortion by giving oil of savin to a woman "with intent to procure miscarriage." Pascoe gave the woman fourteen drops of the oil divided into three doses daily. As an emmenagogue the standard dose of savin oil was from two to six drops, and the court found that Pascoe's dose was within reasonable practice. The case turned not on the dosage but on whether the physician knew or should have known that his patient was pregnant. The woman testified that she had told the physician that she had disease of the heart and liver. The court established that savin oil would not be given for heart and liver problems. The defendant was found guilty because he should have made a pregnancy determination before prescribing savin oil. The legal principle established by this case was summarized by Alfred Swaine Taylor in 1865:

> Every qualified practitioner, acting *bonâ fide*, would undoubtedly satisfy himself that a young female whose menses were obstructed was *not pregnant*, before he prescribed full doses of this oil three times a day, or he would fairly lay himself open to suspicion of criminality. If pregnancy—a frequent cause of obstructed menstruation—were only *suspected*, this would be sufficient to deter a practitioner of common prudence from prescribing, in any dose, a drug which may exert a serious action on the uterine system.[120]

Many physicians welcomed the Catholic Church's new position that defined abortion as any pregnancy termination after conception, because it increased their professional status by giving them the responsibility for determining pregnancy.[121] Even more, the old mark of quickening was subjective and its declaration up to the woman, but physicians who administered menstrual regulators simply because a woman asked were held responsible if it was determined that a pregnancy was terminated.

Neo-Malthusians and the Birth Control Movement

The Neo-Malthusians were persuaded that they were the first in history who had ever thought about birth control. In spite of this, or perhaps because of it, they kept their thoughts private: they would be in danger were their position too vulgarly known.[122]

In counteraction to the state, medical, and ecclesiastical interventions against birth control, a movement began to promote contraception. In 1797 Jeremy Bentham advocated the use of vaginal sponges to curtail the population growth of the poor as a means to relieve their misery.[123] In England the organizer of the movement was Francis Place (1771–1853), "the radical breeches-maker of Charing Cross," a reference to his profession as tailor before becoming a crusader for contraception. In the United States Charles Knowlton (1800–1850), a Massachusetts physician, published a plea for contraception under the title *Fruits of Philosophy: The Private Companion of Young Married People by a Physician* (New York, 1832). Knowlton was up-to-date with his physiology of sexuality, clinical and informative in his descriptions, and desirous of having a practical consequence on society. If population continued rising at its present pace, he saw disaster. He was concerned but not well informed, despite the fact that his work would become celebrated as the best medical advice on the subject of contraception.

Knowlton's advice was withdrawal, "an effect upon the health similar to temperance in eating."[124] He knew of the condom, which he called the "baudruche," but said its use was primarily for syphilis prevention. Another practical suggestion was the vaginal sponge, which could be enhanced by adding a "vegetable astringent" such as an "infusion of white oak bark, of red rose leaves, of nut-galls, and the like."[125] The method he advocated, the last one stated, was douching with cold water, even though there is an "occasional failure."[126]

The very fact that he knew so little about contraception yet was regarded as an authority reflects the ignorance of most physicians in the nineteenth century. Knowlton knew the latest about animalculae (sperm) but not nearly as much about contraception as did ancient physicians. Reprinted in London in 1834, Knowlton's book underwent many printings, until in 1876 one British publisher brought it out with some illustrations. The publisher was fined for the "dirty, filthy book" and withdrew it from the market. Two other publishers, Charles Bradlaugh and Annie Besant, took up the challenge to freedom of speech and the right to disseminate contraceptive information. They reprinted the book—under the title *A Dirty, Filthy Book*—and promptly were indicted with much publicity surrounding the case. Although they were convicted, the sentence was quashed in 1878 on a technicality.[127] So much fuss, while other publishers were printing the texts of classical medical authors, such as Hippocrates and Dioscorides, with far more and better information. They just did not know that the ancients were more reliable than the science of the day when it came to the age-old problem of birth control.

8

Eve's Herbs in Modern America

Ladies in certain situations should not use these.
> Advertisement for Dr. Dacier's Female Pills
> (1859)[1]

Feticide is not a vice of ignorance.
> H. Gibbons, M.D. (1877–1878)[2]

In the nineteenth century, physicians became increasingly aware of their liability when prescribing menstrual regulators, but many, if not all, were also aware that these birth control drugs were taken without a prescription from a trained physician. Around 1800 about two-thirds of those practicing medicine in Philadelphia were neither members of the College of Physicians nor graduates of a medical school.[3] And Philadelphia was better than most places in the quality of professional medical care. Physicians properly trained according to the standards of their times were threatened by irregular practitioners. Their worry about birth control medicines being dispensed outside the Hippocratic chain of professional physicians was basic, genuine concern for their patients, but at the same time they also had a competitive economic motive.[4] Physicians could not readily supply the market for birth control, because their participation in it was barred by their understanding of the Hippocratic Oath, state and religious laws, and the limitations of their formal education in such matters. No wonder, then, that they sought to discredit the birth control peddlers and the efficacy of their wares through laws.[5]

A book by John Burns in 1808 clearly established a position that was shared by many of his colleagues in the early part of the century. Burns's meaning is unambiguous: "Emmenagogues, or acrid substances, such as savin and other irritating drugs, more especially those which tend to excite a considerable degree of vascular action, may produce abortion."[6] He concluded that many physicians "pretend to view attempts to excite abortion as different from murder, upon the principle that the embryo is not possessed of life, in the common acceptation of the world."[7]

Some physicians simply regarded abortion as wrong. One such was Joseph Brevitt, who, in a book advising "female practitioners and intelligent mothers" (1810), stated: "The horrid depravity of human weakness in wretches lost to every sense of religion, morality, and that mutual attachment from a mother to her offspring, and every tender tie in nature, seek the means to procure abortion; nor are there wanting in the other sex, infernals wicked enough to aid their endeavours."[8] These comments were in a footnote. Earlier in the same work, Brevitt described emmenagogues and listed a number: asafetida, black hellebore, bitter apple (colocynth), savin (juniper), cantharides (Spanish fly), and, a new item to the list, electricity![9]

In the early nineteenth century, despite the gradual movement of law in Europe and America to extend protection to the fetus whatever its stage of development,[10] the medical profession continued to recommend emmenagogues, but not as abortifacients. Samuel Jennings's *The Married Lady's Companion or Poor Man's Friend* (New York, 1808) gave three prescriptions in three stages for relief from suppression of the menses, depending on severity. The first was a mild, easy therapy: three grains of chamomile tea. The second stage was six grains of chamomile tea at night or myrrh, nutmeg, cinnamon, rhubarb, rust of iron, all six to eight grains. The third stage, harsh remedies, was chamomile tea, "pretty strong," throughout the day or Peruvian bark (quinine).[11] Earlier, in 1772, a similar treatise prescribed only one remedy for suppressed menstruation, Peruvian bark, because "we know none preferable."[12]

A survey of medical literature of the 1840s through the 1860s indicates awareness of these drugs, despite the fact that many were dropped from the pharmacy and doubt was expressed about the efficacy of the others (as shown in the previous chapter). Immensely popular in the United States through the nineteenth century was Pseudo-Aristotle's *Masterpiece*, which described menstrual stimulators without implicitly referring to birth control (see Chapter 5).[13]

In 1843 Alfred Hall wrote a medical advice book "designed for females only," called *The Mother's Own Book*, published in Rochester. For suppression of menstruation, Hall called for foot baths and "warm drinks taken of either tansy, rue, feverfew (*Chrysanthemum parthenium* L.), southern wood (species of birthwort), motherwort, savin, pennyroyal, thyme, or one of these teas, made strong and drunk profusely with ginger, pepper, or cayenne" (from *Aniba panurense* Meissn.?).[14] In medieval England, the name motherwort was applied to various plants, among them artemisia and squirting cucumber, but in modern times the popular name was applied to *Leonurus cardiaca* L. of the mint family.[15] Presumably Hall intended the latter, which is employed in modern folk medicine as a menstrual regulator. *Leonurus cardiaca* contains rutin, the same substance that makes rue an abortifacient.[16] Hall gave a formula for preparation of savin with Holland gin and mentioned other menstrual drugs, such as black cohosh (*Cimicifuga racemose* Nutt.), bloodroot, and pennyroyal tea warmed with Holland gin.[17] Today's gin is alcohol flavored with juniper berries. The initial inclusion of berries in the recipe truly may have been medicinal.

Frederic Hollick's practical hints for the preservation of female health touched only lightly on the subject of menstrual regulators (New York, 1847). "In commencing to treat amenorrhea, the greatest care and circumspection is required," he wrote.[18] One must make a "careful study of the patient's constitution, habits, and mode of life, before judicious treatment can be recommended."[19] Without stating the obvious, he implied that the physician should make sure the patient was not pregnant before prescribing an emmenagogue. Diet and exercise are the best treatments, but "when such means faile, medicines can be resorted to."[20] The best medicines were iron (especially good was a formula of sulfate of iron), absynthium (4 drachma), syrup of saffron, made into a paste out of which could be made 150 pills, to be taken three times a day. Hollick concluded: "Stronger remedies are of course known, but they are not mentioned here, because they should not be employed except under proper advice."[21] He described a suction device that "*can scarcely fail*" [Hollick's italics], but it also was danger-ous.[22] Electricity ("Galvanism"), newly discovered, was seen to be use-ful in stimulating bad cases of retention.[23]

A year after Hollick wrote, another physician was much less cau-tious in prescribing emmenagogues for menstrual retention. M. K. Hard published in 1848 a woman's guide in which he claimed that drugs were the best treatment for an unhealthy patient. Quite effec-tive were the "emmenagogue pills or emmenagogue syrup."[24] This he wrote matter-of-factly, without stating what the emmenagogues were, the inference being that his reader would know what was available at the store. At the end of the work, however, a glossary told us that the "emmenagogue pills" were an extract of the smartweed *(Polygonum sp.)* and tansy in equal parts, thickened with equal parts of black cohosh and cayenne, formed into pills and given two or three times a day.[25] Substitutes for "the pill" were black cohosh, motherwort *(Leonurus car-diaca* L.), madder *(Rubia tinctorum* L.), tansy, or coltsfoot *(Galax urce-olata* L.?, of the gourd family, related to squirting cucumber), each of which was served in a decoction (a boiled-down preparation). After coltsfoot, he added the symbol for "et cetera," again implying that the reader would know what the other drugs were.[26]

Hard directed physicians to distinguish between amenorrheic pa-tients who were ill and those who were pregnant.[27] Near the end he provided a guide of medicines, including a list of emmenagogues. Jalapa, he said, came from South America and was good for a number of things but never should be given to a pregnant woman, as it caused an abortion. The same was true of aloes. Juniper was a diuretic and stimulant, but he gave no warnings about it or any effects it might have on reproduction![28] The named emmenagogues were black cohosh *(Cimicigua racemosa* L.), blue cohosh *(Caulophyllum thalactroides)*, mad-der, smartweed *(Polygonum sp.)*, and motherwort. Tansy, wild ginger, and pennyroyal "may be used as substitutes for the foregoing articles."[29]

Less knowledgeable was Eastman's medical guide to "diseases pe-culiar to women and girls," published in Cincinnati in 1848, the same year as Hard's work. Eastman called "strong" an emmenagogue tea made of pleurisy root *(Asclepias syriaca* L.) and asafetida.[30] In a way, this recipe symbolizes the old and the new: asafetida has been known since antiquity, but pleurisy root is a more recent folk discovery. Also named in other late-nineteenth- and twentieth-century medical guides, pleurisy root has been reported as a folk remedy in Quebec and among the Hopi Indians in Arizona.[31] As we shall see later in this chapter, pleurisy root will be a part of a well-known American patent medicine.

Other menstrual stimulators named were aloe, rhubarb, camellia alba bark (*Camellia sinensis* L.), cinnamon bark, and anise seed. Camellia bark is used for this purpose in twentieth-century folk medicine.[32] Inasmuch as these plants were not listed in earlier European works, it is probable that they were discovered by Native Americans (in the case of pleurisy root) and Chinese immigrants (in the case of camellia bark). Eastman's list of emmenagogues included balm, catnip, pennyroyal, maidenhair fern, and motherwort, but he also ended the short list with the familiar "et cetera."[33] Intriguingly, ergot (or "rye smut") was not named for birth control but for assistance in bringing on labor, but "the most happy results [are] in the hands of a judicious practitioner."[34]

A. M. Mauriceau's Portuguese Female Pills

A. M. Mauriceau was not his real name; that was Charles R. Lohman, husband to Madame Restell. Restell was not her real name, either. The Madame actually was Ann Lohman, who from the 1830s operated, under her *nom de guerre*, a famous abortion clinic in New York City.[35] In 1847, Ann Lohman's husband published *The Married Woman's Private Medical Companion*. The book advocated abortion quite openly and, unusual for the times, contraception. "Mauriceau" (was it really him or her?) wrote:

> Miscarriage, although attended with but little danger when skillfully effected and properly conducted, can only be considered as an alternative; only a choice of evils ... Thanks to the indefatigable researches of the learned and humane M. M. Desomeaux for his great discovery, ... *pregnancy can be prevented.* By this discovery every woman can have in her own power the means of prevention.[36]

When a woman's life is in danger, the physician whose "profession subserves the amelioration of the suffering" is compelled to assist in preventing pregnancy. This may be achieved "by safe, simple, invariably healthy, and infallibly certain means."[37] "Mauriceau" counters those who argue that, if women had certain knowledge on how to prevent pregnancy, their sexual morals would be destroyed.[38] He or she spoke to the social benefits of limiting family size and justified contraception at length, but no practical methods were revealed.

There were always women, however, who became pregnant and needed help. "Mauriceau" wrote: "The dangers of abortion or miscarriage are often magnificied [*sic*] and exaggerated. It is dangerous if produced by a fall, a blow, a kick from a horse, or any other external bodily violence or injury."[39] Drugs, in contrast, are not dangerous, the author asserted. It is important to note what the book did not do: it did not give specific, how-to-do-it information. At this time, the information was becoming proprietary. What once had been general knowledge now was known only by a limited number of people, some of whom were selling the drugs and keeping the formulas to themselves.

Mauriceau's guide was practical because it told women how to deal with an unwanted pregnancy under the guise of medical advice. Women were told to seek out individuals who sold information together with pills and bottles. For the suppression of menses Mauriceau recommended infusions of "diaphoretic powders" of garden thyme and pennyroyal "freely given."[40] In a lengthy note he or she said that

> the most successful specific, and one almost invariably certain in removing a stoppage, irregularity, or suppression of the menses (monthly turn), is a compound invented by M. M. Desomeaux of Lisbon, Portugal, called the Portuguese Female Pills. It would appear that they are infallible, and would, undoubtedly, even produce miscarriage, if exhibited during pregnancy. And what is equally important, they were always mild, healthy, and safe in their effects.[41]

Testimonials were given to their safety and reliability, and the section concluded with the price ($5 per box, $3 per half-box) and a New York address where they could be ordered by mail.[42] Likely, Dr. Desomeaux and Mauriceau were one and the same. One or both would be called "quacks" by other physicians in their city.[43]

"Female Medicines" and the Power of Advertising

The Lohmans' clever peddling of their Portuguese Female Pills under the mask of helpful medical advice to women tells us what had been missing from the chain of birth control knowledge in the modern period. How were women getting the means to restrict their reproduction? In one generation from 1800 to 1840, the fertility of American women declined dramatically. The birth rate was reduced from 7.04 children per 1,000 women in 1800 to 5.42 in 1850, and declined thereafter to 3.56 by 1900.[44] For certain, these nineteenth-century women knew some things that would control fertility or where to get them.

On one hand, if our interpretation of the evidence is correct, fewer women in the modern period knew about birth control plants because knowledge of antifertility agents was eroded by centuries of laws, religious doctrine, social conventions, and witchcraft suppression. In contrast, birth control seemingly was as prevalent in the nineteenth century as it had been previously. To be sure, what were perceived to be new techniques (but were not)—condoms, vaginal sponges and douches, and coitus interruptus—were available.[45] Various mechanical pessaries for abnormal forward curvature of the uterus are described as "the dread of almost every physician" and a "painful perplexity" to the hapless female.[46] The vaginal sponges were new terms for old concepts, namely the pessaries of the ancient world. Some sponges merely acted as barriers; others delivered chemical agents to the vagina. Douching was increasingly popular (at least, there were more references to it). Women douched with various mineral and vegetable solutions, including one simply consisting of cold water.[47] Generally, douching was considered to be a partial help with both contraception and abortion but not by itself a sure means of birth control. Toward the end of the century, spermicides and diaphragms became popular.[48] Given what the sources say and what our science suggests to be effective, we know that the primary means of birth control still was drugs. How did those women who were cut off from folk traditions but receiving no aid from professional physicians know which drugs to take?

The Lohmans' Portuguese Female Pills tell us: women who did not know which plants to gather knew what products to buy. How the market for birth control drugs disguised as patent medicines developed is not as well known. Its rise was evolutionary, to be sure, but the medicines sold in the nineteenth century could be traced back to the sixteenth-century (and earlier) apothecary shops. An anonymous writer (1752) described the street scene in London, where "young women, whose unhappy minute has been taken advantage of by pretended lovers" go to Ludgate-Hill and St. Martin's Lane and receive "handbills for the cure of all disorders incident to women."[49] The handbills did not cure the women but they told them what to buy, where to buy it, and, last but not least, what it would cost them.

By the nineteenth century, many newspapers carried small advertisements for women's medicines—"in nearly every newspaper in our land" declared a medical editorial in Buffalo in 1859.[50] "Feticide is advertised in our midst and throughout the country," warned fundamental Christians, "Spiritualists," in their annual convention in Chicago in 1873.[51] Examples of medicines included "Farrer's Catholic Pills," "Poudre Unique," "Velnos' Vegetable Syrup," "French Lunar Pills," "Hooper's Female Pills," "Dr. Peter's French Renovating Pills," "Hardy's Woman's Friend," "Colchester's Pennyroyal and Tansy Pills," "Chichester's Pennyroyal Pills," "Dr. Champlin's Red Woman's Relief," "Dr. Monroe's French Periodical Pills," and just plain "Female Monthly Pills."[52] "The very tone of their advertisements . . . call attention to the abortive quality of their drugs," exclaimed in derision a physician of Metamora, Illinois, in 1873.[53]

A single issue of the *Boston Daily Times* (January 4, 1845) carried advertisements for five "medicines" for females. A survey of newspapers in Great Britain during one week showed 100 newspapers with advertisements for abortions thinly disguised.[54] The wording of the promotions was usually clever and seldom direct: "restores female regularity"; "Females laboring under weakness, debility, fluorual bas [vaginal discharge], often so destructive and undermining to health"; "purifying blood, in debilitated and nervous constitutions, and restoring a healthy action to the internal system"; and "removing from the system every impurity."[55] A single issue of the *Central Times* in the small town of Dunn, North Carolina, on Febrary 26, 1891, contained advertisements for three brands of Pennyroyal Pills for four cents.[56]

Typical among the testimonies for such pills was this one from a Mrs. G. of Shelton, England: "Your mixture cured me after *Three Months* last spring . . . *No less than Twelve Times you . . . have Cured me.*"[57] Dr. Peter's French Renovation Pills gave "Authenticated Certificates from ladies who have used them" and gave notice that these pills had "rendered the usual practice of quacks, that of puffing, not only unnecessary but unworthy."[58] An even more revealing certificate was required by a late-nineteenth-century German proprietor. The sale of the medicine required the customer to sign this statement (translated into English): "I hereby declare that I will not take this cure to terminate pregnancy but only to restore monthly cycle, since period disruptions can indeed have several causes."[59]

Many promotions specified the importance of these medicines for married women. Between the 1840s and 1870s the pharmaceutical industry that supplied these medicines experienced dramatic growth.[60] In 1864 a New Hampshire physician reported that 123 different pessaries were sold.[61] In 1872, Ely Van de Warker, M.D., said that he personally knew of "twenty-six different preparations advertised and sold" for abortion.[62] There were many more, he said, and these were primarily oral drugs advertised for abortion (although seldom so blatantly stated). Each druggist also makes up two or three of his own preparations, "which he regards as emmenagogue, in the form of mixture, bolus, or pill."[63] Some few compounds were composed of inert ingredients but most were not, because the druggist wanted a good reputation with returning customers, he said.

Although Van de Warker had difficulty in getting druggists to speak to him about the issue, he compiled a table based on sales in the Syracuse and Troy, New York, areas, with a combined population of 95,000 (see Table 7). Fifteen varieties or brands of pills accounted for most sales. Van de Warker called them "worthless nostrums," decried the needless expenditure of money, and pointed to examples of fatal cases he had known when women took too much. One such example was a Troy woman, advanced in pregnancy in 1860 or 1861, who died from a mixture of oil of savin, ergot, and aloes purchased from a druggist. Oil of savin, of course, was highly concentrated, and the combination was likely to be lethal, if taken in sufficient quantity. Catholics were less likely to take abortion drugs than Protestants, but women from both groups purchased these "nostrums."[64]

Even though Van de Warker called them worthless, inexplicably he related data about the effectiveness of abortifacient drugs. The first (as

Table 7.   Sale of "female pills" in Syracuse and Troy, New York, in 1869

Wholesale drug stores in Syracuse	33 gross packages	=	4952
Retail drug stores in Syracuse	6 gross packages	=	864
Wholesale drug stores in Troy	17 gross packages	=	2498
Retail drug stores in Troy	7 gross packages	=	1008

Source: Ely Van de Warker, "Detection of Criminal Abortion," *Journal of the Gynecological Society of Boston* 4 (1871): 229–245.

ranked by him in importance) was ergot, for which "there are well-grounded doubts as to the power of ergot alone to accomplish an abortion in the early months of pregnancy." It worked for the later stages by its "influence" on causing bleeding within the womb. Cotton root was "the next drug in common use of this type of abortifacients," the type being those that act directly on the womb. Repeating the familiar cliché, Van de Warker said that its properties were discovered by African slaves and brought to the attention of the medical community by Dr. Bouchelle in 1840.[65]

Another class of abortifacients was the group causing reflex irritation. They were aloe (almost never taken by itself but in combination), black hellebore (*Helleborus niger* L., a strong cathartic), savin, tansy ("a potent abortifacient"), and rue. Many case studies where physicians were called after things went wrong were attributable to women taking the concentrated oils—for example, a woman who took five drops of oil of tansy three times a day. The physician was able to rescue her successfully.[66]

Reading the nineteenth-century medical literature reveals a startling contrast: physicians and other medical personnel were increasingly dubious that the medicines women bought on the open market were effective. Many voiced skepticism that the wares sold without their prescriptions could work, and many expressed alarm about harmful side effects. At the same time, these were some of the same recipes they prescribed for menstrual problems. On the other hand, a German rabbi curious about the Talmudic reference to a contraceptive or abortifacient "cup of roots" inquired among physicians about what this drug was. He was told that it was known and "must have been forgotten in the course of time."[67] In 1899 the medical journal *Lancet* said that abortifacient drugs that enjoy a "reputation amongst ignorant persons" are ineffective, but some of the emmenagogic drugs may be effective and should not be taken by pregnant women.[68] If one gives a menstrual stimulant to a woman and it works, it only proves that she was not pregnant in the first place, declared one physician in 1870, who disbelieved the power of herbal drugs to cause an abortion.[69]

Physicians were between the proverbial rock and a hard place. They were held responsible for administering a prescription that caused an abortion, but they were responsible also for addressing a legitimate complaint, the curing of which caused an abortion. Amenorrhea was a true medical problem for some women not pregnant. Considering that neither their education nor their medical books instructed them with detail concerning the pharmacology (in nineteenth-century terms), it is no wonder that physicians were troubled by what women were taking, more often than not without their advice or knowledge.[70]

Medical Statistics from the Nineteenth Century

The experiences of a physician in Manchester, England, provide interesting insight and some rare statistical data. In 1847 James Whitehead, who practiced medicine at the Manchester Lying-in Hospital, published a text on abortion and sterility based on his clinical experiences. He questioned 2,000 women admitted to the hospital. Of the 2,000, 747 said that they had aborted at least once, some many times, for a total number of abortions of 1,222.[71] He neglected to tell us whether he asked a follow-up question about how many abortions were intentional and how many were, in the terminology of his age, "natural." Neither did he inform us about the time period during which the pregnancies were allegedly terminated, nor about the marital status of his patients.

In the section on the causation of abortions, Whitehead said that one cause was "the use of strong purgative, emmenagogue, or mercurial medicines." He expressed some doubt that many of the cathartics and "what are commonly denominated emmenagogue medicines" actually caused abortions, except when "some powerful predisposing cause was already prevailing."[72] He did not specify examples of what these causes might have been. He expressed alarm at the symptoms that he saw when women took medicines that were too strong and gave as examples bitter apple (colocynth), savin, rue, foxglove, and "other drugs, administered with criminal intention."[73] Thus, in mid-nineteenth-century England, we have much the same array of drugs that were taken in antiquity and, in the case of colocynth, in ancient Egypt. Only the foxglove was new and, inasmuch as it contains digitalis, Whitehead was doubtless correct in reporting "alarming symptoms."

There were times, Whitehead admitted, when a competent physician needed to administer an abortive drug. He himself advised a patient with an extremely deformed pelvis to abort. He gave her a standard dosage of ergot of rye in her fifth month of pregnancy, and she safely aborted.[74] Subsequently, three more pregnancies were treated the same way with the same results, except for the last one. In his words, which may hide more than they reveal: "It was perseveringly tried in a fourth pregnancy in the same individual, and failed completely."[75] Left unexplained was whether the woman delivered, died, or had some other form of abortion subsequently administered.

Based on his experiences at Manchester Lying-in Hospital, Dr. Whitehead asked rhetorically in his book: What should a doctor do when he faces the young unmarried female? In his words, the "investigation is often fraught with peculiar difficulty." It is "one of the most delicate positions in which either patient or practitioner can be placed."[76] In such a case he said that a doctor must make every effort to determine pregnancy. The doctor has to discharge a very "disagreeable, difficult and often thankless duty." Dr. Whitehead did not explicitly say what the duty was, but he ended with the enigmatic statement that, I believe, tells us: "It should ever be his aim, however culpable his patient may be, to shield her fame, as far as is practicable, from the censorious taunts of an unfeeling public."[77] Completely omitted from his account is how a physician treated a married woman who asked for an emmenagogue.

Among the 1,000 patients examined in a late-nineteenth- century outpatient clinic in a large London hospital, 183 women had amenorrhea. Twelve were young girls "in whom the question of pregnancy was out of the question," and, among those 171 remaining, 156 were pregnant. Three women had amenorrhea because of anemia, one had "primary amenorrhea," and there were three whose condition was attributed to "no definite causes."[78] Thus, by the end of the century, physicians won the means and the right to determine pregnancy before treating a case of amenorrhea, but still they remained helpless in another area: they could not effectively control a woman's use of menstrual regulators for sale in any drug store. In many cases, physicians doubted the effectiveness of stimulating drugs, just as did the authors of the pharmacy guides, and they therefore thought they had more power than they did. Most women's menstrual problems were due to pregnancy, as the experiences of the London hospital demonstrated, and so the effectiveness of a "menstrual-stimulating" drug would have to be judged by its ability to terminate a pregnancy.

Many physicians were not fooled by what was happening around them. Contrary to the physician quoted above, who said emmenagogues did not work on pregnant women, C. D. Meigs claimed in *Fe-*

males and Their Diseases (1848) that emmenagogues would not cure amenorrhea, but he was certain that such drugs would cause an abortion or induce premature labor. To be deceived by female patients who asked for an emmenagogue was, in Dr. Meigs's opinion, "the stupidest thing a physician can do"![79]

A Maine medical report in 1869 stated that "the criminal practice of abortion is alarmingly prevalent at the present time."[80] The sale of emmenagogues or female medicines on the open market supplied the perceived need for abortifacients. None of the advertised medicines that I researched was explicitly for contraception, but some were contraceptives. In 1857, in pushing for tighter legislation against both abortion and contraception, Henry Brisbane wrote: "It is an undoubted fact that, especially in high life, and in the middle ranks of society, many wives (and often with the connivance of their husbands) take measures of this kind [contraception and abortions]."[81] A late-nineteenth-century medical report claimed that "probably seventy-five or ninety per cent of the abortions of our civilization are committed by the married women of the nation."[82] The sale of these products was as prevalent among married women as it was among single women. The 1886 *Dictionary of Plant-names* said that savin derived its name from its "being able to save a young woman from shame."[83] Compassion made up for what was lacking in linguistic etiology.

There were as many circumstances for taking birth control drugs in the nineteenth century as there were in antiquity, save that in the later period it was probably more difficult to obtain good information. Even so, in 1988, one hundred two years after savin was said to "save" a woman in trouble, a committee of American historians who studied abortion concluded: "Through the 1870s abortion was 'common,' a 'matter of fact' and often 'safe and successful.' "[84] This statement is truer when the contrast is made with the situation in the 1940s than with the level of birth control knowledge in the first century. Physicians of the late nineteenth century were less aware of what women were doing, and women were themselves less knowledgeable, than their forebears thousands of years before. Physicians' contact with antifertility drugs often came only after the medicines were wrongly taken with harmful results, for the medicines were made by druggists who were not attuned to their medicinal actions. In 1911, the *Journal of the American Medical Association* said of Chichester's Pennyroyal Pills in particular and all such "nostrums" in general: "it is well known that there is no drug or combination of drugs which, taken by the mouth, will with certainty produce abortion."[85] The *Journal* was simply repeating the prevailing medical opinion of the early twentieth century: Physicians should not regard these widely available drugs as effective, only as pernicious and dangerous.[86]

Regina v. Wallis: or, Physicians Who Do Not Know

Just how much physicians had forgotten is demonstrated vividly by an English abortion case. In the Winchester Assize in 1871, *Regina v. Mr. Wallis* was an important case in the annals of jurisprudence. At this time Victoria was Queen. Mr. Wallis was accused of "administering or causing to be administered" to a woman, pregnant by him, a "noxious substance." Testimony at the trial quickly established that the noxious substance was an infusion of pennyroyal and a quantity of a drug compound known as Griffith's Mixture, readily available in the stores. The defense did not contest this, nor did they challenge the fact presented by the Queen's prosecution that the woman, then in her sixth month of pregnancy, aborted and "recovered without any bad symptom."[87] Testimony established that she took no other drugs during this period and that no violence or "mechanical" injury had occurred to her body. She was, however, in the habit of horseback riding on a regular basis up to the time of the abortion. Readily she agreed that she took two doses of Griffith's Mixture, which the court was told consisted of iron and myrrh. Witnesses for the Queen's prosecution contended that the ingredients in Griffith's Mixture, although not labeled as such, were "clearly abortive in their character" and that the amount taken of pennyroyal tea was "sufficient to procure abortion."

At this point in the proceedings, the Queen's prosecution and the defense contested the evidence. Medical experts were called by both sides, but neither party could establish whether pennyroyal and Griffith's Mixture could cause an abortion. The defense's experts said that pennyroyal was not a "noxious substance." Three witnesses, Hicks, Tyler Smith, and Barnes, in particular, made an impression on the court. They said that Griffith's Mixture was just a good tonic ("a chalybeate tonic"), although it often was given to women not thought to be pregnant as an emmenagogue. The woman testified that she had asked Mr. Wallis to purchase Griffith's Mixture for her and that she had neither made nor taken the pennyroyal tea. She still had in her possession the dried leaves, she said. Defense witnesses said that there were no instances in medical history of the ingredients in Griffith's Mixture having "any effect on the uterus." Whatever their medical prowess, these experts were poor historians! In contrast, the Queen's prosecution contended that both Griffith's Mixture and pennyroyal (which it believed was taken) were "noxious remedies."

The court became confused. Most witnesses agreed that both substances could be considered emmenagogues and that pennyroyal probably was "used for the purpose by ignorant women, but it had no effect in producing an abortion." The court attempted to find experts who could define the difference between an emmenagogue and an abortifacient. Some witnesses said that any agent that provoked menstruation was synonymous with ecbolic or abortive drugs; others said that they were different. Unable to get medical experts to agree on whether the substances caused an abortion or whether an emmenagogue was the same as an abortifacient, the court ruled that the abortion was caused by the daily horseback rides.[88] In contrast, an interesting corollary was a case of abortive "poisons" before the North Carolina Supreme Court in 1880. Dr. Lyle, described as a medical expert, testified that "the mixture" in question was meant to induce an abortion because he could "tell its ingredients from its smell, taste, and appearance"—"no chemical analysis" was necessary. His testimony was allowed and Jacob Slagle was convicted of abortion.[89]

Regina v. Wallis was an important case in English and American jurisprudence because it demonstrated the difficulty of making legal distinctions between menstrual regulators and abortives, the North Carolina case notwithstanding. The best medical experts could not agree on whether these old herbs worked as antifertility agents; for that matter, they could not even tell whether they were "old" drugs for birth control.

As presented in the law books, *Regina v. Wallis* reveals another important historical event. In *Taylor's Principles and Practices of Medical Jurisprudence* (1865), the possibility that pennyroyal was an abortifacient was accepted. Taylor observed that an infusion of pennyroyal "is more powerful than the decoction since the poison, being a volatile oil, is dissipated by long boiling."[90] By the 1905 edition of the same work, Frederick J. Smith, its new editor, said that while pennyroyal may have been a popular emmenagogue and abortifacient, it is, "we believe, never used at the present day by medical men. It has neither emmenagogue nor ecbolic properties."[91] A superstition about pennyroyal did not develop between 1865 and 1905. No, this is a case of unwitting ignorance; medical professionals came to view all nonprescription drugs—patent medicines, women's remedies, anything available by mail order or from a traveling salesman—as superstitious nonsense. Hardly a hint is found in the pharmacy and medical guides in the latter half of the nineteenth century that abortion drugs were being taken and were effective, at least to some degree. Contraceptive drugs were even more difficult to find.

The Law in the United States, 1855–1870s

Whereas physicians may have been ignorant of what was going on in their own society, lawmakers were not. Lawmakers had little professional conflict over the availability of medicinal products. Unlicensed lawmakers were not competing for their services and causing liability problems for them. Doctors' motives were not entirely mercenary. After all, they saw the results of botched abortions and were legitimately concerned for their patients. Lawmakers were responding to the complaints of physicians as well as to those concerned that birth control encouraged immorality, restricted men's rights over their progeny, and kept the state and community from growing in population.[92]

In 1859, a legislator in Indiana called attention to the sale of thinly disguised birth control drugs. He showed the Indiana House "A Card to the Ladies" that proclaimed the virtues of Dr. Duponco's Golden Periodical Pills for Females, sold through the mail. He proposed to charge with a misdemeanor

> any person as druggist, apothecary, physician, or other person selling medicine, whether he be a merchant or pedlar, who shall sell any medicine in the form of pills, powders, fluid, or in any other form, which from its character by advertisement or otherwise is known to be capable of producing abortion or miscarriage with intent to produce abortion, not withstanding any caution given in the advertisement of such medicine, or contained in the directions accompanying the same.[93]

A not-so-friendly amendment slipped in the phrase "with intent to procure abortion."[94] Passed and signed into law, the legislation was to have little effect because of the burden of proving intent. Just the same, the movement to outlaw abortion drugs had begun.

From the 1850s, aggressive anti-abortion laws were passed in every state and most jurisdictions. *State of New Jersey v. Cooper* (1849) represents an important case in judicial thinking. While conceding that procuring an abortion was not "an indictable offence at common law," the decision stated, nevertheless, that abortions were "offences against the person of the child."[95] The court was taking a step toward regarding a fetus as a person or, in the court's words, "whether the child be *in esse*."[96] Eight years later another New Jersey court (in *State v. Murphy*, 1858) said of a woman who took a drink for an abortion, "Her offence at the common law is against the life of the child."[97]

In Texas in 1857 a provision was added to an abortion law that anyone who "furnishes the means for procuring an abortion knowing the purpose intended is guilty as an accomplice."[98] North Carolina followed the example in 1881.[99] Like many others, the Texas law did not define abortion by making a distinction between quickening and non-quickening but only employed the single word *abortion*. The North Carolina law declared an abortion given to "any woman, either pregnant or quick with child," to be a felony and an abortion given to "any pregnant women" (in other words, before quickening) to be a misdemeanor. Not until 1953 was the distinction modified by making both acts a felony. A North Carolina judge in 1880 said that "abortion was a flagrant crime at common law . . . because it interferes with and violates the mysteries of nature . . . It is not the murder of a living child which constitutes the offense, but the destruction of gestation by wicked means and against nature."[100] Neither courts nor legislatures pointed explicitly to the protection of the fetus as a human life, but the direction the arguments are taking is unmistakable.

Furthermore, all the laws specified drugs and instruments as the means of abortion. A Nebraska law in 1873 employed similar words regarding "any medicine, drug, or substance whatever . . . [used for] any pregnant woman with a vitalized embryo, or fetus, at any stage of utero gestation."[101] The expected means were drugs and, secondarily, surgery.[102]

Connecticut in 1860 passed an anti-abortion law that became a model because it combined several elements: (1) an abortionist was guilty of a felony, punished by up to $1,000 in fines and up to five years in prison; (2) those aiding and abetting an abortion were felons as well, but the sentence was left to the discretion of the court.[103] A woman receiving an abortion was adjudged a criminal too, but she received a less severe penalty because of "the protection due to the woman, protection against her own weakness as well as the criminal lust and greed of others." Finally, the Connecticut law fined ($300–$500) those who engaged in advertising for the dissemination of abortifacient information or materials.[104]

At the same time that the law was turning against the provision of antifertility agents, the sale of birth control drugs received two boosts from unwitting governmental action. First, a federal copyright law in 1831 licensed brand names, which led to increased public confidence in medicines with a familiar trademark. Second, in the late 1840s, Congress reduced postal rates to such a degree that ordering by mail became a practical and inexpensive way to obtain goods, particularly drugs.[105]

In most states, local government was dealing with the issue of birth control, because abortion, which was usually conducted away from licensed physicians, was not regulated by the medical profession. Inasmuch as physicians were criminally liable and prohibited by the Hippocratic Oath (which was increasingly cited) from participating in abortion, they turned to pressuring legislators to control the illegal abortions.[106] The advertisement and sale of birth control medicines caused an enormous gap between capital and medical interests. No wonder physicians sought solution in the law, not the clinic.

The Comstock Act of 1873

Anthony Comstock (1944–1915) was the leader of the New York Society for the Suppression of Vice. He supposed that only the federal government could control the trade in pornography because the U.S. Mail was being used both to advertise and deliver the wares. In 1873 his lobbying resulted in an act, named after him, that reads as follows:

> That no obscene, lewd, or lascivious book, pamphlet, picture, paper, print, or other publication of an indecent character, or any article or thing designed or intended for the prevention of conception or procuring of abortion, nor any article or thing intended or adapted for any indecent or immoral use or nature, nor any written or printed card, circular, book, pamphlet, advertisement or notice of any kind giving information, directly or indirectly, where, or how, or of whom, or by what means either of the things before mentioned may be ob-

tained or made, nor any letter upon the envelope of which, or postal-card upon which indecent or scurrilous epithets may be written or printed, shall be carried in the mail, and any person who shall knowingly deposit, or cause to be deposited, for mailing or delivery, any of the hereinbefore-mentioned articles or things, . . . shall be deemed guilty of a misdemeanor . . .[107]

The law was strong and tightly reasoned. The federal government was involved for the first time against contraception as well as abortion. The lawmakers must have been aware that some of the medicines were contraceptive as well as abortifacient but, whatever the intent, the law was passed and enforced.

Comstock had more to do: in 1878 he had arrested Madame Restell (the famous abortionist discussed above) after she allegedly purchased from herself an abortion preparation. Her establishment was patronized by "the most wealthy and fashionable women of this metropolis," or so said a contemporary who knew of her famous "Female Pills."[108] One must say she "allegedly" took her own pills because she was never tried. She committed suicide the day before the trial, not by taking pills but by cutting her wrist in a bath.[109] The newspapers handled the news with gusto; one cartoon shows New York's Fifth Avenue packed with so many children that traffic could hardly move.[110] Abortion was an issue for public discourse. The newspapers saw some good from the Madame Restells of this world. Before Comstock's campaign, New York City reportedly had two hundred full-time abortionists and, one would suppose, many more who were part-time or occasional.[111]

Midwives continued to be a major source for birth control in the United States, and presumably elsewhere. "The practice of abortion has become a very great evil, largely as a result of a lack of midwife control," declared the president of Chicago's obstetrical staff for the Health Department in 1896.[112] Other countries had similar problems with midwives.[113] In seeking to solve "the midwife problem" in Chicago, lawmakers forbade its practitioners to possess "any drug or instrument . . . which may be used to procure an abortion."[114] Despite suppression, torture, and extermination of midwives as witches at modernity's dawn, midwives were recognized into the twentieth century as providers of information and wares about how to control fertility. The presumption is that, after centuries of suppression, the midwives' knowledge had deteriorated in quality, which may explain some of the bad public relations midwives suffered. We need to learn more about what nineteenth- and early-twentieth-century midwives knew and how they knew it.

Allen's Mixture and England's Law on Advertisements

In England in 1898 the proprietors of "Allen's Mixture" were prosecuted. The mixture was advertised as "Important to Ladies—Especially to those who require an ABSOLUTELY CERTAIN and speedy remedy; a remedy which in thousands of cases has never failed to afford COMPLETE RELIEF."[115] When the newspaper that ran this ad changed owners, its new owners took the money but refused to publish the advertisement because they maintained it was illegal. Justice Darling, who presided, reported to the *Times* on the question that was raised to the jury:

> It was said that the advertisements [of Allen's Mixture] were of an illegal and immoral nature . . . The question was, Was it intended by the advertisements to convey that the medicine would procure miscarriage or abortion? To procure abortion or to attempt, or counsel, or assist to procure it was a criminal offense and therefore you would expect any advertisement relating to it to be in very guarded terms. If the advertisement advised the taking of something for the purpose of procuring abortion it was undoubtedly forbidden by law.[116]

An analysis of Allen's Mixture revealed very little, but it was sufficient for the court; it contained 82.67 percent water, chloroform 1.66 percent, mineral matter 0.73 percent, and unknown "organic substances."[117] Biochemistry was yet to be born, as the elementary chemical analysis shows. The jury found that the advertisements did imply that the mixture could be used for abortion and found in favor of the defendants, the newspaper owners who refused to run the ad.

Abortion Laws in the United States

Most of the states' laws passed in the late nineteenth century regarded pregnancy as any period of fetal development. Many contained anti-advertising provisions for the sale or dissemination of information about abortion drugs or procedures. Generally these laws remained in force until the 1960s.[118] In practically every law in every state until 1960, the means specified for an abortion were drugs, first, and surgery. The usual phrase was that anyone who administers "any drug or substance or [anyone who] uses or employs any instrument or other means" to procure an abortion is criminally liable.[119] Some law texts substituted medicine for drug and a few gave both names.

The territory of Arizona's law of 1865 referred to the drugs only as "poisons," and the Rhode Island law (1956) borrowed from the Lord Ellenborough Act the words "any poison or other noxious thing."[120] Going back to the Bible, Illinois's law of 1833 merely said "killing poison," and Pennsylvania (1945) combined the old and new terms: "any poison, drug or substance" or unlawful uses of any instrument or other means.[121] Only the District of Columbia (1960) and Mississippi (1956) specified instruments or surgery before drugs, as "any instrument, medicine or drug or other means" (Mississippi).[122] Wisconsin's law of 1958 defined "unborn child" as "a human being from the time of conception until it is born alive," but it does not name any specific means; it states only that abortion was criminal. Wisconsin did provide for therapeutic abortion, however. Even so, the older Wisconsin law (1858) specified drugs as the primary, expected means.[123]

Though these laws against abortion were the states' responsibility, the federal government became involved as a reaction to concerns of a different sort. A number of publicized scandals about drug quality led to a call for federal action in regulating drugs, and in 1906 Congress passed the Federal Food and Drug Act. With this act, all birth control drugs were automatically illegal inasmuch as their usage was for a criminal act.[124] The difficulty that remained in enforcing the law was determining the intent of the seller. Four types of medicines continued to be sold for women only, except in those few states that prohibited them. One type, such as "Female Remedy," was usually called a tonic and advertised as a pick-me-up or a stimulant. Generally, alcohol accounted for the bulk of the content of the tonic. The second group was the pain relievers or analgesics. The third group was emmenagogues, pills and potions for the relief of menstrual problems. The fourth was contraceptives, but they were very heavily disguised because of the laws against them. The euphemism by which these drugs were called was usually "feminine hygiene product."

Between 1919 and 1934 the U.S. Department of Agriculture issued legal restraints, called "Notices of Judgment," against fifty-seven medicines for women. Among them were:

Apgo Capsules (with savin and celery, unstated but probably seeds, 1934)
Blair's Female Tablets ("plant drugs, incl. a bitter drug," 1932)
Dupree's French Specific Pills (aloes, iron sulfate, cotton-root bark, tansy, and other alkaloids, 1921)
Ergot-Apoil (plant materials including celery [seed?] and savin [but no ergot alkaloids!], 1933)
Madame LeRoy's Regulative Pills (aloe with pennyroyal and tansy, 1922)
Premo Ergot-Apoil Capsules (aloin from aloe, oils of celery and savin and traces of ergot alkaloids, 1934)[125]

Many content reports simply specified "plant substances." The chemistry was incomplete, even according to the standards for the time. Two fairly obvious contraceptive medicines were Womanette and Wycones, each of which appears to have as its only active ingredient willow bark or salicylic acid.[126] To be sure, the intended action could only have been to relieve pain, but willow was used, as discussed in the first chapter, as a contraceptive drug from ancient times. In addition to the Department of Agriculture, the Post Office was active in bringing criminal charges against the mail-order drug salesmen.[127]

Obviously, some of the state legislators were aware that the drugs could be contraceptive and sought to legislate against contraception by banning the drugs. In 1876 a federal court, in *U.S. v. Foote*, rejected a request by physicians to disseminate *information* about contraception.[128] A Colorado law of 1921 made it a misdemeanor to dispense or advise or even publish information of "recipes or prescriptions for drops, pills, tinctures, or other compounds, designed to prevent inceptions, or tending to produce miscarriage or abortion."[129] Kansas had a similar law.[130] In 1924, the State of Iowa was much more specific; the law actually specified the drugs:

No person shall sell, offer or expose for sale, deliver, give away, or have in his possession with intent to sell, except upon the original written prescription of a licensed physician, dentist, or veterinarian any cotton root, ergot, oil of tansy, oil of savin [juniper], or derivatives of any said drug.[131]

The same wording was included in a revision made in 1946.[132] The drugs named in the Iowa law were abortifacients, not contraceptives.

Louisiana's law (1924) against contraception and abortion was more vague in one way, more precise in another. It did not specify the drugs but made it a misdemeanor to provide for the "sale or advertisement of . . . any *secret* drug or nostrum purporting to be *exclusively for the use of females* or *for preventing conception* or for procuring abortion or miscarriage" (italics added).[133] The medieval "secrets of women" were known to Louisiana legislators. Too, the law's fathers must have been cognizant of the use of menstrual regulators, because it forbade the sale or advertisement of any drug for female use only. In a revision in 1950, the provisions were dropped against contraception and drugs intended only for females.[134]

These laws are extraordinary. At a time when medical books had dropped all learning about contraceptive and abortion drugs, when physicians considered their use only superstitious folk medicine, Iowa's and probably Louisiana's legislators knew what the drugs were being used for and they aimed to stop the practices. The Iowa solons even knew what the principal drugs were, but they failed to name them all.

In 1938 the federal Food, Drug, and Cosmetic Act greatly strengthened the law against illegal drug sales, although there was some opposition from women's groups. The strongest fear was that Lydia E. Pinkham's Vegetable Compound would be removed from the market. The original formula for this medicine, mixed in Lydia Pinkham's kitchen, was taken from or inspired by a formula published in John King's *American Dispensatory*. Pinkham's Vegetable Compound, first sold around 1875, consisted in its original formula of the following:

Unicorn Root (*Aletris farinosa* L.), 8 oz.
Life Root (*Senecio aureus* L.), 6 oz.
Black Cohosh (*Cimicifuga racemosa* [L.] Nutt.), 6 oz.
Pleurisy Root (*Asclepias tuberosa* L). 6 oz.
Fenugreek Seed (*Trigonella foenum-graecum* L.), 12 oz.
Alcohol [18–19 percent] to make 100 pints[135]

The life root was one of two species of ambrosia or *Senecio aureus* L., the latter known in modern science as an abortifacient alkaloid.[136] The pleurisy root and fenugreek were used in the old recipes, as we saw, with the former having a strong estrogenic effect on animals.[137] A 1989

German Federal Health Commission concluded that 40 milligrams of an alcohol extract of black cohosh root is good for treatment of dysmenorrhea (dysfunctional menstruation), the amount being comparable to the quantity in Lydia Pinkham's recipe.[138]

Pinkham's compound was widely advertised as a "Blood Purifier" for women, but it sold also for birth control, or so it would seem (because it did have antifertility properties). Women took the mixture for contraception and abortion. Some of the advertisements hinted at abortion—"dissolves and expels tumors . . . , cures irregularity." Also it was supposed to "cure" sterility: "There's a Baby in Every Bottle."[139] Women's protests were successful in saving it. One person wrote her congressman, who pushed the legislation, "The women of America will show you."[140] Another letter said that "you cannot deprive them [women] of Lydia E. Pinkham's Vegetable Compound without hearing from us at election time."[141] Never was it entirely banned; in fact, Lydia Pinkham's Vegetable Compound is sold today. The 1930s formula contains the same original ingredients, save for fenugreek seed, but other ingredients, primarily vitamins, are added.[142] The modern notion that all the medicine did was give the ladies an alcoholic lift deserves a smile—not at the medicine's takers but its unknowing critics.

Modern studies of the movement to regulate drugs and to eliminate the entrepreneurial sales of patent medicines regard the medicines as inert at best, and harmful at worst, and its salespeople as "quacks" and "charlatans." A publication of the American Medical Association in 1936 said of the medicines for females: "The facts are, practically none of these preparations will reestablish the menstrual flow when its cessation has been due to pregnancy. There is, in fact, no drug or medicine known that will terminate pregnancy without seriously endangering the woman's life."[143] In the same year a researcher on abortions declared that he doubted the efficacy of drug abortifacients, which "belong more properly in a volume on toxicology."[144]

Quite possibly some of these medicines were, as stated, inert, harmful, even potentially fatal. No quality controls were followed in the manufacture of these products and many were mixed by people, likely men, who lacked the knowledge, once better known, of amounts and effective combinations. More apt, however, is the assumption that most were effective enough to maintain women's confidence in the drugs. The median age of pregnant brides in Medmenham, England, 1854–1927, was exactly the same as the median age for non-pregnant brides, 23 years of age.[145] This indicates that women were using pregnancy as a marriage strategy (forcing a "shotgun wedding"). As the decades went by, pregnant women who were unable to effect a marriage were increasingly likely to end up "in trouble," as abortifacient drug-store remedies became less readily available in the twentieth century.

According to nineteenth-century reports, it was not only desperate single women who were driven to take these patent medicines because of indiscreet moments; married women, too, who for whatever reasons did not want a pregnancy, also relied on them. For suppliers to married women, repeat business would be important. Nevertheless, steady pressure from state and federal governmental agencies and law enforcement officers combined to eradicate natural-product birth control medicines first from the drug stores, then from catalogues and the advertisement sections of newspapers.

Margaret Sanger and the Birth Control Movement without Herbs

Ads for these same drugs were also banned, surprisingly, from the journal of Margaret Sanger's birth control movement. Sanger is almost universally known as the pioneer of the American birth control movement, and in the journal she founded, *The Birth Control Review*, she began the first issue with an editorial on "Shall we break this law?" and a later editorial calling for "a birth strike to avert world famine."[146] This modern Lysistrata did not advocate abortion, only contraception.[147] She was particularly incensed when a New York State court (January 8, 1918) enjoined physicians not to give out information for the prevention of disease if the information also could be used to promote contraception. Before the court was Sanger herself.[148]

Sanger distrusted drugs and her journal, therefore, did not have information about them. Advertisers of other wares were welcomed, however. For example, an advertisement ran for "3-in-One Oil" for lubricating sewing machines and vacuum cleaners.[149] The symbolism is significant: the mother of the American birth control movement promoted sewing but demoted abortion.

Still, Margaret Sanger's relentless campaign between 1916 and 1945 succeeded in legalizing contraception. In 1937 the American Medical Association recognized contraception as a legitimate part of medical practice, provided patients requested the information.[150] By 1945 there

were more than eight hundred clinics available. Sanger and her followers separated contraception, which they supported, from abortion,
which they regarded as politically unwise and, in many cases, im-
moral.[151] In her memoirs, Sanger wrote of the terrible experiences of
women who had "cheap abortions," especially abortions by mechanical means. Also she wrote disapprovingly of those who drank "various
herb-teas" without specifying the herbs or the results.[152] Sanger and
her organization were responsible for the dissemination of a great deal
of information on birth control—but none of it continued the tradition of using natural products as antifertility agents.

Folk Medicine and Birth Control in the Twentieth Century

Many of Eve's herbs were forgotten by the 1900s, but not all. An account from Germany in 1907 shows that there were women who kept
alive the old knowledge. In Herzegovina some women took St. John's
wort (*Hypericum perforatum* L.) to prevent conception.[153] It is
Frauenkraut or *Johanniskraut* in German, the first name betraying its
use. In the sixth century the medical writer Paul of Aegina named this
plant as a menstrual regulator.[154] In all probability, however, the classical Greek text was not the source of the practice; the plant's effect
was known through oral tradition. Tansy is associated with sexual activity in other folk medicines from Germany.[155]

English ivy was known as an abortifacient in German folk medicine,
whereas in classical medicine it was used for both contraception and
abortion.[156] Ivy also was employed in modern African folk medicine as
an abortifacient.[157] Laurel was used for sterility.[158] Pomegranate was
associated in German culture as an "erotic, sexual fruit tree," and the
fruit was eaten to prevent fertility.[159] In Iceland willow is believed to
hinder the conception of children, as it was said to do by Dioscorides
in the first century.[160] In Thüringia, a province of Germany, the black
poplar was regarded as an abortion tree.[161] The hazelnut (*Coryllus avel-
lana* L.) was used for an abortion along the Danube in Germany.[162]
Apiol made from parsley, which was particularly important, was sold
by pharmacists until 1931, when the German health law forced it off
the shelves and it became available by prescription only.[163]

Finally, the use of the fern *filix* remained in popular German folk
medicine until the twentieth century, when Dr. Aigremont wrote of

its use both as a contraceptive and as an abortifacient. Interestingly, he said that this fern was a witch's drug *(Hexenkraut)* and a prostitute's drug *(Hurenkraut)!*[164] The names preserve the history of a thousand years.

James Woycke's study of birth control in Germany, 1871–1933, discloses that, although the traditional birth control herbs were still known during these years, their use probably declined. In Woycke's words, "not every weed growing in the cemeteries of Germany could be effective."[165] People moving to the cities lost touch with the lore. Perhaps as a consequence, oral and anal sex, mutual masturbation, and various variants of coitus (including the so-called *coitus saxonicus)*[166] became increasingly popular means of satisfying the urges of married and unmarried couples.[167]

Never has the old herbal knowledge entirely left this world, despite the medicalization of birth control. In the last part of the twentieth century, anthropologists and ethnopharmacists report folk usage of contraceptive and abortifacient plant drugs. One recent survey found plants used as contraceptives among the peoples of New Guinea, the Eddystone Islands, the Peruvian jungles, and in the southwestern United States (among Navahos).[168] Studies conducted in Nigeria,[169] China,[170] Korea,[171] the Soviet Union,[172] Haiti,[173] New Mexico,[174] Paraguay,[175] Egypt,[176] Malaysia,[177] and India[178] reveal that contemporary traditional societies employ a variety of antifertility agents. Some are new, such as the papaya. Most of the plant drugs are the same as those discussed in this book. Even when the plants are not still used to limit fertility, a faint echo of ancient practices is heard still: in modern Lithuania a mother gives a pot of rue to her daughter on her wedding day.[179] The reason has been forgotten, but the custom remains.

In the 1970s, when James C. Mohr was researching his book, *Abortion in America*, he encountered references to women in the nineteenth century who took abortifacient drugs. Baffled by the discrepancy between the historical documents and modern medical authorities, he asked colleagues at the Johns Hopkins Medical Center about the possible efficacy of the abortifacient drugs. He was told, among other things, that the psychological pressure on some women who took these agents was probably sufficient to induce abortion, but the drugs themselves could not have been effective.[180]

In the second half of the twentieth century, our modern culture came to the mistaken conclusion that plants were not effective for birth control. Scientists and medical personnel rejected techniques that had been within the cognitive terrain of their professional ancestors, including their Hippocratic forefathers. Historians were led to disbelieve their documents because they were unwilling to ascribe to earlier ages that which modern science did not deem possible. Equally discouraging is the fact that scientists would not trust folklore well enough to test its practices. I write this book not from a mistaken belief in historical positivism but in its opposite. It is perfectly possible that people in past ages knew some aspects of science better than we do in the modern age.

Modern science has been cautious about birth control, especially since the nineteenth century, when abortion became a criminal offense and contraception was associated with moral and religious interdictions. The trend toward limiting the choices in birth control techniques seemingly would have been countered by the Malthusian movement, which saw danger in population growth. The early Malthusian movement was partly countered by a realization that some modern industrial states had achieved population stability or, in some cases, a decline that alarmed leaders in Western Europe and North America. These conditions pushed lawmakers to legislate against birth control. In the twentieth century Chinese lawmakers took the opposite stance: alarmed by population density, they restricted the number of children a woman may have. West or East, now the state defines the rules of reproduction.

In addition to complex economic factors, deep, new religious concerns shaped the history of birth control in the past two centuries. The new science of embryology made untenable the old notion of ensoulment during the second trimester of fetal development. In place of the old doctrine there arose the idea that life begins at conception. At the same time, pregnancy became an event determined by a physician, not by the woman, and woman's role in her own sexuality underwent significant changes. Nevertheless, whatever the age, and however the age put restraints on pregnancy, always women retained some say about whether to bear children.

By the twentieth century, some people regarded the fetus as "life" itself and referred to the fetus as a "human," in the imagery of language that Barbara Duden calls the "iconography of pregnancy."[181] Just as quickening was once a nebulous, pseudo-scientific term that was thought to describe a critical stage in fetal development, so the notion of a separate "life" within the womb was derived from popular conceptions and misconceptions of what science was thought to have said. Today fertilization and "conception" are defined not as a single event but as a number of stages; it is recognized that genetic identity does not occur at the moment the sperm enters the ovum.[182] In 1987, the proposal was made (but not accepted) that the "killing of human life" replace the words "abortion" and "termination of pregnancy" in the federal statutes of Germany.[183]

By the second part of the nineteenth century aggressive secular legislation and public policy were pursued to remove abortive and contraceptive medicines from the marketplace. It was feared that contraceptive drugs encouraged sexual immorality in single women. As a result of these economic, social, and religious trends, birth control had become a matter of state policy by the early twentieth century. By voting, the individual could influence the making of public policy, but not every woman could necessarily make an individual decision. The twentieth-century woman in western society was far removed from the thirteenth-century Béatrice, who decided with her lover when she wished to have children. As the century closes, many societies have concluded that the fetus requires protection and that women's reproductive rights are not absolute. Other societies establish limits on the number of children permitted. Confusion clouds our judgments while the silent armies of popular opinion clash by night.

Epilogue

If you are pregnant or nursing a baby, seek the advice of a
health professional before using this product.

Label on *Lydia Pinkham Herbal Compound*,
May 1995

I learned many surprising things as I researched this book, but what
seemed truly astonishing was that knowledge about herbal medicines
is not entirely lost in our day (although it is not very prominent either). While having dinner in the Appalachian mountains of North
Carolina, I described my work on ancient drugs to an old friend, Peter Reichle, and his wife, Mary, a public health nurse in Watauga
County. She said that she had some clients who were taking an herb
as a contraceptive and were pleased with the results. My interest
piqued. I inquired what part of the plant was eaten and whether it was
ingested pre- or post-coitus. Told that the seed was ingested after intercourse, I guessed that they were taking Queen Anne's lace, about a
tablespoon. It was then Mary's turn to be surprised, and she asked how
I knew. Ignoring her question for a moment, I told her, "Thank you,
you have just provided me with my only source since the seventeenth
century for its use!"

Queen Anne's lace appeared in medical records until the early modern period, when it dropped out of the medical literature. One woman
Mary knew had taken the seeds (gathered in the fall) for ten years, but
she had recently become pregnant. She had taken a trip with her husband and neglected to take her Mason jar of seeds. It seems that near
my home there were women who took the herb much as ancient women
did, but the herb (or any drug made from it) does not appear in modern western medical manuals for this use.

257

Since that evening's disclosure I have acquired more anecdotal information from others in the mountain regions of North Carolina, Virginia, and Tennessee, and in New York City. A student from rural Indiana told me that her grandmother told her that the seeds of Queen Anne's lace were what "nasty girls took not to have a baby." From one person I learned something very important for interpreting the historical sources. Before the seeds are taken, I learned, they must be crushed. Otherwise they go through the alimentary canal without absorption, or, in her words, they "go right through you." That is in keeping with the report that in India women chew the seeds. Nothing in the historical sources specified this critical piece of information. Experienced herbalists may know instinctively to crush the seeds. It makes me all the more aware that the medical writings themselves were not sufficient to explain the continuous use of natural products over many centuries. By and large, information about these drugs has been transmitted orally.

While writing this book, I received a catalogue from a mail-order firm, the Health Center for Better Living of Naples, Florida, that sells herbs. In the United States the herbs can be sold but not as medicines, only as nutritional supplements. Without giving any hint either of birth control or menstrual regulation—circumlocutions commonly used to refer to abortifacients—the catalogue, entitled "A Useful Guide," listed the same familiar herbs that I had found in records of two thousand years or more ago. Some of the herbs, such as aloe, angelica, catnip, coltsfoot, feverfew, hyssop, juniper berries, mint, myrrh, pennyroyal, pleurisy root, sage, spikenard, tansy, and wormwood, are found in both ancient written accounts and in contemporary oral sources.

Harking back to the past, however, were descriptions of six herbs that the catalogue explained were useful in regulating menstruation ("will correct irregular menstruation"; "for suppressed menstruation"; "regulate menstrual flow and for menstrual cramps"). Those herbs were black and blue cohosh, motherwort (*Leonurus cardiaca* L.), mugwort (artemisia), rue, and St. John's wort. In many health food stores, one finds many of the same drugs formerly sold in drug stores and by medieval apothecaries, and some are labeled with the "recommended" uses that appear in early modern written works. Since these products cannot legally be sold as drugs, the labels can only advertise how some people have used them.

A problem arises when some of these drugs are sold with no warnings attached. For example, the catalogue I just mentioned (which is undated) described tansy as "An old, well-known remedy used to tone up the system and soothe the bowels. Strengthens weak veins. Will expel worms. Very good for the heart." What happens to a pregnant woman who wants to deliver but who takes too much tansy tea to strengthen her veins? As long ago as 1499, an anonymous woman before the Inquisition spelled out what we see now as a warning: one who knows how to cure also knows how to kill.

At the end of the twentieth century, we know more natural-product drugs that affect fertility than did ancient women. What's more, our science has an explanation for many of the drugs' actions. What separates us from our ancestors is that today this knowledge is mainly in the hands of the experts: there are few modern women who know the antifertility plants in their environment, whereas women in the past did know them. In ancient and medieval days, many women employed them. Whatever we decide on the morality of contraception and abortion, we must recognize that women in the past made deliberate decisions about whether to have children and when to have them. These decisions, and the knowledge behind them, left their mark on human history.

Notes

Introduction

1. David Garrow, *Liberty and Sexuality: The Right to Privacy and the Making of Roe vs. Wade* (New York, 1994), pp. 389–407 *et passim;* Macian Faux, *Roe vs. Wade: The Untold Story of the Landmark Supreme Court Decision That Made Abortion Legal* (New York, 1988).

2. *Roe v. Wade*, 410 U.S. 113, pp. 120 and 125.

3. Ibid., p. 119, n. 3.

4. Ibid., pp. 129–130, 117.

5. Ibid., p. 116.

6. A. Castiglioni, *History of Medicine*, trans. E. B. Krumbhaar, 2d ed. (New York, 1958), p. 84, calls the period of around 1000 A.C.E. "early Persian," a misnomer.

7. Ibid., p. 131.

8. I base this claim, in part, on a recent survey made by Dr. Jonathon Erlen (University of Pittsburgh), who received from all the medical schools in the United States copies of the oath and how it is administered at graduation. Dr. Erlen kindly made copies available to me. See report of the survey by Emil Dickstein, Jonathon Erlen, and Judith A. Erlen, "Ethical Principles Contained in Currently Professed Medical Oaths," *Academic Medicine* 66 (1991): 622–624.

9. Such as J. Chadwick and W. N. Mann, *Hippocrates* (Harmondworth, England, 1978), p. 67; L. Edelstein, "The Hippocratic Oath: Text, Translation and Interpretation," in *Ancient Medicine*, ed. Oswei Temkin and C. Lilian Temkin (Baltimore, 1967), p. 6.

10. Emile Littré, *Oeuvres complètes d'Hippocrate*, 10 vols. (Paris, 1839–1861), 4 (1844): 631: "je ne remettrai à aucune femme un pessaire abortif."

11. Ibid., 4: 620–621.

12. Edelstein, "Hippocratic Oath," pp. 3–63.

13. *Roe v. Wade*, 410 U.S. 113, p. 132.

14. Ibid., pp. 166–167.

15. Ibid., p. 135, n. 26; see Cyril C. Means, "The Phoenix of Abortional Freedom: Is a Prenumbral or Ninth-Amendment Right About to Arise from the Nineteenth-Century Legislative Ashes of a Fourteenth-Century Common-Law Liberty?" *New York Law Forum* 17 (1971): 335–410.

16. *Roe v. Wade*, 410 U.S. 113, p. 136.

17. Ibid., p. 136.

18. Ibid., p. 170.

19. Ibid., pp. 169–170.

20. Ibid., pp. 71ff.

21. Eric M. Matsner, "Contraceptives and the Consumer," *Consumers Defender* 1 (1935): pp. 9–10.

22. Bernard Asbell, *The Pill: A Biography of the Drug That Changed the World* (New York, 1995).

23. Brief 281, American Historians as Amici Curiae, Supporting Appellees, in Webster v. Reproductive Health Service, No. 88–605, Supreme Court of the United States, October Term, 1988, p. 22 (brief separately paged as pp. 1–31; pp. 339–369 in volume).

24. Ibid., p. 30.

25. *Roe v. Wade*, 410 U.S. 113, p. 165.

26. Ibid., pp. 117, 165.

27. Ibid., pp. 141–147.

28. Ibid., p. 160.

29. Ibid., p. 161.

30. Daniel Callahan, *Abortion: Law, Choice, and Morality* (New York, 1970), pp. 409–447.

31. From *Discorsi e radio messagi di Sua Santita Pio XII 13.415*, November 26, 1951, in T. J. O'Donnell, "Abortion, II (Moral Aspect)," *New Catholic Encyclopedia* (New York, 1967) 1: 29.

32. *Roe v. Wade*, 410 U.S. 113, pp. 174–177; see also Phillip A. Rafferty, *Roe v. Wade: The Birth of a Constitutional Right*, 2 vols. (Ann Arbor: University Microfilms, 1992) 1: 9, 251–253; and Mark Tushnet, "The Supreme Court on Abortion: A Survey," in *Abortion, Medicine, and the Law*, 3d ed., ed. J. Douglas Butler and David F. Walbert (New York: Facts on File Publications, 1986), p. 167.

33. *Roe v. Wade*, 410 U.S. 113, pp. 154, 162–166.

34. Tushnet, "Supreme Court," pp. 161–177; Hans Lotstra, *Abortion: The Catholic Debate in America* (New York: Irvington Publishers, 1985), pp. 32–36; Michael Tooley, *Abortion and Infanticides* (Oxford, 1983), pp. 87–302.

35. Stephen M. Krason and William B. Hollberg, "The Law and History of Abortion: The Supreme Court Refuted," in *Abortion, Medicine, and the Law*, 3d ed., ed. J. Douglas Butler and David F. Walbert (New York, 1986), pp. 196–225 at 197.

36. *Roe v. Wade*, 410 U.S. 113, pp. 201–202.

37. Ibid., p. 160: "Viability is usually placed at about seven months (28 weeks) but may occur earlier, even at 24 weeks." The Court was conscious of a return to "Aristotelian theory of 'mediate animation.' " (See also p. 160.) On the law in the post–*Roe v. Wade* period, see Butler and Walbert, *Abortion, Medicine, and the Law.*

38. A number of science writers published favorable reviews in various newspapers, and I wrote an article summarizing the thesis for the *American Scientist* (80 [1992]: 226–233]), the second-largest science journal in the United States.

39. Bruce W. Frier, "Natural Fertility and Family Limitation in Roman Marriage," *Classical Philology* 89 (1994): 318–333.

40. A. J. Coale and T. J. Trussell, "Model Fertility Schedules: Variations in Age Structure of Childbearing in Human Populations," *Population Index* 44 (1974): 185–258; and "Technical Note: Finding the Two Parameters That Specify a Model Schedule of Marital Fertility," *Population Index* 44 (1978): 203–213.

41. Colin Newell, *Methods and Models in Demography* (New York, 1988), p. 35.

42. *Taber's Cyclopedic Medical Dictionary*, 16th ed. (Philadelphia, 1989).

1. A Woman's Secret

1. *Aucassin and Nicolette*, 6.

2. Emmanuel Le Roy Ladurie, *Montaillou: The Promised Land of Error*, trans. Barbara Bray (New York, 1978), p. 157.

3. Vatican Ms. lat. 4030, fol. 43va.

4. Norman Edwin Himes, *Medical History of Contraception* (Baltimore, 1936); Emmanuel Le Roy Ladurie, "Demographie et 'funestes secrets' le Languedoc (fin XVIIIe–début XIXe siècle)," in *Le territoire de l'historien*, 2 vols. (Paris, 1973), 1: pp. 316–330.; Angus McLaren, *Birth Control in Nineteenth-Century England* (New York, 1990); John E. Knodel and Etienne van de Walle, "Lessons from the Past: Policy Implications of Historical Fertility Studies," *Population and Development Review* 5 (1979): 217–245 at 227; Ansley Coale, "The Demographic Transition Reconsidered," in *International Population Conference, Liège* 1 (1973): 53–72 at 54, quoting and accepting Frank Notestein.

5. As cited in Chapter 8.

6. Colin McEvedy and Richard Jones, *Atlas of World Population History* (New York, 1978), p. 21; contrary to most demographers, McEvedy and Jones regard the fourteenth century as the only period of *global* population decline, but this does not mean that regions such as Europe could not have experienced declines.

7. Josiah C. Russell, *The Control of Late Ancient and Medieval Population* (Philadelphia, 1985), p. 36; and "Population in Europe, 500–1500," in *The Fontana Economic History of Europe*, ed. Carlo M. Cipolla (Sussex and New York, 1976), 25–70 at 39; for slightly different but generally similar data, see McEvedy and Jones, *World Population*, pp. 21–24.

8. See the recent account by Joel E. Cohen, *How Many People Can the Earth Support?* (New York, 1995), pp. 32–42.

9. Plato, *Laws*, 5.740 (Trevor J. Saunders trans., 1970).

10. Plato, *Theaetetus*, 149c–d (Harold North Fowler trans., 1952).

11. Polybius, *Histories*, 36.17.5–12.

12. Aristotle, *Politics*, 7.16.15.1335b19–26.

13. Musonius, *Fragments*, 15a (Keith Hopkins, ed., *Classical Quarterly* 15 [1965]: 72–74).

14. David Herlihy, "The Tuscan Town in the Quattrocentro: A Demographic Profile," *Medievalia et humanistica* n.s. 1 (1970): 81–109 at 96; and "The Population of Verona in the First Century of Venetian Rule," in *Renaissance Venice*, ed. J. Hale (London, 1973), pp. 113–114. The average life span for the friars of Santa Maria Novella declined from 31.78 years in the period 1276–1300 to 26.51 in 1376–1400, according to Herlihy and Christiane Klapisch-Ziber, *Tuscans and Their Families* (New Haven, 1985), p. 85.

15. Herlihy, "Verona," pp. 101, 113.

16. Barbara Hanawalt, *The Ties That Bound: Peasant Families in Medieval England* (New York, 1986), p. 229; late sixteenth and early seventeenth century parish records show roughly between 8 and 15 percent of the population over sixty.

17. Russell, *Late Ancient and Medieval Population*, pp. 146–148.

18. Ibid., pp. 146–147; for a recent discussion of reproductive rates in a quasi-stable population, see Jean Bourgeois-Pichat, *La dynamique des populations: Populations stables, semi-stables et quasi-stables* (Paris, 1994), pp. 169–190, 249.

19. R. S. Bagnall and Bruce Frier, *The Demography of Roman Egypt* (Cambridge, England, 1994), pp. 138–139. The authors follow the methodology suggested by Colin Newell, *Methods and Models in Demography* (New York, 1988), and the model by Coale and Russell cited in note 40 to the "Introduction," above. Another estimate of constant population size is "no more than 30 percent of all married couples must have families of 4 or more children" (see Coale, "Demographic Transition," p. 59).

20. Bagnall and Frier, *Demography of Roman Egypt*, p. 145; see also Newell, *Methods and Models in Demography*, pp. 38–44.

21. H. W. F. Saggs, *The Might That Was Assyria* (London, 1984), pp. 137–138.

22. Bruce W. Frier, "Natural Fertility and Family Limitation in Roman Marriage," *Classical Philology* 89 (1994): 318–333.

23. Russell, *Late Ancient and Medieval Population*, p. 147.

24. Richard R. Ring, "Early Medieval Peasant Households in Central Italy," *Journal of Family History* 4 (1979): 2–21 at 12; Barbara C. Beuys, *Familienleben in Deutschland: neue Bilder aus der deutschen Vergangenheit* (Reinbeck, 1980), p. 72 (reporting 2.4 per family in Fulda); Gunnar Heinsohn and Otto Steiger, "The Elimination of Medieval Birth Control and the Witch Trials of Modern Times," *International Journal of Women's Studies* 5 (1982): 193–214 at 195.

25. Herlihy, "Verona," pp. 110–111.

26. Ibid.

27. Danielle Jacquart and Claude Thomasset, *Sexuality and Medicine in the Middle Ages* (Princeton, 1988), p. 134.

28. Herodotus (*Histories* 1.61.1) believed that Peisistratus anally penetrated his wife to avoid children; for the Assyrian sources on the same, see Gwendolyn Leick, *Sex and Eroticism in Mesopotamian Literature* (London, 1944), pp. 218–219; on perverse practices as a means of birth control, see Philippe Ariès, "Sur les origines de la contraception en France," *Population* 8 (1953): 465–472 at 467; and, in general, Michel Foucault, *Histoire de la sexualité* (Paris, 1984).

29. On infanticide, see Richard C. Trexler, "The Foundlings of Florence, 1395–1455," *History of Childhood Quarterly* 1 (1973): 259–284; Yves Brissaud, "L'infanticide à la fin du moyen âge, ses motivations psychologiques et sa repression," *Revue historique de droit français et étranger* 50 (1972): 229–256; Barbara Kellum, "Infanticide in England in the Later Middle Ages," *History of Childhood Quarterly* 1 (1973–74): 367–388; Russell, *Late Ancient and Medieval Population*, p. 222; Peter C. Hoffer and N. E. H. Hull, *Murdering Mothers: Infanticide in England and New England* (New York, 1981). Hanawalt, *Ties That Bound*, and Bagnall and Frier, *Demography of Roman Egypt*, pp. 151–153, disparage the idea that infanticide had much influence on population size.

30. Russell, *Late Ancient and Medieval Population*, p. 222; Brissaud, "L'infanticide," p. 251, n. 91; Kellum, "Infanticide in England," p. 367.

31. See the references cited and the novel theory presented by Vern Bullough and C. Campbell, "Female Longevity and Diet in the Middle Ages," *Speculum* 55 (1980): 317–325.

32. Hanawalt, *Ties That Bound*, pp. 101–103.

33. I say people did both despite an assertion made by Knodel and van de Walle ("Lessons," pp. 219, 226–7) that premodern people may have engaged in some birth control for premarital situations but did not limit family size after marriage; see also Frier, "Natural Fertility," pp. 318–319.

34. Doubt about the accuracy of estimating ancient life spans is expressed by Tim G. Parkin, *Demography and Roman Society* (Baltimore, 1992).

35. Bagnall and Frier, *Demography of Roman Egypt*, pp. 84, 90.

36. D. Gentry Steele and Claud A. Bramblett, *The Anatomy and Biology of the Human Skeleton* (College Station, Texas, 1988), p. 203.

37. Judy Myers Suchey et al., "Analysis of Dorsal Pitting in the Os Pubis in an Extensive Sample of Modern American Females," *American Journal of Physical Anthropology* 51 (1979): 517–540 at 517–523.

38. I say "family size" not unmindful of distinguishing between total fertility rates and family limitation but rather because I assume that most births were within families. Lacking other plausible reasons, I concluded that family limitation was necessary for the aggregate results.

39. Ariès, "Origines de la contraception," p. 465.

40. Ansley Coale, basing his argument on Louis Henry's work, distinguishes between parity-specific limitation ("folk methods, such as withdrawal, or more modern techniques, such as condoms, diaphragms, IUDs, or pills")— Henry's "controlled fertility"—and non-parity-specific limitation (reliance on behavioral methods, such as celibacy and restraint, and the natural decrease in fertility for a period after giving birth)—Henry's "natural fertility." Ansley J. Coale, "The Decline of Fertility in Europe since the Eighteenth Century as a Chapter in Demographic History," in *The Decline of Fertility in Europe*, ed. Ansley J. Coale and Susan Cotts Watkins (Princeton, 1986), 1–30 at 9; Louis Henry, "Some Data on Natural Fertility," *Eugenics Quarterly* 8 (1961): 81–91. Coale (p. 44) concedes that some populations may have discovered and used from time to time effective birth-control techniques only for its practitioners "to die out."

41. Dioscorides, *De materia medica*, 1.185 (Max Wellmann ed., in 3 vols.); Nosher N. Dastur, "Milk-Clotting Enzymes from Plants," *Indian Farming* 9 (1949): 451–453, cited in *Chemical Abstracts* 46 (1949): 2706.

42. Dastur, "Milk-Clotting Enzymes," pp. 451–453; Torald Sollmann, *A Manual of Pharmacology and Its Applications to Therapeutics and Toxicology*, 8th ed. (Philadelphia, 1957), p. 230.

43. Dioscorides, *De materia medica*, 1.185.

44. Norman R. Farnsworth, Audrey S. Bingel, Geoffrey A. Cordell, Frank A. Crane, and Harry H. S. Fong, "Potential Value of Plants as Sources of New Antifertility Agents," *Journal of Pharmaceutical Sciences* 64 (1975): 552 [pt. 1: 535–598; pt. 2: 717–754]; Adelina de S. Matsui, Somsong Hoskin, Midori Kashiwagi, Bonnie W. Aguda, Barbara E. Zegart, T. R. Norton, and W. C. Cutting, "A Survey of Natural Products from Hawaii and Other Areas of the Pacific for an Antifertility Effect in Mice," *Internationale Zeitschrift für klinische Pharmakologie, Therapie und Toxikologie* 1 (1971): 65–69 at 66.

45. Vatican Ms. lat. 4030, fol. 43vb.

46. Emmanuel Le Roy Ladurie, *Montaillou: village occitan de 1294 à 1324* (Paris, 1975), pp. 248–249; Jean Duvernoy, ed., *Inquisition Pamiers, interrogatoires de Jacques Fournier, 1318–1325*, 2 vols. (Paris, 1965), 1: 280–281.

47. Vatican Ms. lat. 4030, fol. 43vb.

48. Marbode of Rennes, *De lapidibus*, No. 43, p. 80 (Riddle ed.).

49. Helen Rodinte Lemay, *Pseudo-Albertus: Women's Secrets; A Translation of Pseudo-Albertus Magnus'* De secretis mulierum *with Commentaries* (Albany, 1992).

50. Pseudo-Albertus, *De secretis mulierum*, pp. 74, 76, 78 (Lemay ed.).

51. Ibid., p. 138.

52. Ibid.

53. Ibid.

54. Ibid., p. 140.

55. *Useful Plants of India*, "Wealth of India" series (New Delhi, 1986), p. 544; C. D. Casey, "Alleged Anti-fertility Plants of India," *Indian Journal of Medical Sciences* 14 (1960): 590–600 at 597; R. N. Chopra, S. L. Nayar, and I. C. Chopra, *Glossary of Indian Medicinal Plants* (New Delhi, 1956), p. 220; for recent discoveries in chemistry, see Z. Darmati, R. M. Jankov, Z. Vujcic, J. Csanadi, E. Svirtlih, A. Dordevic, and K. San, "Natural Terpenoids Isolated from the Grown Variety of Sage," *Journal of the Serbian Chemical Society* 58 (1993): 515–523.

56. Audrey Eccles, *Obstetrics and Gynaecology in Tudor and Stuart England* (Kent, Ohio, 1982), p. 58.

57. Paul Schauenberg and Ferdinand Paris, *Guide to Medicinal Plants*, trans. Maurice Pugh-Jones (New Canaan, Conn., 1977), p. 257; Julia Morton, *Atlas of Medicinal Plants of Middle America: Bahamas to Yucatan* (Springfield, 1981), p. 781; G. F. Asprey and Phillis Thornton, "Medicinal Plants of Jamaica," *West Indian Medical Journal* 4 (1953–55): 69–82, 145–468 at 81.

58. Vatican Ms. lat. 4030, fol. 37vb.

59. Albertus, *De animalibus*, 9.1.3 (Stadler ed., 15: 687); cf. Luke Demaitre and Anthony A. Travill, "Human Embryology and Development in the Works of Albertus Magnus," in *Albertus Magnus and the Sciences: Commemorative Essays 1980*, ed. James A. Weisheipl (Toronto, 1980), 405–440 at 427.

60. Aristotle, *On the Generation of Animals*, 2.3.736b27–28.

61. Albertus, *De animalibus*. 16.1.11 (Stadler ed., 15: 1094); cf. discussion in Pamela M. Huby, "Soul, Life, Sense, Intellect: Some Thirteenth-Century Problems," in *The Human Embryo: Aristotle and the Arabic and European Traditions*, ed. G. R. Dunstan (Exeter, 1990), 113–122 at 116.

62. Albertus, *De animalibus*, 16.1.11 (Stadler ed., 15: 1093–94.

63. Thomas, *Summa Theologica*, Ia.118.1–2 (M. J. Charlesworth ed.).

64. Huby, "Soul, Life," pp. 120–121.

65. Burchard, *Decretum*, 17.57 *(Patrologiae Cursus Completus . . . Series Latina*, 140: 933).

66. Albertus, *De vegetabilibus, libri VII*, 6.2.2, 273, 278 (Jessen ed.).

67. Farnsworth et al., "Potential Value of Plants," p. 736; A. Sharaf and N. Goma, "Phytoestrogens and Their Antagonism to Progesterone and Testosterone," *Journal of Endocrinology* 31 (1965): 289–290; James Duke, *Handbook of Medicinal Herbs* (Boca Raton, 1985), p. 375.

68. Henry De Laszlo and Paul S. Henshaw, "Plants Used by Primitive Peoples to Affect Fertility," *Science* 119 (1954): 626–631 at 627; V. J. Brondegaard, "Contraceptive Plant Drugs," *Planta Medica* 23 (1973): 167–172 at 168; Farnsworth et al., "Potential Value of Plants," p. 542; L. Palma, *Le piante medicinale d'Italia: botanica, chimica, farmacodinamica, terapia* (Rome, 1964), p. 166; J. C. Saha, E. C. Savini, and S. Kasinathan, "Ecobolic Properties of Indian Medicinal Plants," *Indian Journal of Medical Research* 49 (1961): 132, 150; L. T. Angeles et al., "Toxicity Studies on Aristolochic Acid Isolated from *Aristolochia tagala* Cham.," *Acta Medica Philippina* 6 (1970): 139–148; Yun Cheung Kong, Jing-Xi Xie, and Paul Pui-Hay But, "Fertility Regulating Agents from Traditional Chinese Medicines," *Journal of Ethnopharmacology* 15 (1986): 1–44 at 5–6.

69. Albertus, *De vegetabilibus, libri VII*, 6.1.16, 85.

70. I am aware that a controversy exists about whether "Trotula" was a woman, as legend so ascribes. For my purposes it is enough to know that in the Middle Ages it was believed Trotula was a female. Trotula's writings influenced patients who believed the legend, and that is sufficent fact upon which to proceed.

71. Trotula, *Gynaecology*, in *Gynaeciorum hoc est De mulierum tum aliis*, ed. Conrad Gesner and Caspar Wolf (Basel, 1566), cols. 222–223.

72. *Aemilius Macer De herbarum virtutibus cum Joannis Atrocian commentariis* ([Basel], 1530), fol. 1. The poem is usually attributed to a person called Macer but I have argued elsewhere that the author is Marbode.

73. Peter of Spain [Petrus Hispanus *or* Johanness XXI], *Thesaurus Pauperum* (Frankfurt, 1578), fol. 66v.

2.   The Herbs Known to the Ancients

1. Papyrus Ebers, in *Papyros Ebers das hermetische Buch über die Arzneimittel der alten Ägypter in hieratischen Schriften*, trans. George Ebers (Leipzig, 1875).

2. Ebers 783.

3. Kahun, No. 21, 22 [3,7], in *Grundriss der Medizin der alten Ägypter*, ed. Hildegard von Deines, Herman Graprow, and Wolfhart Westendorf, 7 vols. (Berlin, 1954–1962), vol. 4, pt. 1, p. 277; note pt. 2, p. 211; vol. 5, p. 477.

4. K. Gopinath and K. Raghunathan, "Historical Significance of Contraception," *Bulletin of the Indian Institute for the History of Medicine* 15 (1985): 17–45 at 22–23.

5. Adelina de S. Matsui, Somsong Hoskin, Midori Kashiwagi, Bonnie W. Aguda, Barbara E. Zegart, T. R. Norton, and W. C. Cutting, "A Survey of Natural Products from Hawaii and Other Areas of the Pacific for an Antifertility Effect in Mice," *Internationale Zeitschrift für klinische Pharmakologie, Ther-*

apie und Toxikologie 1 (1971): 65–69 at 67–68; Norman R. Farnsworth, Audrey S. Bingel, Geoffrey A. Cordell, Frank A. Crane, and Harry H. S. Fong, "Potential Value of Plants as Sources of New Antifertility Agents," *Journal of Pharmaceutical Sciences* 64 (1975): 535–598 (pt. 1), 717–754 (pt. 2), at 550, 565.

6. R. L. Bardhwar, I. C. Chopra, and S. L. Nayar, "Reputed Abortifacient Plants of India," *Indian Journal of Agricultural Science* 16 (1946): 342–355 at 348.

7. Varro E. Tyler, Lynn R. Brady, and James E. Robbers, *Pharmacognosy*, 9th ed. (London, 1981), pp. 191–192.

8. Soranus, *Gynaecology*, 1.60.

9. Soranus, *Gynaecology*, 1.61–63 (Temkin trans. with modifications).

10. Loren C. MacKinney, "Medical Ethics and Etiquette in the Early Middle Ages: The Persistence of Hippocratic Ideals," *Bulletin of the History of Medicine* 26 (1952): 1–31; Oswei Temkin, *Hippocrates in a World of Pagans and Christians* (Princeton, 1991) p. 252; for other evidence, see that presented in subsequent chapters of this volume.

11. L. Edelstein, "The Hippocratic Oath: Text, Translation and Interpretation," in *Ancient Medicine*, Oswei Temkin and C. Lilian Temkin, eds. (Baltimore, 1967); Charles Lichtenthaeler, *Der Eid des Hippokrates: Ursprung und Bedeutung* (Cologne, 1984).

12. Scribonius, *Compositiones*, Praef., 5.20–23.

13. Soranus, *Gynaecology*, 1.60.

14. Ibid.

15. Theodorus Priscianus, *Euporiston*, 3.6 (Rose ed., pp. 240–241).

16. Hesiod, *Work and Days*, 513.

17. See references, John M. Riddle, *Contraception and Abortion from the Ancient World to the Renaissance* (Cambridge, Mass., 1992), pp. 25–26, 32–33, 51–53, 57, 88–89, 94–97, 102, 120, 126, and 132.

18. Iraq Museum, Baghdad, and described by Friedrich Muthmann, *Der Granatapfel: Symbol des Lebens in der alten Welt* (Bern, 1982), p. 13.

19. Louvre, Paris, Inv. S. 1208 (Bj.2169), described by Muthmann, *Granatapfel*, pp. 35–38.

20. Athens National Museum 484 and reproduced in Jane Harrison, *Prolegomena to the Study of Greek Religion* (London, 1961), p. 275. Harrison (p. 274) believes that Demeter and Persephone are combined in one representation.

21. For numerous other examples of the use of pomegranate in association with fertility, see Muthmann, *Granatapfel*.

22. Ibn Sīnā, *Liber canonis*, ii.2.578 (translated from Arabic by Meyerhof, in Norman Edwin Himes, *Medical History of Contraception* [Baltimore, 1936], pp. 142–143; Latin translation by Gerard of Cremona, *Avicenna: Canon* [Venice, 1507], fol. 146v).

23. Adolf Butenandt and H. Jacobi, "Über die Darstellung eis krystallisierten pflanzlichen Tokokinins (Thelykinins) und seine Identifizierung mit dem α-Follikelhormon," *Zeitschrift für physiologische Chemie* 218 (1933): 104–112.

24. Eric Heftmann, Shui-Tze Ko, and Raymond D. Bennett, "Identification of Estrone in Pomegranate Seeds," *Phytochemistry* 5 (1966): 1337–1339.

25. H. W. Bennetts, E. J. Underwood, and F. L. Shier, "A Specific Breeding Problem of Sheep on Subterranean Clover Pastures in Western Australia," *Australia Veterinary Journal* 22 (1946): 2–12; see also John R. Lacey, Lynn F. James, and Robert E. Short, *The Ecology and Economic Impact of Poisonous Plants on Livestock Production* (Boulder, Colo., 1988).

26. Heftmann et al., "Estrone in Pomegranate," pp. 1337–1339; P. D. G. Dean, D. Exley, and T. W. Goodwin, "Steroid Oestrogens in Plants: Reestimation of Oestrone in Pomegranate Seeds," *Phytochemistry* 10 (1971): 2215–2216.

27. M. L. Gujral, D. R. Varma, and K. N. Sareen, "Oral Contraceptives. Part I: Preliminary Observations on the Antifertility Effect of Some Indigenous Drugs," *Indian Journal of Medical Research* 48 (1960): 46–51 at 50.

28. Anand O. Prakash, "Potentialities of Some Indigenous Plants for Antifertility Activity," *International Journal of Crude Drug Research* 24 (1986): 19–24 at 21, 23.

29. Anand O. Prakash et al., "Anti-implantation Activity of Some Indigenous Plants in Rats," *Acta Europaea Fertilitatis* 16 (1985): 441–448 at 447.

30. J. J. Segura, L. H. Morales-Ramos, J. Verde-Star, and D. Guerra, "Inhibicion del orecimiento de *Entamoeba histolytica* y *E. invandens* producida por la raiz del granado (*Punica granatum* L.)," *Archivos Investigacion Medica* 21 (1990): 235–239.

31. Yūhannā ibn Sarafyun (Serapion), *De simplicibus medicinis*, in *Practica* (Lyon, 1525), fol. 140r&v.

32. *Knights*, 893–894; another comment about its high cost is found in Plautus, *Plutus*, 4.

33. Theophrastus, *Enquiry*, 6.3.3.; Hippocrates, *De morbis*, 2.4.3.

34. Soranus, *Gynaecology*, 1.63.

35. Dioscorides, *De materia medica*, 3.48, 80; Pliny, *Natural History*, 22.48.100.

36. Pliny, *Natural History*, 19.15.40–41.

37. Synesius, *Letters*, 106, 135 (A. Fitzgerald trans., 1926, pp. 202, 228); on the history of the plant, see Alfred C. Andrews, "The Silphium of the Ancients: A Lesson in Crop Control," *Isis* 33 (1941–42): 232–236; Chalmers L. Gemmill, "Silphium," *Bulletin of the History of Medicine* 40 (1966): 295–313; John M. Riddle and J. Worth Estes, "Oral Contaceptives in Ancient and Medieval Times," *American Scientist* 80 (1992): 226–233.

38. Prakash, "Potentialities of Indigenous Plants."

39. M. M. Singh et al., "Contraceptive Efficacy and Hormonal Profile of Ferujol: A New Coumarin from *Ferula jaeschkeana*," *Planta Medica* 51 (1985): 268–270.

40. Farnsworth et al., "Potential Value of Plants," pp. 554, 590.

41. Ibid., p. 576; J. C. Saha, E. C. Savini, and S. Kasinathan, "Ecobolic Properties of Indian Medicinal Plants," *Indian Journal of Medical Research* 49 (1961): 136.

42. Bamberg Ms med. 1, fol. 17 (in Ulrich Stoll, ed., *Das 'Lorscher Arzneibuch,'* Sudhoffs Archiv, vol. 20 [Stuttgart, 1992], p. 103; see p. 459 for identification of *lasar* with asafetida); also, I have found in manuscripts of drug substitutes that asafetida is the substitute for *silphium*.

43. Aristophanes, *Lysistrata*, 87–89 (Rogers trans.).

44. D. Thomassen, J. T. Slattery, and S. D. Nelson, "Menthofuran-dependent and Independent Aspects of Pulegone Hepatotoxicity: Roles of Glutathione," *Journal of Phamacology and Experimental Therapy* 253, no. 2 (1990): 567–572; D. Thomassen, P. G. Pearson, J. R. Slattery, and S. D. Nelson, "Partial Characterization of Biliary Metabolites of Pulegone by Tandem Mass Spectrometry Detection of Glucuronide Glutathione and Glutathionyl-glucuronide Conjugates," *Drug Metabolism and Disposition* 19 (1991): 997–1003; O. Froelich and T. Shibamato, "Stability of Pulegone and Thujone in Ethanolic Solution," *Journal of Agricultural and Food Chemistry* 38 (1990): 2057–2560; W. P. Gordon, A. C. Huitric, C. L. Seth, R. H. Mc-Clanahan, and S. D. Nelson, "The Metabolism of the Abortifacient Terpene, (R)-(+)-Pulegon, to a Proximate Toxin, Menthofuran," *Drug Metabolism and Disposition* 15 (1987): 589–594.

45. John B. Sullivan, Jr., Barry H. Rumack, Harold Thomas, Jr., Robert G. Peterson, and Peter Bryson, "Pennyroyal Oil Poisoning and Hepatotoxicity," *Journal of the American Medical Association* 242 (1979): 2873–2874; W. P. Gordon, A. J. Forte, R. J. McMurtry, J. Gal, and S. D. Nelson, "Hepatoxity and Pulmonary Toxicity of Pennyroyal Oil and Its Constituent Terpenes in the Mouse," *Toxicology and Applied Pharmacology* 65 (1982): 413–424.

46. See Dioscorides, *De materia medica*, 3.113; see also Helen Lemay, "Women and the Literature of Obstetrics and Gynecology," in *Medieval Women and the Sources of Medieval History*, ed. Joel T. Rosenthal (Athens, Ga., 1990), p. 194.

47. James Duke, *Handbook of Medicinal Herbs* (Boca Raton, 1985), p. 66; Farnsworth et al., "Potential Value of Plants," p. 549; B. Weniger, H. Haag-Berrurier, and R. Anton, "Plants of Haiti Used as Antifertility Agents," *Journal of Ethnopharmacology* 6 (1982): 67–84 at 73–74.

48. Nimmi Chandhoke, "Scoparone: Effect of Reproductive Processes in Rats," *Indian Journal of Experimental Biology* 17 (1979): 740–742.

49. Riddle and Estes, "Oral Contraceptives," p. 231.

50. Jessica Kerr, *Shakespeare's Flowers* (New York, 1969), p. 50.

51. Yun Cheung Kong, C. P. Lau, K. H. Wat, K. H. Ng, P. P. H. But, K. F. Cheng, and P. G. Waterman, "Antifertility Principle of *Ruta graveolens*," *Planta Medica* 55 (1989): 176–178; see also Farnsworth et al., "Potential Value of Plants," p. 572; B. N. Dhawan and P. N. Saxena, "Evaluation of Some Indigenous Drugs for Stimulant Effect on the Rat Uterus: A Preliminary Report," *Indian Journal of Medical Research* 46 (1958): 808–811.

52. Yun Cheung Kong, Jing-Xi Xie, and Paul Pui-Hay But, "Fertility Regulating Agents from Traditional Chinese Medicines," *Journal of Ethnopharmacology* 15 (1986): 1–44].

53. *Merck Index* (1960), p. 818.

54. George A. Conway and John C. Slocumb, "Plants Used as Abortifacients and Emmenagogues by Spanish New Mexicans," *Journal of Ethnopharmacology* 1 (1979): 241–261 at 247–248; Farnsworth et al., "Potential Value of Plants," p. 576.

55. M. O. Guerra and A. T. L. Andrade, "Contraceptive Effects of Native Plants in Rats," *Contraception* 2 (1974): 191–199.

56. M. M. Sharma, G. Lal, and D. Jacob, "Estrogenic and Pregnancy Interceptory Effects of Carrot *Daucus carota* Seeds," *Indian Journal of Experimental Biology*, 14 (1976): 506–508.

57. B. B. Kaliwal, R. Nazeer Ahamed, and M. Appaswomy Rao, "Abortifacient Effect of Carrot Seed *(Daucus carota)* Extract and Its Reversal by Progesterone in Albino Rats," *Comparative Physiology and Ecology* 9 (1984): 70–74; B. B. Kaliwal and R. Nazeer Ahamed, "Maintenance of Implantation by Progesterone in Carrot Seed *Daucus carota* Extracted Treated Albino Rats," *Indian Journal of Physical and Natural Sciences*, Section A7 (1987): 10–14.

58. This information was related to me by Mary Reichle, a public health nurse. She says that she has other clients who report its use. Since then I have received reports of women in Virginia and Tennessee who use Queen Anne's lace seeds for contraception.

59. Hippocrates, *De mulierum affectibus*, 1.78 (Littré ed., 8: 184, 15–18).

60. Dioscorides, *De materia medica*, 3.72; Scribonius, *Compositiones*, 121 (Sconocchia ed., p. 64); Marcellus, *De medicamentis*, 20.33 (Niedermann ed., pt. 2, 340); Pliny, *Natural History*, 26.90.157.

61. Pliny, *Natural History*, 29.27.85.

62. Ibid., 25.64.112.

63. There are various versions of the story, some of which have Myrrha being the recipient of Aphrodite's spell and the agressor with her father. Marcel Detienne (*The Gardens of Adonis: Spices in Greek Mythology*, trans. Janet Lloyd [Atlantic Highlands, N.J., 1977; French ed., 1972], pp. 1–4, 60–66) interprets the myth's meaning as the association of perfumes, sweet smells, and

seductive power. While I accept her association, I see more than that in the story.

64. Myrrh is mentioned elsewhere in the New Testament: anointing the body of Jesus (John 19:39), in connection with its use in embalming; and in a drink with wine before the cross (Mark 15:23), as an anodyne.

65. Dioscorides, *De materia medica*, 1.64.

66. Mieczaslaw Mazur et al., "Pharmacology of Lupanine and 130 Hydroxylupanine," *Acta Physiologiae Polononica* 17, no. 2 (1966): 299–309 (*Chemical Abstracts*, 65 [1966]: 11163q); P. I. Sizov, "Experimental Parturifacient Action of Pachycarpine Brevicolline and Thalictrimine," *Zdravookhranenie Belorusii* 15 (1969): 44–6 (*Chemical Abstracts* 72 [1970]: 119957u); Farnsworth et al., "Potential Value of Plants," p. 566.

67. A. K. Reynolds, "Uterine Stimulants," *The Alkaloids*, 5 (1955): 163–209 at 178–179.

68. Hippocrates, *De mulierum affectibus*, 1.78 (Littré ed, 8: 188, 18–21); Pliny, *Natural History*, 26.90.154; Galen, *De simplicium medicamentorum temperamentis ac facultatibus*, 9.18.30–31 (Kuhn ed., 12:127).

69. See references to works of al-Razi (Rhases) in B. F. Musallam, *Sex and Society in Islam: Birth Control before the Nineteenth Century* (Cambridge, 1983), p. 77; and Najib al-Din Muhammad ibn 'Ali Samarquandi, *The Medical Formulary*, trans. Martin Levy and Noury al-Khalady (Philadelphia, 1967), pp. 333–334.

70. Trotula, *Gynaecology*, in *Gynaeciorum hoc est De mulierum tum aliis*, ed. Conrad Gesner and Caspar Wolf (Basel, 1566), col. 223.

71. Arnald de Villanova [pseudo], *Breviarum practice*, 3.7, in *Articella* (Venice, 1483).

72. R. Claeson, R. Aandersson, and G. Samuelson, "T-cadinol, a Pharmacological Active Constituent of Scented Myrrh: Introductory Pharmacological Chacterization and High Field 1H- and 3C-NMR Data," *Planta Medica* 57 (1992): 352–356; Pier Dolara et al., "Analgesic Effects of Myrrh," *Nature* 379 (1996): 29.

73. Hippocrates, *De mulierum affectibus*, 1.78 (Littré ed., 8: 178, 11–14).

74. Dioscorides, *De materia medica*, 4.150; Galen, *De simplicium medicamentorum*, 8.18.15 (Kühn ed., 12: 122); Mustio, *Pessaria* (Rose ed., pp. 123–125).

75. Oribasius, *Euporistes*, 2.1.3 (Daremberg-Bussemaker, eds., 5: 635); Paul of Aegina, *Epitomae medicae*, 7.3 s.v. (Heilberg ed., 2: 209, 11.6–7).

76. Pseudo-Apuleius, *Herbarius*, 114 (Howald and Sigerist, eds., p. 199).

77. Farnsworth et al., "Potential Value of Plants," p. 549.

78. Pliny, *Natural History*, 24.11.18.

79. Dioscorides, *De materia medica*, 1.77.

80. Galen, *De simplicium medicamentorum*, 6.2.15 (Kühn ed., 11: 854).

81. N. Pages, G. Fournier, G. Chamorro, M. Salazar, M. Paris, and C. Boudene, "Teratological Evaluation of *Juniperus sabina* Essential Oil in Mice," *Planta Medica* 55 (1989): 144–146.

82. Duke, *Handbook of Medicinal Herbs*, pp. 256–257.

83. Prakash et al., "Anti-implantation Activity," pp. 441, 447; Prakash, "Potentialities of Indigenous Plants," p. 23.

84. Riddle, *Contraception and Abortion*, pp. 9–12.

85. For example, Galen, *De remediis parabilibus*, 2.020 (Kühn ed., 14: 480–481), but aloe is not a named antifertility drug in Dioscorides (*De materia medica*, 3.22).

86. Theodorus, *Euporiston*, 3.6 (Rose ed., 241–244).

87. Aëtius, *Biblia iatrika*, 16.17 (Zervòs ed., pp. 18–19).

88. Saha, Savini, and Kasinathan, "Ecobolic Properties," pp. 149–150.

89. S. K. Bhargava, "Antifertility Agents from Plants," *Filoterapia* 59 (1988): 163–177 at 166.

90. Pliny, *Natural History*, 26.90.153.

91. Wolfgang Jöchle, "Menses-Inducing Drugs: Their Role in Antique Medieval and Renaissance Gynecology and Birth Control," *Contraception* 10 (1974): 425–439 at 434.

92. Won Sick Woo et al., "Antifertility Principle of *Dictamnus albus* Root Bark," *Planta Medica* 53 (1987): 399–401.

93. Hippocrates, *De mulierum affectibus*, 1.78 (Littré ed., 8: 180, 14–18).

94. Dioscorides, *De materia medica*, 3.32; Thomas Oswald Cockayne, *Leechdoms, Wortcunning and Starcraft of Early England*, 3 vols. (1864; reprinted London, 1965), 1: 164–169.

95. Aspasia through Aëtius, *Biblia iatrika*, 16.18 (Zervòs ed., p. 22).

96. Ibn Sarafyun [Serapion], *De simplicium medicamentorum* (Venice, 1552), 1 (fol. 8).

97. Galen, *De sanitate tuenda*, 1.36 (Kühn ed., 6: 446). For citations and interpretations on the chaste tree, see Heinrich von Staden, "Spiderwoman and the Chaste Tree: The Semantics of Matter," *Configurations* 1 (1992): 23–56.

98. Galen, *De locis affectis*, 6.6 (Kühn ed., 8: 439).

99. Von Staden, "Spiderwoman and the Chaste Tree," p. 41.

100. *Hymn to Hermes*, 409–413, through von Staden, "Spiderwoman and the Chaste Tree," pp. 44–45.

101. Von Staden, "Spiderwoman and the Chaste Tree," p. 45.

102. For example, Dioscorides, *De materia medica*, 1.103; Hippocrates, *De mulierum affectibus*, 1.79 (Littrè ed., 8: 184, 2–5).

103. C. D. Casey, "Alleged Anti-fertility Plants of India," *Indian Journal of Medical Sciences* 14 (1960): 590–600 at 594; V. P. Kamboj and B. N. Dhawan, "Research on Plants for Fertility Regulations in India," *Journal of Ethnopharmacology* 6 (1982): 191–226 at 192.

104. S. K. Bhargava, "Estrogenic and Pregnancy Interceptory Effects of the Flavoids [VI–VII) of *Vitex negundo* L. Seeds in Mice," *Plantes médicinales et phytothérapie* 18 (1984): 74–79 at 78.

105. S. K. Bhargava, "Antiandrogenic Effects of a Flavonoid-rich Fraction of *Vitex negundo* Seeds: A Histological and Biochemical Study in Dogs," *Journal of Ethnopharmacology* 27 (1989): 327–339 at 338; also Bhargava, "Antifertility Effects of the Flavonoids (VI–VII) of *Vitex negundo* L. Seeds in Dogs," *Plantes médicinales et phytothérapie* 20 (1986): 188–198.

106. Von Staden, "Spiderwoman and the Chaste Tree," pp. 47–48.

107. Ibid., p. 40.

108. Jacques Gélis, *History of Childbirth, Fertility, Pregnancy and Birth in Early Modern Europe* (Boston, 1991), p. 29.

109. Henry De Laszlo and Paul S. Henshaw, "Plants Used by Primitive Peoples to Affect Fertility," *Science* 119 (1954): 626–631 at 627; V. J. Brøndegaard, "Contraceptive Plant Drugs," *Planta Medica* 23 (1973): 167–172 at 168; Farnsworth et al., "Potential Value of Plants," p. 542.

110. L. Palma, *Le piante medicinale d'Italia: botanica, chimica, farmacodinamica, terapia* (Rome, 1964), p. 166; Saha, Savini and Kasinathan, "Ecobolic Properties," pp. 132, 150; L. T. Angeles et al., "Toxicity Studies on Aristolochic Acid Isolated from *Aristolochia tagala* Cham.," *Acta Medica Philippina* 6 (1970): 139–148.

111. Kamboj and Dhawan, "Research on Plants," pp. 194, 206.

112. Saha, Savini, and Kasinathan, "Ecobolic Properties," p. 150.

113. Kong, Xie, and But, "Fertility Regulating Agents," pp. 5–6; W. H. Wang and J. H. Zheng, "The Pregnancy Terminating Effect and Toxicity of an Active Constituent of *Aristolochia mollissima* Hance, Aristolochic Acid α" [in Chinese], *Yao Hsueh Pao* 19 (1984): 405–409; Chung-Tao Che et al., "Studies on Aristolochia III: Isolation and Biological Evaluation of Constituents of *Aristolochia indica* Roots for Fertility-Regulating Activity," *Journal of Natural Products* 47 (1984): 331–341.

114. Dioscorides, *De materia medica*, 3.7.

115. Galen, *De antidotis*, 2.1 (Kühn ed., 14: 109–110).

116. Petrus Maranchus, *Tabula* (in Salvatore DeRenzi, ed., *Storia documentata della scuola di Salerno* [Naples, 1852–59], 4: 564) calling it an "earth apple"; Abu l-Fadl Dawud ibn Abi l-Bayan al-Isra'ili, *Al-Dustur al-bimaristani fi l-adwiya al-murakkada*, 8.124 (trans. José Luis Valverde Carmen Peña Muñoz, in *El formulario de los hospitales de ibn Abi l-Baya* [Granada, 1981], p. 87).

117. Farnsworth et al., "Potential Value of Plants," p. 542; de Laszlo and Henshaw, "Plants Used by Primitive Peoples," p. 627; and Brøndegaard, "Contraceptive Plant Drugs," p. 168.

118. Dioscorides, *De materia medica*, 1.10.

119. Hildegard, *Physica*, 4, in *Patrologiae Cursus Completus . . . Series Latina*, ed. J. P. Migne (Paris, 1879–1890), 197: 1148, calling it by its German name, Haselwurtz.

120. Serapion, *De simplicium medicamentorum*, 1 (fol. 8).

121. Dioscorides, *De materia medica*, 3.134.

122. R. S. R. Murthy, D. K. Basu, and V. V. S. Murti, "Anti-implantation Activity of Isoadiantone," *Indian Drugs* 21, no. 4 (1984): 141–144, reported through *Chemical Abstracts* Ca 101(3): 17582t.

123. Dioscorides, *De materia medica*, 4.184; Al-Razi cited by Musallam, *Sex and Society in Islam*, p. 77; Pliny, *Natural History*, 27.17.34, 55.80.

124. Kong, Xie, and But, "Fertility Regulating Agents," p. 22.

125. Brøndegaard, "Contraceptive Plant Drugs," p. 168.

126. Kong, Xie, and But, "Fertility Regulating Agents," p. 16.

127. George Usher, *A Dictionary of Plants Used by Man* (London, 1974), p. 260.

128. *Dispensatory of the United States of America*, 25th ed. (Philadelphia, 1955), pp. 121–122; Kong, Xie, and But, "Fertility Regulating Agents," p. 16.

129. William of Saliceto, *Summa conservationis et curationis* (Venice, 1502), chap. 175.

130. Hildegard, *Physica*, 47 (Migne ed., 197: 1148).

131. Boleslaw, "An Oestrogenic Substance from Plant Material," *Nature* 131 (1933): 766; Skarzynski, "Recherches sur les corps oestrongènes d'origine végétale," *Zoologischer Bericht* 35 (1933): 323 [abstracts of paper].

132. Guerra and Andrade, "Contraceptive Effects of Native Plants," pp. 191–199; Prakash et al., "Anti-implantation Activity," pp. 447–448; see also J. B. Harborne, *Introduction to Ecological Biochemistry* (London, 1977), p. 85.

133. For example, Dioscorides, *De materia medica*, 1.104.

134. Aetius, *Biblaa iatrika*, 16.17.

135. Constantine, *De gradibus*, in *Opera* (Basel, 1536), p. 358.

136. Oribasius, *Book of Eunapius*, 4.114.777–778 (Raeder ed., 6/3: 489–489).

137. Dioscorides, *De materia medica*, 1.81; Aetius, *Biblia iatrika*, 16.17.

138. Galen, *De compositione medicamentorum secundum locus*, 9.4 (Kühn ed., 13: 283–284); Pliny, *Natural History*, 24.37.56–58 (willow); 24.32.47 (poplar).

139. Dioscorides, *De materia media*, 1.4; Oribasius, *Synopsis ad Eunapium*, 2.53 (Daremberg-Bussemaker ed., 5: 68; Raeder ed., 6/3: 43); Macer, *Herbarius*, in *Aemilius Macer De herbarum virtutibus cum Joannis Atrociani Commentarius* (Basel, 1530), fol. 76v; William of Saliceto, *Summa*, chap. 163 (fol. 60 r&v).

140. A. Dini, E. Ramundo, P. Saturnino, A. Scimone, and Stagno d'Alcontres, "Isolation, Characterization and Antimicrobial Activity of Coumarian Derivatives from *Cyperus incompletus*," *Bollettin società italiana di biologia sperimentale* 68 (1992): 453–460; Farnsworth et al., "Potential Value of Plants," p. 735.

141. P. Arenas and R. Moreno Azorero, "Plants Used as Means of Abortion, Contraception, Sterilization and Fecundation by Paraguayan Indigenous People," *Economic Botany* 31 (1977) 302–306 at 304.

142. Dini et al., "Coumarian Derivatives from *Cyperus incompletus,*" p. 453.

143. Aretino, *Dialogues* (Raymond Rosenthal trans., New York, 1971), p. 85.

144. Macer, *De herbarum virtutibus,* fol. 75v.

145. Farnsworth et al., "Potential Value of Plants," pp. 539, 550 (with references).

146. Hippocrates, *De mulierum affectibus,* 1.78 (Littré ed., 8:184).

147. Duangta Kanjanapothi et al., "Postcoital Antifertility Effect of *Mentha arvensis,*" *Contraception* 24 (1981): 559–567.

148. Kapoor, Garg, and Mathur, "Antiovulatory Activity," pp. 1225–1227; Bhargava, "Antifertility Agents from Plants," p. 168.

149. Berlin 192 (Rs. I, 2–20), in von Deines, Graprow, and Westendorf, *Grundriss der Medizin der alten Ägypter,* vol. 4, pt. 1, p. 277; pt. 2, pp. 211–221; vol. 5, p. 478; and Lise Manniche, *An Ancient Egyptian Herbal* (Austin, 1989), pp. 76, 152.

150. Casey, "Alleged Anti-fertility Plants," p. 592; R. R. Chaudhury, "Plants with Possible Antifertility Activity," *Indian Council for Medical Research: Special Reports Series* 55 (1966): 4, 14; J. M. Watt and M. G. Breyer-Brandwijk, *The Medicinal and Poisonous Plants of Southern and Eastern Africa,* 2d ed. (Edinburgh, 1962), p. 1033.

151. Farnsworth et al., "Potential Value of Plants," p. 554.

152. B. B. Sharma et al., "Antifertility Screening of Plants. Part I: Effect of Ten Indigenous Plants on Early Pregnancy in Albino Rats," *International Journal of Crude Drug Research* 21 (1983): 183–187 at 185.

3.   Ancient and Medieval Beliefs

1. Plato, *Theaetetus,* 149c–d (Fowler trans.).

2. Hippocrates, *On Generation,* 5.1.

3. Aristotle, *Historia animalium,* 8.1.21–38 [608a–b]; cf. G. E. R. Lloyd, *Science, Folklore and Ideology* (Cambridge, 1983), pp. 98–99.

4. Hippocrates, *Regimen,* 1.28.

5. Diogenes Laertius, *Lives,* 2.26.

6. Plato, *Laws,* 5.740.

7. Plato, *Charmides,* 157b.

8. Aristotle, *Politics,* 7.14.10.1335b.

9. Plato, *Charmides,* 155e.

10. Peter V. Taberner, *Aphrodisiacs: The Science and the Myth* (Philadelphia, 1985).

11. Qustā ibn Lūqā, "On Physical Ligatures," 1995.

12. Dioscorides, *De materia medica,* 1.93.

13. Arthur Osol et al., eds., *Dispensatory of the United States of America,* 25th

ed. (Philadelphia, 1955), p. 1710; R. Ullsperger, "Die Entwicklung der Crataegusforschung," *Planta Medica* 1 (1953): 43–50; A. S. Abdul-Ghani, R. Amin, and M. S. Suleiman, "Hypotensive Effect of *Crataegus oxyacantha*," *International Journal of Crude Drug Research* 25 (1987): 216–220.

14. Dan Bensky and Andrew Gamble, *Chinese Herbal Medicine Materia Medica* (Seattle, 1986), p. 320.

15. *Grundriss der Medizin der alten Ägypter*, ed. Hildegard von Deines, Herman Graprow, and Wolfhart Westendorf, 7 vols. (Berlin, 1954–1962), vol. 4, pt. 1, p. 277.

16. J. C. Pangas, "Notas sobre el aborto en la antigua Mesopotamia," *Aula orientalis* 7 (1990): 213–218 at 214–215.

17. R. Campbell Thompson, *A Dictionary of Assyrian Botany* (London, 1949), p. 315.

18. See Mott T. Greene, *Natural Knowledge in Preclassical Antiquity* (Baltimore, 1992), pp. 125 ff.; Mary Kilbourne Matossian, *Poisons of the Past: Molds, Epidemics, and History* (New Haven, 1989).

19. Robert D. Biggs, "Ergotism and Other Mycotoxicoses in Ancient Mesopotamia," *Aula Orientalis* 11 (1991): 15–21 at 20.

20. Ibid.

21. Marie Delcourt, *Stérilité mystérieuses & naissances maléfiques dans l'antiquité classique* (Liège, 1938).

22. H. W. F. Saggs, *The Might That Was Assyria* (London, 1984), p. 138.

23. *Ancient Near Eastern Texts Related to the Old Testament*, 2d ed., ed. J. B. Pritchard (Princeton, 1955), p. 525 (hereinafter cited as *ANET*).

24. Hammurabi, *Laws*, 209–214 (Pritchard ed., p. 162).

25. Law 50 (*ANET*, p. 184).

26. Ibid.

27. *Babylonia Laws* (Driver and Miles ed., 1: 313).

28. For a review of the ancient West Asian laws, see Stephen D. Ricks, "Abortion," in *Anchor Bible Dictionary* 1 (1992): 31–32.

29. Ibid., p. 31; *ANET*, pp. 525 (Sumerian Laws 4.1–2), 181, 184–185 (Middle Assyrian 50).

30. Ricks, "Abortion," p. 31; Emiel Eyben, "Family Planning in Graeco-Roman Antiquity," *Ancient Society* 11 (1980–1981): 81 ff.

31. *Hittite Laws*, 1.17–18 (*ANET*, p. 180).

32. Elaine Adler Goodfriend, "Prostitution (OT)," in *Anchor Bible Dictionary* 5 (1992): 505.

33. W. H. House, "Miscarriage or Premature Birth: Additional Thoughts on Exodus 21: 22–25," *Westminister Theological Journal* 41 (1978–79): 108–123.

34. Ibid., pp. 117–120; Meredith G. Kline, "*Lex talionis* and the Human Fetus," *Journal of the Evangelical Theological Society* 20 (1977): 194–201; for other references, see Ricks, "Abortion," p. 32.

35. Daniel B. Sinclair, "The Legal Basis for the Prohibition on Abortion in Jewish Law," *Israel Law Review* 15 (1980): 109–130 at 112–113.

36. For example, *TB Bava Kamma* 78a; *Sanhedrin* 80b (Epstein trans., 3: 535), and elsewhere; see D. Feldman, *Birth Control in Jewish Law: Marital Relations, Contraception, and Abortion as Set Forth in the Classic Texts of Jewish Law* (New York, 1968), p. 253.

37. Arguments summarized and referenced in *Anchor Bible Dictionary* 1 (1992): 31–32.

38. Sinclair, "Legal Basis."

39. Feldman, *Birth Control in Jewish Law*, p. 254.

40. Immanuel Jakobovits, "Jewish Views on Abortion," in *Jewish Bioethics*, ed. Fred Rosner and J. David Bleich (New York, 1979), p. 120; Feldman, *Birth Control in Jewish Law*, pp. 255–257.

41. Sinclair, "Legal Basis," p. 111.

42. *Sanhedrin* 72b (Babylonian Talmud, Epstein trans., *Seder Nazikin*, 3: 494).

43. John T. Noonan, Jr., *Contraception: A History of Its Treatment by the Catholic Theologians and Canonists*, enlarged ed. (Cambridge, Mass., 1986), p. 33.

44. *Yebamoth* 62b (Babylonia Talmud, Epstein trans., *Seder Nashim*, 1: 426–427); *Yebamot* 6:6 (Jerusalem Talmud, vol. 21, Neusner trans.); see also Fred Rosner, "Contraception in Jewish Law," in Rosner and Bleich, *Jewish Bioethics*, p. 89.

45. For example, Genesis 1:22, 15:5, 22:17, 9:1, 26:4, 16:10; Deuteronomy 7:13–14; Ruth 4:11; Job 1:2, 42:13.

46. Noonan, *Contraception*, p. 32; on mutual pleasure, see Rosner, "Contraception in Jewish Law," p. 90.

47. Rosner, "Contraception in Jewish Law," pp. 91 ff.; Jakobo-vits, "Jewish Views on Abortion," pp. 120–122.

48. *Yebamoth* 12b (Babylonia Talmud, Epstein trans., *Seder Nashim*, 1: 62).

49. Although Feldman, *Birth Control in Jewish Law* (p. 170), says wool or cotton.

50. Rosner, "Contraception in Jewish Law," p. 94.

51. *Niddah* 3a–3b (Epstein ed., *Tohoroth*, 1: 10).

52. *Yebamoth* 65b (Babylonian Talmud, Epstein ed., *Seder Nashim*, 1/3: 436–437).

53. *Yebamoth*, 8.4; on meaning of *ikarin*, see Marcus Jastrow, *A Dictionary of the Targumim, the Talmud Babli and Yershalmi, and the Midrashic Literature*, 2 vols. (New York, 1903), 2: 1074. I am grateful to Samuel Levin and to Josef Statzmiller for assistance in translating this passage. The translation by Noonan (*Contraception*, p. 51) incorrectly says that a woman *is* permitted to take the drug. For a discussion of the Talmudic passage, see Feldman, "Birth Control in Jewish Law," pp. 235–244.

54. *Yebamoth*, 65b.

55. Rosner, "Contraception in Jewish Law," p. 93; Feldman, *Birth Control in Jewish Law*, pp. 240–243.

56. Dioscorides, *De materia medica*, 4.14.

57. *Jasher*, 20 (Goldschmidt ed., *Sepher Hajaschar* [Berlin, 1923]). I am grateful to C. Dailey for calling my attention to this passage and to Samuel Kottek for the Hebrew translation into English.

58. Plato, *Republic*, 5.9 (460e).

59. Hesiod, *Work and Days*, 375.

60. Richard Feen, "Abortion and Exposure in Ancient Greece: Assessing the Status of the Fetus and 'Newborn' from Classical Sources," in *Abortion and the Status of the Fetus*, ed. William B. Bonderson et al. (Dordrecht, 1983), p. 287; William Harris, "The Theoretical Possibility of Extensive Infanticide in the Graeco-Roman World," *Classical Quarterly* 32 (1982): 114–116; Donald Engels, "The Problem of Female Infanticide in the Greco- Roman World," *Classical Philology* 75 (1980): 112–120; Engels, "The Use of Historical Demography in Ancient History," *Classical Quarterly* 34 (1984): 386–389; another form of infanticide, ritual sacrifice, is discussed by Aline Rouselle, *Porneia: On Desire and the Body in Antiquity* (Oxford, 1988), pp. 107–121.

61. Claudius Aelian, *Varia historia*, 2.7 (Mervin Dilts ed., pp. 19–20); translated by Feen, "Abortion and Exposure," p. 289 [citation in error].

62. Yves Brissaud, "L'infanticide à la fin du moyen âge, ses motivations psychologiques et sa repression," *Revue historique de droit français et étranger* 50 (1972): 229–256.

63. See references in Enzo Nardi, *Procurato aborto nel mondo greco romano* (Milan, 1971).

64. Hippocrates, *Epidemics*, 5.53.

65. Nancy Demand, *Birth, Death, and Motherhood in Classical Greece* (Baltimore, 1994), p. 58.

66. M. Moïssidés, "Contribution à l'étude de l'abortement dans l'antiquité grecique," *Janus* 26 (1929): 59–85.

67. Tertullian, *A Treatise on the Soul*, 25 (Holmes trans., in *Ante-Nicene Fathers: Translation of the Writings of the Fathers Down to A.D. 325*, ed. A. Roberts and J. Donaldson, 10 vols. [Grand Rapids, Mich., 1950–], 3: 206).

68. Hippocrates, *On the Nature of the Child*, 13 (Lonie trans., pp. 325–326).

69. Aristotle, *Politics*, 7.14.10 (1335b).

70. Demand, *Birth, Death, and Motherhood*, pp. 55–57, 103–107.

71. See P. Prioreschi, "Quandoque bonus dormitat Hippocrates: Induced Abortion and Embryos' Age in the Hippocratic Corpus," *Acta belgicae historicae medicinae* 5, no. 4 (1992): 181–184; and Demand, *Birth, Death, and Motherhood*.

72. [Pseudo-]Galen, *An animal sit quod est in utero*, 5 (Kühn ed., 19: 179).

73. Eyben, "Family Planning," p. 21 (with references to various opinions).

74. Fragments of Aelius Theon and Soprato as printed by Nardi, *Procurato aborto*, pp. 82–83, 87–88.

75. Demand, *Birth, Death, and Motherhood*, p. 61.

76. Homer, *Odyssey*, 14.426.

77. Plato, *The Republic*, 4.435–442.

78. Stanley W. Jackson, "Galen—On Mental Disorders," *Journal of the History of Behavioral Sciences* 5 (1969): 365–384 at 367; Walter Riese, "Introduction," in *Galen On the Passions and Errors of the Soul*, trans. Paul W. Harkins (Columbus, Ohio, 1963), pp. 15–16.

79. Aristotle seems to suggest the gender-staged development; see Feen, "Abortion and Exposure," pp. 293–294, based on *Generation of Animals*, 736a–b, and various passages in *Politics*; see also Wolfgang Jöchle, "Menses-Inducing Drugs: Their Role in Antique Medieval and Renaissance Gynecology and Birth Control," *Contraception* 10 (1974): 425–439 at 426.

80. Aistotle, *Historia animalium*, 7.1 (588b).

81. Pindar, Fragment 133.3 (Maehler ed., 2: 119).

82. Jan Bremmer, *The Early Greek Concept of the Soul* (Princeton, 1983).

83. For a background on the pre-Galenic views regarding the soul's connection with the body, see Heinrich von Staden, *Herophilus: The Art of Medicine in Early Alexandria* (Cambridge, 1989).

84. Francisziek Sokolowski, *Lois sacrées des cités grecques* (Paris, 1955), no. 115, p. 189.

85. Philo, *Special Laws*, 3.108–9 (F. H. Colson trans., 7: 545).

86. Jakobovits, "Jewish Views on Abortion," p. 130; Feldman, "Birth Control in Jewish Law," pp. 65, 258–262.

87. Josephus, *Jewish Antiquities*, 4.278.

88. Josephus, *Against Apion*, 2.202; cf. Feldman, "Birth Control in Jewish Law," pp. 258–259.

89. Francisziek Sokolowski, *Lois sacrées de l'asie mineure* (Paris, 1955), no. 20, pp. 553–555.

90. Porphyry, *To Gauros*, 1–2, through Feen, "Abortion and Exposure," p. 294.

91. Read with caution Michael Gorman, *Abortion and the Early Church: Christian, Jewish and Pagan Attitudes in the Greco-Roman World*, (Downers Grove, Ill., 1982), regarding Christian views; regarding pagan opinion, see Daniel Callahan, *Abortion: Law, Choice, and Morality* (New York, 1970), p. 410, who quotes Athenagoras' letter to Marcus Aurelius as saying, "all who use abortifacients are homicides and will account to God for their abortion as for the killing of men."

92. See Noonan, *Contraception*, esp. pp. 72–106; Joyce E. Salisbury, "The Latin Doctors of the Church on Sexuality," *Journal of Medieval History* 12 (1986): 279–289.

93. Plato, *Charmides*, 157b.

94. Noonan, *Contraception*, p. 91; see also *Didache* 2:2.

95. *Gospel of the Egyptians*, through Clement of Alexandria, *Stromata*, 3.66 (John Ferguson trans., 85: 297).

96. Ricks, "Abortion," pp. 31–34; Gorman, *Abortion and the Early Church*, pp. 47–62.

97. Samuel Laeuchli, *Power and Sexuality: The Emergence of Canon Law at the Synod at Elvira* (Philadelphia, 1972), p. 92.

98. Ibid., p. 47.

99. Athenagoras, *Embassy for the Christians*, in *Patrologiae Cursus Completus . . . Series Graeca*, ed. J. P. Migne, 161 vols. (Paris, 1857–1866), 6: 91); translated by John T. Noonan, Jr., in "Abortion and the Catholic Church: A Summary History," *Natural Law Forum* 12 (1967): 92.

100. Minucius, *Octavius*, 30:2, in *Corpus Scriptorum Ecclesiasticorum Latinorum*, ed. J. Zyche (Vienna and Prague, 1887–), 2: 43; Tertullian, *Apology*, 9.8, in *Corpus Scriptorum*, 69: 24.

101. Tertullian, *Apology*, 9 (Thelwall trans., 3: 25).

102. Clement of Alexandria, *Paedagogus*, 2.10.96.1.

103. Gorman, *Abortion and the Early Church*, p. 57.

104. Tertullian, *De anima*, 26.5 (P. Holmes trans., 3: 207).

105. Augustine, *Questiones Exodi*, 80.1439–1445 in *Corpus Christianorum: Series Latina* (Turnhout, 1958–), vol. 33, pt. 5.

106. Quoted in G. R. Dunstan, ed., *The Human Embryo: Aristotle and the Arabic and European Traditions* (Exeter, 1990), p. 44, citing Gregory's *Adversus Macedonianos*.

107. On Jewish interpretation, see *Yebamoth* 4:11, in *The Talmud* (Neusner trans., 21: 158–159).

108. Basil, *Epistolarum*, 188.2, in Migne, *Patrologiae Cursus Completus . . . Series Graeca*, 32: 671.

109. Ibid.

110. Angus McLaren, *History of Contraception from Antiquity to the Present* (Oxford, 1990), p. 48.

111. The most recent confirmation of an early age for marriage for females is found in R. S. Bagnall and Bruce Frier, *The Demography of Roman Egypt* (Cambridge, 1994), p. 136.

112. Ibid., p. 51.

113. Paul Veyne, "The Roman Empire," in *A History of Private Life*, vol. 1, ed. Paul Veyne (Cambridge, 1987), pp. 9–233; McLaren, *History of Contraception*, p. 44; among other sources who said that marriage was for procreation were Aulus Gelius (*Attic Nights*, 4.3) and Soranus (*Gynaecology*, 1.9.34).

114. Cicero, *Pro Marcello*, 8.

115. Polybius, *Histories*, 36.17.5.12.

116. Harris, "Theoretical Possibility of Extensive Infanticide," pp. 114–116.

117. Richard Duncan-Jones, *The Economy of the Roman Empire: Quantitative Studies* (Cambridge, 1974), pp. 294–300 (esp. 295n), 333–335.

118. P. A. Brunt, *Italian Manpower, 225 B.C.–A.D. 14* (London, 1971); Noonan, "Abortion and the Catholic Church," p. 88.

119. Translated by Keith Hopkins, "A Textual Emendation in a Fragment of Musonius Rufus," *Classical Quarterly* 15 (1965–66): 141, based on text in Musonius, Fragment 15a (Hopkins ed., pp. 72–74).

120. Juvenal, *Satires*, 6.595–596.

121. Lucretius, *De rerum natura*, 4.1277.

122. Jerome, *Letter* 22, *to Eustochium*, 13, in *Patrologiae Cursus Completus . . . Series Latina*, ed. J. P. Migne (Paris, 1879–1890), 22: 401.

123. Paulus, *Digest*, 48.19.38.5 (Scott trans., 11: 123).

124. Cicero, *Pro Cluentio*, 11.32; Paulus, *Digest*, 47.11.4; 48.8.8, 19.39.

125. Pseudo-Bede, *Order for Giving Penance*, 30; cited in Noonan, *Contraception*, p. 156.

126. See Eyben, "Family Planning," pp. 30–32.

127. L. Lewin, *Die Fruchtabtreibung durch Gifte und andere Mittel: Ein Handbuch für Ärtze und Juristen* (Berlin, 1922), p. 85.

128. *Lex Alamannorum*, 91, in Lewin, *Fruchtabtreibung*, p. 85.

129. C. S. F. Burnett, "The Planets and the Development of the Embryo," in Dunstan, *Human Embryo*, pp. 95–112 at 100, 102.

130. *Lex Bajuvariorum*, 7.18, in Lewin, *Fruchtabtreibung*, p. 86.

131. *Leges Visigothorum*, 6.3.1–7, in Lewin, *Fruchtabtreibung*, p. 87.

132. Burchard, *Decretum*, 19, in Migne, *Patrologiae Cursus Completus . . . Series Latina*, 140: 972); Pseudo-Bede, *Penitential*, 2.11 (see also Noonan, *Contraception*, p. 160).

133. Noonan, *Contraception*, p. 220.

134. Bamberg Ms med. 1, in Ulrich Stoll, ed., *Das 'Lorscher Arzneibuch,'* Sudhoffs Archiv, vol. 20 [Stuttgart, 1992], p. 116.

135. Paris BN Ms gr. 2179 (critical apparatus, Max Wellmann ed., *Dioscorides*, 3 vols. [Berlin, 1906–1914, reprint, 1958], 2: 59).

4.   From Womancraft to Witchcraft, 1200–1500

1. Dante, *Purgatorio*, 25.130–140 (Sinclair ed.); interpretation by John T. Noonan, Jr., *Contraception: A History of Its Treatment by the Catholic Theologians and Canonists*, enlarged ed. (Cambridge, Mass., 1986), p. 214; for Dante's views on birth control, see Stephen Bemrose, " 'Come d'animal divegna fante': The Animation of the Human Embryo in Dante," in *The Human Embryo: Aristotle and the Arabic and European Traditions*, ed. G. R. Dunstan (Exeter, 1990), pp. 123–135.

2. Chaucer, *Persones Tales*, 575–580.

3. *Leechbook*, nos. 237, 245–250, in Warren R. Dawson, *Leechbook or Collections of Medical Recipes of the Fifteenth Century; the Text of Ms no. 136 of the Medical Society of London* (London, 1934), pp. 89, 92–95.

4. Augustine, *Marriage and Concupiscence*, 1.15.17, in *Corpus Scriptorum Ecclesiasticorum Latinorum*, ed. Joseph Zyche (Vienna and Prague, 1887–), 42: 229–230.

5. Sylvie Laurent, *Naître au moyen age. Da la conception a la naissance: La gorssesse et l'accouchement (XIIe–XVe siècle)* (Paris, 1989), esp. pp. 150–167.

6. Noonan, *Contraception*, p. 95, citing Epiphanius, *Panarion* ("Medicine Chest"), 63.1.4. See also *Patrologiae Cursus Completus . . . Series Graeca*, 161 vols., ed. J. P. Migne (Paris, 1857–1866), 41: 1063.

7. Regino, *Church Disciplines*, 2.89, in *Patrologiae Cursus Completus . . . Series Latina*, 221 vols., ed. J. P. Migne (Paris, 1879– 1890), 132: 301; translated in Noonan, *Contraception*, p. 168.

8. James Brundage, "Concubinage and Marriage in Medieval Canon Law" (pp. 120–128), "Adultery and Fornication: A Study in Legal Theology" (pp. 129–143), and "Rape and Seduction in the Medieval Canon Law" (pp. 141–148) in *Sexual Practices and the Medieval Church*, ed. Vern L. Bullough and James Brundage (Buffalo, 1982).

9. Burchard, *Decretum*, in Migne, *Patrologiae Cursus Completus . . . Series Latina*, 140: 972.

10. For the medieval understanding of *maleficus, -a*, see Edward Peters, *The Magician, the Witch, and the Law* (Philadelphia, 1978), p. 68.

11. Noonan, *Contraception*, pp. 167–197.

12. For an understanding of how people in the Middle Ages viewed premature births and infants born dead and prior to baptism, see Pierre André Sigal, "La grossesse, l'accouchement et l'attitude envers l'enfant mort-né à la fin du moyen âge d' après les récits de miracles," in *Santé, médecine et assistance au moyen âge*, Actes du 110e Congrès National de Sociétes Savantes, Montpellier (Paris, 1987), pp. 23–35.

13. Peter Cantor, *Summa theologica*, III², 463–464, cited by Noonan, *Contraception*, p. 177.

14. John T. Noonan, Jr., "Abortion and the Catholic Church: A Summary History," *Natural Law Forum* 12 (1967): 104.

15. Ibid.

16. Frederick Pollock and Frederic William Maitland, *The History of English Law Before the Time of Edward I*, 2d ed., in 2 vols. (Cambridge, 1968), 1: 175–176; Ralph V. Turner, *The English Judiciary in the Age of Glanvill and Bracton, c. 1176–1239* (Cambridge, 1985), p. 239.

17. Bracton, *De legibus*, fol. 121 (Thorne ed. and trans., 2: 341).

18. *Fleta*, 1.23 (Richardson-Sayles, ed. 1, pp. 60–61; see also L. Lewin, *Die Fruchtabtreibung durch Gifte und andere Mittel: Ein Handbuch für Ärtze und Ju-*

risten (Berlin, 1922), p. 89; and Leonard Arthur Parry, *Criminal Abortion* (London, 1932), p. 95. *Fleta* was written in Latin by an unknown writer who sought to modernize Bracton by extending the legislation of Edward I.

19. *Fleta*, 1.23.

20. For tracing the concept of quickening in English thought, see Barbara Duden, *Disembodying Women: Perspectives on Pregnancy and the Unborn*, trans. Lee Hoinacke (Cambridge, Mass., 1993).

21. Year Book Mich. 1 Edward 3, on vol. 1, fol. 214, of Anthony Fitzherbert, *Le graunde abridgment . . .* , 2 vols. (London, 1577); see translation by Cyril C. Means, "The Phoenix of Abortional Freedom: Is a Prenumbral or Ninth-Amendment Right About to Arise from the Nineteenth-Century Legislative Ashes of a Fourteenth-Century Common-Law Liberty?" *New York Law Forum* 17 (1971): 335–410 at 337, based on text of earlier editions (1516, 1565). A translation from the Plea Roll, published by Phillip A. Rafferty, *Roe v. Wade: The Birth of a Constitutional Right*, 2 vols. (Ann Arbor, 1992), pp. 516–519, supplies the names of the people involved with various readings of Jane and John.

22. *Calendar of the Patent Rolls Preserved in the Public Record Office: Edward III, A.D. 1327–1330*, 16 vols. (London, 1891), 2: 113.

23. Means, "Phoenix of Abortional Freedom," p. 337.

24. Robert A. Destro, "Abortion and the Constitution: The Need for a Life-Protective Amendment," *California Law Review* 63 (1975): 1250–1351 at 1269–70.

25. Published by Rafferty, *Roe v. Wade*, 2: 519–520.

26. Year Book Mich., 22 Edw. 3, in Fitzherbert, *Le graunde abridgement*, 2: fol. 217, no. 263; translated by Means, "Phoenix of Abortional Freedom," p. 339, from earlier edition.

27. Translated and printed by Rafferty, *Roe v. Wade*, 2: 541.

28. Just. Itin., Somersetshire Roll 756, membrane 25d, no. 1243, published in *Somersetshire Pleas (Civil and Criminal)*, ed. Charles E. H. Chadwyck Healey, *Somerset Record Society Publications* 11 (1897): 321.

29. For example, see *Rex vs. Le Gaoeler* (Kent, 1279); *Pekering vs. Swynestone* (Kent, 1279); *Sorel vs. Hakeney* (London, 1276); *Orscherd vs. Trenchard et al.* (Wiltshire [?], 1230s or 1240s); *Merchant vs. Andvere* (1249); *Sauter vs. Ferur* (Gloucester, 1221); *Placita Corone de Comitatu Gloucestrie*, 69, in *Pleas of the Crown for the County of Gloucester . . . 1221)*, ed. F. W. Maitland (London, 1884), p. 16 [warrant for arrest in last two but their outcome not known]. See also discussion of these cases in Rafferty, *Roe v. Wade*, 2: 555–556, 559–560, 565–566, 569–570.

30. Harold N. Schneebeck, Jr., "The Law of Felony in Medieval England from the Accession of Edward I until the Mid-Fourteenth Century," Ph.D. diss., University of Iowa, Iowa City (1973), p. 234.

31. *Calendar of Inquisitions Miscellaneous (Chancery) Preserved in the Public Records Office (1399–1422)*, 16 vols. (London, 1968), no. 523, 7: 296.

32. London, Public Record Office, Eyre Rolls, Just. Itin. 1, Roll 369, membrane 36, Eyre of 1279 (7 Edw. 1); see also Schneebeck, "Law of Felony," p. 236.

33. London, Public Record Office, Just. Itin. 1, Roll 369, membrane 37d; Schneebeck, "Law of Felony," p. 238.

34. London, Public Record Office, Just. Itin. 1, Roll 186, membrane 3r, 9–10 Edw. 1, Eyre of 1281–2, Rochester Assize Rolls; Schneebeck, "Law of Felony," pp. 238–239.

35. Schneebeck, "Law of Felony," pp. 239–240; Rafferty, *Roe v. Wade*, 2: 551. The roll for the case (Just. Itin. 1, Roll 789, membrane 1; Eyre Rolls, Assize Rolls; Eyre of Hampshire, 1281) was missing from the Public Records Office when I was there in September 1995.

36. London, Public Record Office, Just. Itin. 1, Roll 112, membrane 9v, 7 Edw. 1, Eyre of 1279, Rots 46; see also Schneebeck, "Law of Felony," pp. 236–237.

37. Schneebeck, "Law of Felony," p. 241; Rafferty, *Roe v. Wade*, 2: 531, raises the question whether Maud was hanged for this offense but believes that she was. The document (London, Public Record Office, Just. Itin. 1, Roll 547a, membrane 20d) containing Maud's case was missing when I looked for it on September 4, 1995.

38. *R. vs. Ragoun* (London, 1321); *R. vs. Eppinge* (London, 1321); *R. vs. Scot* (London, 1321); *R. vs. Dada* (London, 1321); *R. vs. Hervy* (London, 1321); *R. vs. Mercer* (Oxford, 1285); *Swayne vs. Fuatard* (1230s or 1240s); see also discussion of these cases in Rafferty, *Roe v. Wade*, 2: 532–536, 549–550, 569; see also Schneebeck, "Law of Felony," pp. 240–242.

39. *R. vs. Cobbeham* (London, 1321); *R. vs. Godesman* (Kent, 1313); see also discussion of these cases in Rafferty, *Roe v. Wade*, 2: 535–537.

40. Andrew Horne, *The Mirrour of Justices Written Originally in the Old French, Long Before the Conquest; and Many Things Added* (Washington, 1903), 4.16, p. 209.

41. Britton, *Britton: An English Translation and Notes*, ed. Francis Morgan Nichols (Washington, 1901), 1.45.7, pp. 95–96.

42. Although Schneebeck, "Law of Felony," p. 241, presents two cases in which women accused of causing an abortion were acquitted: Just. Itin. 1, Roll 1011, membrane 56 (Wilts., p. 1289); Just Itin. 1, Roll 383, membranes 18d., 96 (Kent, 1312–13), where the same case is recorded both in the crown pleas division and the jail delivery division of the Eyre roll.

43. *Placita Corone*, no. 69, p. 16.

44. Mesue (the Younger), *Opera medicinalis* (Venice, 1484), fols. 199v–200.

45. B. F. Musallam, *Sex and Society in Islam: Birth Control before the Nineteenth Century* (Cambridge, 1983), p. 54.

46. B. F. Musallam, "The Human Embryo in Arabic Scientific and Religious Thought," in Dunstan, *Human Embryo*, pp. 36–43.

47. The subject is well treated by Mussalam, *Sex and Society.*

48. Michael Scot, *De secretis mulierum libellus* (Strassbourg, 1615), p. 52.

49. Raymond Lull, *De secretis naturae sive quinta essentia libri duo* (Venice, 1542), pp. 63–64.

50. Ibid., pp. 72–73.

51. Michael R. McVaugh, *Medicine Before the Plague: Practitioners and Their Patients in the Crown of Aragon, 1285–1345* (Cambridge, 1993), pp. 113, 121, 127, 135, although McVaugh sees physicians and surgeons as having a somewhat "live-and-let-live" attitude toward irregular medical providers.

52. Haly Abbas [Abu'l 'Ali- ibn 'Abbas], *Pantegni* (Venice, 1515), pt. 2, fol. 1; published under the name of Isaac Israeli.

53. Ibid., pt. 2, fol. 57.

54. Ibid., pt. 2, fol. 69.

55. Ibid., pt. 2, fol. 84.

56. Translated from Arabic by Max Meyerhof, in Himes, *Medical History of Contraception* (Baltimore, 1936), pp. 142–143.

57. Avicenna, *Canon*, 3.21.1, chaps. 9–11 (on contraception) and 12–14 (on abortion).

58. Helen Lemay, "William of Saliceto on Human Sexuality," *Viator* 12 (1981): 165–181.

59. [Pseudo-]Arnald, *Breviarum practice*, 3.6, in *Articella* (Venice, 1483).

60. Platearius, *Circa instans, ad passim*, in *Das Arzneidrogenbuch Circa instans*, ed. Hans Wölfel (Berlin, 1939).

61. See references in Chalmers L. Gemmill, "Silphium," *Bulletin of the History of Medicine* 40 (1966): 295–313 at 307.

62. *Antidotarium Nicolai*, fols. 263vb, in Mesue, *Opera*. Queen Anne's lace is called *daucus creticus*, according to medieval usage; see Hermann Fischer, *Mittelalterliche Pflanzenkunde* (Munich, 1929), p. 267.

63. Nicholaus of Salerno, *Antidotarium* (1471 ed.; no pagination provided but by count, pp. 24, 39, 57); reproduced in fascimile in Dietlinde Goltz, *Mittelalterliche Pharmazie und Medizin* (Stuttgart, 1976), pp. 145–147.

64. Ibid., p. 65.

65. Ibid., p. 67.

66. Gundolf Keil, "magister giselbertus de villa parisiensi: Beobachtungen zu den Kranewittbeeren und Gilberts pharmakologischen Renommé," *Sudhoffs Archiv* 78 (1994): 80–89 at 87.

67. ADBR 56 H 955, fols. 6–8, published by Joseph Shatzmiller, ed., *Médecine et justice en Provence médiévale: Documents de Moanosque, 1262–1348* (Provence, 1989), pp. 80–83; discussed by Joseph Shatzmiller, *Jews, Medicine, and Medieval Society* (Berkeley, 1994), p. 84.

68. Gerd Dähn, "Zur Geschichte des Abtreibungsverbots," in *Das Abtrei-*

bungsverbot des § StGB: Eine Vorschrift, die mehr schadet als nützt, ed. Jürgen Bauman (Neuwied, 1971), 329–339 at 333.

69. Christina Larner, *Enemies of God: The Witch-hunt in Scotland* (Baltimore, 1981), p. 94.

70. Carolyn Merchant, *The Death of Nature: Women, Ecology, and the Scientific Revolution* (San Francisco, 1979), p. 138.

71. Wolfgang Behringer, *Hexenverfolgung in Bayern: Volksmagie, Glaubenseifer und Staatsräson in der Frühen Neuzeit* (Munich, 1988), p. 52.

72. Francesco-Maria Guazzo, *Compendium maleficarum* (Milan, 1608), 2.4; trans. Montague Summers (London, 1929), p. 92.

73. Henry Boguet, *An Examen of Witches Drawn from Various Trials* (New York, 1971), p. 88.

74. Heinrich Kramer and James Sprenger, *Malleus Maleficarum* (1487), 1.6; trans. Montague Summers (New York, 1971), p. 41.

75. Ibid., pp. 47 *et passim*; cf. Gunnar Heinsohn and Otto Steiger, *Die Vernichtung der weisen Frauen: Beiträge zur Theorie und Geschichte von Bevölkerung und Kindheit* (Herbstein, 1985), pp. 77–78; Gregory Zilboorg, *The Medical Man and the Witch during the Renaissance* (New York, 1969), pp. 37–38; Selma R. Williams, *"Riding the Nightmare": Women and Witchcraft from the Old World to Colonial Salem* (New York, 1978), pp. 35–45.

76. Barbara Ehrenreich and Deirdre English, *Witches, Midwives, and Nurses: A History of Women Healers* (Old Westbury, N.Y., 1973), p. 10, summarize witch crimes in three categories: female sexuality, magical powers affecting health, and possession of various medical and obstetrical skills.

77. Jean Bodin, *De la démonomanie des sorciers* (Paris, 1580), and discussed by Gunnar Heinsohn and Otto Steiger, "Inflation and Witchcraft: The Case of Jean Bodin Reconsidered," paper first presented at *Det fjärde nordisak forskarmötet om ekonomisk idè historia* (Aabo, Finland, October 10–13, 1996), 48 pp. An abridged French version will be published in Jean-Michel Servet, ed., *L'oeuvre de Jean Bodin 1596–1996* (Lyon: Centre Walras, 1997), forthcoming.

78. Margaret Alic Murray, *The Witch-cult in Western Europe: A Study in Anthropology* (Oxford, 1921), p. 170.

79. Alan Macfarlane, *Witchcraft in Tudor and Stuart England: A Regional and Comparative Study* (New York, 1970), pp. 97–98.

80. Richard Kieckhefer, *European Witch Trials: Their Foundations in Popular and Learned Culture, 1300–1500* (Berkeley, 1976), p. 96.

81. Silvia Bovenschen, "The Contemporary Witch, the History Witch and the Witch-Myth," *New German Critique* 15 (1978): 83–119 at 92; reprinted in Brian Levack, *Witchcraft, Women and Society* (New York, 1992), pp. 131–167.

82. Rosemary Ruether, "The Persecution of Witches: A Case of Sexism and Agism?" *Christianity and Crisis* 34 (1974): 291–295, argues that the persecution of witches was discrimination against both women and the aged.

83. Lyndal Roper, *Oedipus and the Devil* (London, 1994), pp. 1–3.

84. Soranus, *Gynaecology*, 1.2.4.

85. Thomas Forbes, *The Midwife and the Witch* (New Haven, 1966), p. 127.

86. H. C. Erik Midelfort, *Witch-Hunting in Southwestern Germany, 1562–1684: The Social and Intellectual Foundations* (Stanford, 1972), pp. 172, 195.

87. Dähn, "Zur Geschichte des Abtreibungsverbots," p. 333.

88. Jean Bodin, *The Six Books of a Commonwealth* (English translation of 1606; reprinted in fascimile by Harvard University Press, 1962), p. 571.

89. Heinsohn and Steiger, "Bodin Reconsidered."

90. Manfred Hammes, *Hexenwahn und Hexenprozesse* (Frankfurt am Main, 1977), p. 62, whose context suggests that the city was Cologne; I was unable to verify these figures from Hammes's apparent source: Wilhelm G. Soldan-Soldan, *Geschichte der Hexenprozesse*, 2 vols. (Munich, [1912]), 2: 17–20. These pages have a list of witches burned in Würzburg, but 1: 537 and 554 discuss a connection between witches and midwives.

91. Larner, *Enemies of God*, p. 101.

92. Williams, *"Riding the Nightmare,"* p. 135.

93. Carol F. Karlsen, *The Devil in the Shape of a Woman: Witchcraft in Colonial New England* (New York, 1989), pp. 40, 142.

94. Henry Charles Lea, *A History of the Inquisition of the Middle Ages*, 3 vols. (New York, 1888); Joseph Hansen, *Quellen und Untersuchungen zur Geschichte des Hexenwahns und der Hexenverfolgung im Mittelalter* (reprint of 1901 ed., Hildesheim, 1963); Hansen, *Zauberwahn, Inquisition und Hexenprozess im Mittelalter und die Entstehung der grossen Hexenverfolgung* (Aalen, 1964).

95. Louis Ginzberg, *The Legends of the Jews*, trans. Henrietta Szold, 4 vols. (Philadelphia, 1909), 1: 65–66; Williams, *"Riding the Nightmare,"* p. 76. Talmudic references to Lilith are: *Nid.* 24b; *B. Bat.* 73a; *Sabb.* 151b; *'Erub*, 100b.; see other ancient references in Lowell K. Handy, "Lilith," *Anchor Bible Dictionary* 4 (1992): 324–325.

96. Kramer and Sprenger, *Malleus maleficarum*, 1.11 (Summers trans., p. 66).

97. Kramer and Sprenger, *Malleus maleficarum*, 1.8 (Summers trans., pp. 54–55); Lea, *History of the Inquisition*, 1: 144–146, 240, 256, 262, 269, 274–275 et passim; Ginzburg, "Witches' Sabbat," pp. 188–189.

98. Guazzo, *Compendium maleficarum*, 2.3 (Summer trans., p. 90).

99. Kramer and Sprenger, *Malleus maleficarum*, 1.8 (Summers trans., p. 55).

100. Lea, *Materials* 1: 231.

101. Ibid., 1: 240 et passim; for example, the first Irish witch, Alice Kyteler (d. 1324), was accused of boiling the brains and clothes of a boy who died without baptism. See L. S. Davidson and J. O. Ward, *The Sorcery Trial of Alice Kyteler: A Contemporary Account (1324)* (Binghampton: Medieval and Renaissances Texts and Studies, 1993), p. 63.

102. Reginald Scot, *Discoverie of Witchcraft* (fascimile repr. of London ed., 1584, New York, 1971) 2. 9, p. 33.

103. Richard C. Trexler, "Infanticide in Florence: New Sources and First Results," *History of Childhood Quarterly* 1 (1973): 98–116 at 103; and Trexler, "The Foundlings of Florence, 1395–1455," *History of Childhood Quarterly* 1 (1973): 259–284.

104. See Alan C. Kors and Edward Peters, *Witchcraft in Europe, 1100–1700: A Documentary History* (Philadelphia, 1972), pp. 93–97.

105. Quoting from Forbes, *Midwife and the Witch*, p. 120.

106. Ibid.

107. Fletcher, "Witches' Pharmacopoeia."

108. On cinquefoil as an antidote, see Dioscorides, *De materia medica*, 4.42. Interestingly, the text of Dioscorides had added to it by a scribe (published in Frankfurt, 1598) a statement that cinquefoil stimulates menstrual flow.

109. Thomas Middleton, *The Witch* (Oxford, 1963), p. 87.

110. Fletcher, "Witches' Pharmacopoeia," p. 150.

111. Margaret B. Kreig, *Green Medicine: The Search for Plants That Heal* (Chicago, 1964), p. 93; Michael J. Harner, "The Role of Hallucinogenic Plants in European Witchcraft," in *Hallocinogens and Shamanism* (New York, 1972), pp. 139–140.

112. Cited from Porta (1562), xxvii, pp. 197–198, by Harner, "Hallucinogenic Plants," p. 138; see also Forbes, *Midwife and the Witch*, p. 120.

113. Andreas De Laguna's commentary to Dioscorides, cited by Theodore Rothman, "De Laguna's Commentaries on Hallucinogenic Drugs and Witchcraft in Dioscorides' Materia Medica," *Bulletin of the History of Medicine* 46 (1972): 562–567 at 562.

114. Guazzo, *Compendium maleficarum*, 1.12 (Summers trans., p. 34).

115. Zilboorg, *Medical Man and the Witch*, pp. 144–145.

116. Gordon R. Forrer, "Psychodynamic Factors in Atropine Toxicity Therapy," *Journal of Nervous and Mental Diseases* 120 (1946): 40–43 at 41.

117. Marcos R. Ferraz and Ricardo Santos, "Amantadine Stimulates Sexual Behavior in Male Rats," *Pharmacology, Biochemistry and Behavior* 51 (1995): 709–714; T. Y. Chang, "Anticholinergic Poisoning Due to Chinese Herbal Medicines," *Veterinary and Human Toxicology* 37 (1995): 156–157.

118. Jole Agrimi and Chiara Crisciani, "Medici e 'vetulae' dal Duecento al Quattrocento: problemi di una ricera," in *Cultura popolare e cultura dotta nel seicento*, ed. Paolo Rossi, Lucilla Borselli, Chiaretta Poli, and Giancarlo Carabelli, (Milan, 1983), p. 147, citing Henri de Mondeville's *Cyrurgia* (1892), pp. 67–68.

119. E. Mansell Pattison, "Psychosocial Interpretations of Exorcism" *Journal of Operational Psychiatry*, 7 (1977): 5–19; reprinted in Levack, *Possession and Exorcism* (New York, 1992), pp. 203–217.

120. R. I. Moore, *The Formation of a Persecuting Society: Power and Deviance in Western Europe, 950–1250* (Oxford, 1987), pp. 134–139.

121. For a medieval view, see Helen Lemay, "Anthonius Guainerius and Medieval Gynecology," in *Women of the Medieval World* (Oxford, 1985), 317–336 at 330; and Lemay, "Women and the Literature of Obstetrics and Gynecology," in *Medieval Women and the Sources of Medieval History*, ed. Joel T. Rosenthal (Athens, Ga., 1990), 189–209, esp. p. 193; for early modern views, see Heinsohn and Steiger, *Vernichtung der weisen Frauen.*

122. Scot, *Discoverie of Witchcraft*, 8.1, p. 158.

123. Ibid., 3.7, p. 50.

124. Ibid.

125. For the perspective of women as victims of changing attitudes, see Roper, *Oedipus and the Devil.*

126. Keith Thomas, "An Anthropology of Religion and Magic, II," *Journal of Interdisciplinary History* 6 (1975): 91–109 at 100; reprinted in Levack, *Witchcraft*, vol. 1.

127. Quoted from Inquisition documents by Carlo Ginzburg, *The Night Battles: Witchcraft and Agrarian Cults in the Sixteenth and Seventeenth Centuries*, trans. John and Anne Tedeschi (Baltimore, 1983), p. 78; also see Irma Naso, *Medici e strutture sanitarie nella società tardo-medievale: Il Piemonte dei secoli XIV e XV* (Milan, 1982), p. 132.

128. Agrimi and Crisciani, "Medici e 'vetulae,' " p. 159.

129. Larner, *Enemies of God*, pp. 122–123.

130. Andrew Blaikie, *Illegitimacy, Sex and Society* (Oxford, 1993), p. 211.

131. Formicarius, *De visionibus ac revelationibus*, in Lea, *Materials* 1: 261.

132. Brian P. Levack, *The Witch-hunt in Early Modern Europe* (London, 1987), pp. 127–128; David Harley, "Historians as Demonologists: The Myth of the Midwife-witch," *Social History of Medicine* 3 (1990): 1–26 at 6–7.

133. Everett M. Rogers and Douglas S. Solomon, "Traditional Midwives and Family Planning in Asia," *Studies in Family Planning* 6 (1975): 126–133.

134. Juan Flavier and Charles H. C. Chen, "Induced Abortion in Rural Villages of Cavite, the Philippines: Knowledge, Attitudes, and Practice," *Studies in Family Planning* 11 (1980): 65–71.

135. For a picture of the old wives in practice, see Mary Chamberlain, *Old Wives' Tales: Their History, Remedies, and Spells* (London, 1981), pp. 50–62.

136. A. D. J. MacFarlane, "Witchcraft in Tudor and Stuart Essex," in *Witchcraft in England*, vol. 6 of Levack, *Witchcraft* (New York, 1992), p. 12.

137. Leslie J. Reagan, "Linking Midwives and Abortion in the Progressive Era," *Bulletin of the History of Medicine* 69 (1995): 569–598 at 569.

138. Trexler, "Foundlings of Florence," pp. 259–284.

139. John Pechey, *The Compleat Herbal of Physical Plants*, 2d ed. (London, 1707), p. 86.

140. Bamberg Ms med. 1 (in Ulrich Stoll, ed., *Das 'Lorscher Arzneibuch,'* Sudhoffs Archiv, vol. 20 [Stuttgart, 1992], p. 116); Macer, *De herbarum virtutibus,* fol. 45v.

141. Adolf Wuttke, *Der deutsche Volksaberglaube der Gegenwart,* 3d ed., by Elard H. Meyer (Leipzig, 1900), pp. 101, 419, 435; Ginzburg, *Night Battles,* p. 24 et passim. Dioscorides (*De materia medica,* 3.70) speaks highly of its qualities in eye medicines.

142. Ginzburg, *Night Battles,* p. 24.

143. A. K. Reynolds, "Uterine Stimulants," *The Alkaloids,* 5 (1955): 163–209 at 196 (under "alkaloid hordenina"); Norman R. Farnsworth, Audrey S. Bingel, Geoffrey A. Cordell, Frank A. Crane, and Harry H. S. Fong, "Potential Value of Plants as Sources of New Antifertility Agents," *Journal of Pharmaceutical Sciences* 64 (1975): 535–598 (pt. 1), 717–754 (pt. 2), at 563.

144. Ginzburg, *Night Battles,* p. 4.

145. Murray, *Witch-cult,* pp. 12 ff.

146. Grete Jacobsen, "Pregnancy and Childbirth in the Medieval North: A Topology of Sources and a Preliminary Study," *Scandinavian Journal of History* 9 (1984): 91–111 at 102.

147. Geoffrey Robert Quaife, *Godly Zeal and Furious Rage: The Witch in Early Modern Europe* (New York, 1987), p. 93.

148. Monica Green, "Documenting Medieval Women's Medical Practice," in *Practical Medicine from Salerno to the Black Death,* ed. Luius Garcia-Ballester, Roger French, John Arrizabalaga, and Andred Cunningham (Cambridge, 1994), p. 336.

149. Jacques Gélis, *History of Childbirth, Fertility, Pregnancy and Birth in Early Modern Europe* (Boston, 1991), p. 105.

150. Michael R. McVaugh, *Medicine Before the Plague,* pp. 98–103.

151. Lewin, *Fruchtabtreibung,* p. 138.

152. Ehrenreich and English, *Witches, Midwives, and Nurses,* p. 12; these authors did not give references. Their evidence is more speculative than certain.

153. The difficulty of knowing women's culture as a subset of popular culture is discussed by Peter Burke, *Popular Culture in Early Modern Europe* (London, 1978), pp. 49 ff.

154. Roper, *Oedipus and the Devil,* p. 136.

155. Jerry Stannard, "Medieval Arzneitaxe and Some Indigenous Plant Species," in *Orbis Pictus: Kultur- und pharmaziehistorische Studien* (Frankfurt, 1985), 267–272 at 268.

156. This observation was made to me by Jerry Stannard. For an assessment of medieval knowledge of plants see Stannard, "Botanical Data and Late Mediaeval Rezeptliteratur," in *Fachprosa-Studien* (Berlin, 1982), pp. 371–395.

157. On the importance of *secreta* literature, see William Eamon, *Science and the Secrets of Nature: Books of Secrets in Medieval and Early Modern Culture* (Princeton, 1994).

158. Pliny, *Natural History*, 20.51.143.

159. Soranus *Gynaecolgy*, 1.64.

160. Presented in a paper by Herbert N. Nigg, University of Florida, at State College, Pennsylvania, May 20, 1995, and in subsequent personal correspondence. Professor Nigg says that the 30 percent figure "has been bandied about in meetings for 10 years."

161. Theophrastus, *Enquiry into Plants*, 9.20.5.

5. Witches and Apothecaries in the Sixteenth and Seventeenth Centuries

1. In Alan C. Kors and Edward Peters, *Witchcraft in Europe, 1100–1700: A Documentary History* (Philadelphia, 1972), p. 108.

2. Günter Jerouschek, *Lebensschutz und Lebeensbeginn: Kulturgeschichte des Abtreibungsbungsverbotes* Medizin in Rechte und Ethik, vol. 17 (Stuttgart, 1988), pp. 5–6.

3. Ibid., p. 6.

4. Gunnar Heinsohn and Otto Steiger, *Die Vernichtung der weisen Frauen: Beiträge zur Theorie und Geschichte von Bevölkerung und Kindheit* (Herbstein, 1985), p. 117, believe that contraception itself was treated as a homicide.

5. Quoted from manuscript of a Gray's Inn lecture by Phillip A. Rafferty, *Roe v. Wade: The Birth of a Constitutional Right*, 2 vols. (Ann Arbor, 1992), 2: 597.

6. William Staunford, *Les Plees del Coron* (London, 1557; facsimile ed., London, 1971), 1: 13 (p. 21). Staunford cited the two cases according to the pagination in Anthony Fitzherbert, *Le graunde abridgment. . .*, 2 vols. (London, 1577). On Staunford and Bracton, see D. E. C. Yale, " 'Of No Mean Authority': Some Later Uses of Bracton," in *On the Laws and Customs of England: Essays in Honor of Samuel E. Thorne* (Chapel Hill, 1981), p. 385.

7. Staunford, *Plees del Coron*, 1: 13 (pp. 21r&v), cited and translated (from the 1568 edition) by Cyril C. Means, "The Phoenix of Abortional Freedom: Is a Prenumbral or Ninth-Amendment Right about to Arise from the Nineteenth-Century Legislative Ashes of a Fourteenth-Century Common-Law Liberty?" *New York Law Forum* 17 (1971): 335–410 at 340–341.

8. Rafferty, *Roe v. Wade*, 2: 601.

9. Ibid., 2: 602.

10. Robert A. Destro, "Abortion and the Constitution: The Need for a Life-Protective Amendment," *California Law Review* 63 (1975): 1250–1351 at 1271, believes that Staunford's citation of the cases was an argument about difficulty of proof, not whether abortion was a crime. Means's argument ("Phoenix of Abortional Freedom," pp. 337–339, nn. 3, 6) is much more straightforward; not only does Means provide a reading of the two Edwardian cases and Staunford's interpretation, but he also cites the Massachusetts Crim-

inal Law Commissioners (1844), who used a French text for their decision although they slightly mistranslated the text.

11. Ralph A. Houlbrooke, *Church Courts and the People during the English Reformation, 1520–1570* (Oxford, 1979), p. 78.

12. Ibid.

13. Rafferty, *Roe v. Wade*, 2: 504–505.

14. Means, "Phoenix of Abortional Freedom," pp. 344–345; for a different view, see Destro, "Abortion and the Constitution," p. 1272n.

15. Edward Coke, *Third Part of the Institutes of the Laws of England Concerning High Treason and Criminal Cases*, chap. 7, p. 50 (London, 1747).

16. Means, "Phoenix of Abortional Freedom," p. 346.

17. Ibid., pp. 345–348.

18. Destro, "Abortion and the Constitution," p. 1272.

19. See discussion by Rafferty, *Roe v. Wade*, 1: 161–210, regarding how quickening came to be regarded as the period of ensoulment in English common law.

20. Means, "Phoenix of Abortional Freedom," p. 349.

21. Matthew Hale, *Pleas of the Crown: or, A Methodical summary of the Principal Matters Relating to that Subject* (London, 1682; facsimile ed., London, 1972), p. 53; in a later, expanded edition, Hale says that administering a potion that kills a fetus and not the mother is not a felony, although "by the judicial law of Moses [Exodus 21:22] [the act] was punishable with death" (*History of the Pleas of the Crown*, 2 vols. [Dublin, 1778], 1: 433.)

22. Hale, *History of the Pleas*, 1: 429–430.

23. Nadia Maria Filippini, "The Church, the State and Childbirth: The Midwife in Italy during the Eighteenth Century," in *The Art of Midwifery: Early Modern Midwives in Europe*, ed. Hilary Marland (London: Routledge, 1993), p. 155; Thomas G. Benedek, "The Changing Relationship between Midwives and Physicians during the Renaissance," *Bulletin of the History of Medicine* 51 (1977): 550–564.

24. Teresa Ortiz, "From Hegemony to Subordination: Midwives in Early Modern Spain," in Marland, *Art of Midwifery*, pp. 95–114.

25. Ibid.

26. Margaret Alice Murray, *The Witch-cult in Western Europe: A Study in Anthropology* (Oxford, 1921), p. 170; see also David Harley, "Historians as Demonologists: The Myth of the Midwife-witch," *Social History of Medicine* 3 (1990): 1–26 at 19.

27. Mary Chamberlain, *Old Wives' Tales: Their History, Remedies, and Spells* (London, 1981), p. 56.

28. Harley, "Historians as Demonologists," p. 19; also skeptical of the generalization that midwives should be closely identified with witchcraft is Monica Green, "Women's Medical Practice and Health Care in Medieval Europe," *Signs: Journal of Women in Culture and Society* 14 (1989): 434–473 at 451.

29. Harley, "Historians as Demonologists," p. 18.

30. Irma Naso, *Medici e strutture sanitarie nella società tardo-medievale: Il Piemonte dei secoli XIV e XV* (Milan, 1982), p. 133.

31. E. William Monter, "Protestant Wives, Catholic Saints, and the Devil's Handmaid: Women in the Age of Reformations," in *Becoming Visible: Women in European History*, 2nd ed., ed. Renate Bridenthal, Claudia Koonz, and Susan Stuard (Boston, 1987), 203–219 at 216.

32. Peter C. Hoffer and N. E. H. Hull, *Murdering Mothers: Infanticide in England and New England* (New York, 1981), p. 28.

33. Marcianus, in *Digest*, 47.11.4 (Mommsen-Watson ed., *Corpus Iuris Civilis*, 4: 820, 854).

34. Joanne K. Kuemmerlin-McLean, "Magic O.T.," in *Anchor Bible Dictionary*, 4 (1992): 468.

35. Benedek, "Changing Relationship," p. 561.

36. Ludwig Knapp, *Theologie und Geburtshilfe nach F. E. Cangiamila's Sacra Embryologia (Editio Latin, MDCCLXIV mit aktuellen Bemerkungen)* (Prague, 1908), p. 61.

37. Ortiz, "Hegemony to Subordination," p. 101.

38. J. H. Aveling, *English Midwives: Their History and Prospects* (London, 1872), p. 91. The text is from the 1662 oath but, according to Aveling, the sixteenth-century text is similar.

39. Quoted by Barbara Ehrenreich and Deirdre English, *Witches, Midwives, and Nurses: A History of Women Healers* (Old Westbury, N.Y., 1973), p. 19.

40. Merry E. Wiesner, "The Midwives of South Germany and the Public/Private Dichotomy," in Marland, *Art of Midwifery*, p. 87.

41. Ibid.

42. H. C. Erik Midelfort, *Witch-Hunting in Southwestern Germany, 1562–1684: The Social and Intellectual Foundations* (Stanford, 1972), p. 23.

43. 33 Hen. 8, c. 8 (*Statutes of the Realm*, 3: 837).

44. 1 Edw. 6, c. 12 (*Statutes of the Realm*, 4, pt. 1: 446–447).

45. 1 Jac. 1, c. 12 (*Statutes of the Realm*, 4, pt. 2: 1028–29).

46. Aveling, *English Midwives*, pp. 90–91. Wiesner, *Working Women*, p. 64, observes that city ordinances in Germany did not mention the superstitious or magical practices to be avoided.

47. Mark Jackson, "Suspicious Infant Deaths: The Statute of 1624 and Medical Evidence at Coroners' Inquests," in *Legal Medicine in History*, ed. Michael Clark and Catherine Crawford (Cambridge, 1994), pp. 64–69.

48. Stanislav Andreski, "The Syphilitic Shock: A New Explanation of the Witch-Burnings," *Encounter* 58 (1982): 7–26 at 15.

49. Allison P. Coudert, "The Myth of the Improved Status of Protestant Women: The Case of Witchcraze," in *Politics of Gender in Early Modern Europe*, 12 (1989): 61–89 at 85; reprinted in Brian Levack, *Witchcraft, Women and Society* (New York, 1992), pp. 85–113 (I was unable to verify Coudert's citation).

50. E. William Monter, *Witchcraft in France and Switzerland: The Border-lands during the Reformation* (Ithaca, N.Y., 1976), p. 196; Midelfort, *Witch-Hunting,* p.181.

51. Wolfgang Behringer, *Hexenverfolgung in Bayern: Volksmagie, Glauben-seifer und Staatsräson in der Frühen Neuzeit* (Munich, 1988), p. 158, excerpting from Jakob Vallick's *Tractat von Zauberern, Hexen und Unholden* (Cologne, 1576).

52. Andreski, "Syphilitic Shock," p. 18.

53. Cited by Chamberlain, *Old Wives' Tales,* p. 45.

54. Silvia Bovenschen, "The Contemporary Witch, the History Witch and the Witch-Myth," *New German Critique* 15 (1978): 83–119 (with review of lit-erature).

55. Andreski, "Syphilitic Shock," pp. 22–26.

56. Jane Crawford, "Evidences for Witchcraft in Anglo-Saxon England," *Medium Aevum,* 32 (1963): 99–116 at 105.

57. Keith Thomas, *Religion and the Decline of Magic* (New York, 1971), p. 192.

58. John T. Noonan, Jr., *Contraception: A History of Its Treatment by the Catholic Theologians and Canonists,* enlarged ed. (Cambridge, Mass., 1986), pp. 344, 350.

59. Scot, *Discoverie of Witchcraft,* 10.5 (1584 ed., p. 181).

60. Quoted by Scot (ibid., 12.7, p. 225) from an English translation of Vergil's *Aeneid* (4).

61. Johann Weyer, *De praestigiis daemonum,* translation of 1583 edition by John Shea, in *Witches, Devils, and Doctors in the Renaissance* (Binghamton, N.Y., 1991), p. 264.

62. Ibid., p. 395.

63. *Tractatus de fascinatione,* cited in Thomas Forbes, *Midwife and the Witch* (New Haven, 1966), p. 127.

64. Forbes, *Midwife and the Witch,* p. 128.

65. Ritta Jo Horsley and Richard A. Horsley, "On the Trail of the 'Witches': Wise Women, Midwives and the European Witch Hunts," in *Women in German Yearbook 3: Feminist Studies and German Culture,* ed. Mar-ianne Burkhard and Edith Waldstein (Lanham, Md., 1986), 1–28 at 7–9.

66. Ibid., pp. 6–7.

67. As cited by Chamberlain, *Old Wives' Tales,* p. 49.

68. Monter, "Protestant Wives," pp. 216–218.

69. Grete Jacobsen, "Pregnancy and Childbirth in the Medieval North: A Topology of Sources and a Preliminary Study," *Scandinavian Journal of His-tory,* 9 (1984): 91–111 at 102.

70. English edition of Achillini's recension of Pseudo-Aristotle, *Secretum secretorum* (Paris, 1520; rpt., London, 1702), pp. 33–34.

71. *Rex vs. Lichefeld* (Nottinghamshire, 1505), King's Bench 27/974, cited in Rafferty, *Roe v. Wade*, 2: 507.

72. Geoffrey Robert Quaife, *Godly Zeal and Furious Rage: The Witch in Early Modern Europe* (New York, 1987), p. 93.

73. Vivian Nutton, "The Anatomy of the Soul in Early Renaissance Medicine," in *The Human Embryo*, ed. G. R. Dunstan (Exeter, 1990), 136–157 at 140.

74. John M. Riddle, *Contraception and Abortion from the Ancient World to the Renaissance* (Cambridge, Mass., 1992), pp. 144–153.

75. Maurice De l'Corde (translator and commentator), *Hippocratis Coi, medicorum principis, Liber prior de morbus mulierum* (Paris, 1585), p. 308.

76. Hermolaus Barbarus, *Pedacii Dioscorides Anazarbei de medicanale materia* (Venice, 1516), fol. 92.

77. *Tractatus de virtutibus herbarum* (Venice, 1499), nos. 11, 15, 33, 75, 102, 12, 117.

78. Ibid., 13, 14.

79. Ibid., 34, 140.

80. Ibid., 77, 99, 101, 106.

81. Ibid., 43.

82. Ibid., 132.

83. Ibid., 106 (on pennyroyal, citing Pliny), 136 (on willow), and 111 (on poplar).

84. Dioscorides, *De materia medica*, 1.81.

85. *Herbolarium de virtutibus herbarum* (Vicenza, 1491).

86. *Gart der Gesundheit*, as *In diesem Buch ist der Herbary: oder Kreuterbuch: ganant der Gart der Gesundheit* (Strassburg, 1515), fol. bii; the Mainz edition (1485), chap. 1 (no numbering), has a slightly different text; for the references to birth control in Wonnecke von Cube, see Sylvie Laurent, *Naître au moyen age. De la conception a la naissance: La gorssesse et l'accouchement (XIIe–XVe siècle)* (Paris, 1989).

87. Ibid., fol. biiii.

88. Ibid., fol. 10.

89. Ibid., fol. 73v.

90. Ibid., fol. 126v.

91. Hieronymus Bock (H. Tragus), *Kreütterbuch . . .* (Strassburg, 1595), fols. 96, 98r&v; Latin ed., *De stirpium* (Strassburg, 1552), pp. 336, 341.

92. Ibid. (1595 ed., p. 27v; 1552 ed., p. 68).

93. This appeared in the 1551 edition (fol. 403v), cited by Larissa Leibrock-Plehn, *Hexenkräuter oder Arznei: Die Abtreibungsmittel im 16. und 17. Jahrhundert* (Stuttgart, 1992), pp. 103–104, but it was dropped from the 1595 edition that I saw. Robert Jütte, "Die Persistenz des Verhütungswissens in der Volkskultur," *Medizinhistorisches Journal* 24 (1989): 214–231 at 220, cites Bock as

saying that priests and prostitutes regarded juniper as the best birth control drug.

94. Otto Brunfels, *Herbarum vivae eicones ad natura imitationem* (Strassburg, 1554), vol. 3, appendix (no pagination).

95. Ibid., 2: 53–54, 74.

96. Ibid., 2: 237.

97. Ibid. 2: 16–17.

98. Ibid., 2: 251.

99. Fuchs, *De historia stirpium* (Basel, 1542), p. 618.

100. Ibid., p. 93.

101. Ibid., p. 585.

102. Josse de Harchies, *Enchiridion* (Basel, 1573), pp. 144–145 (juniper), 229 ("sabina"), 102 (dittany), 211 *(Ferula)*, and 257 (death carrot).

103. Ibid., pp. 82, 154, 156, and 182, in order.

104. Ibid., p. 147.

105. Ibid., p. 115.

106. Karen Meier Reeds, *Botany in Medieval and Renaissance Universities* (New York, 1991).

107. Valerius Cordus, *Dispensatorium* (Nüremberg [?], 1546), col. 44.

108. Ibid., cols. 14–15.

109. Bamberg Ms med. 1, in Ulrich Stoll, ed., *Das 'Lorscher Arzneibuch,'* Sudhoffs Archiv, vol. 20 (Stuttgart, 1992), p. 116.

110. Valerius Cordus, *Dispensatorium*, cols. 20–23.

111. Ibid., col. 184.

112. Ibid., cols. 44, 61–63, 76–79, 111–113, 145–147, 63–72, 137–138, 184.

113. Ibid., cols. 145–147.

114. Ibid., col. 234.

115. Ibid., col. 237.

116. Ibid., col. 10.

117. *Enchiridion* (facsimile edition of *Pharmacopoeia Augustana* [Augsburg, 1564; Madison, 1927]), p. 110.

118. Ibid., p. 37.

119. Ibid., p. 68.

120. Ibid., pp. 119–120; cf. Cordus, *Dispensatorium*, cols. 145–147.

121. *Pharmacopoeia Augustana* (Augsburg, 1597), p. 228, cited by Leibrock-Plehn, *Hexenkräuter*, p. 38.

122. Ibid., p. 286, in Leibrock-Plehn, *Hexenkräuter*, p. 39n.

123. Leibrock-Plehn, *Hexenkräuter*, pp. 42–43.

124. Anutius Foesius, *Pharmacopoeia* (Basel, 1561), p. 566, cited by Leibrock-Plehn, *Hexenkräuter*, p. 46n.

125. Franciscus Alexander, *Phoebus medicorum* (Frankfurt, 1613), p. 281, as cited by Leibrock-Plehn, *Hexenkräuter*, p. 49n.

126. As surveyed by Leibrock-Plehn, *Hexenkräuter*, pp. 48–60.

127. Johann Jakob Wecker, *Antidotarium generale et specilae* (Basel, 1595), pp. 215, 243, 271, 315.

128. Ibid., p. 823.

129. Johann Schroeder, *Pharmacopoeia medico-chymica sive thesaurus pharmacologicus* (Ulm 1641, 1655, 1662, and Lyon 1649).

130. Doubt about Eucharius's originality has recently come to light, as an earlier manuscript in the possession of his family contains some of the same material published under his name. See Britta-Juliane Kruse, "Neufund einer handschriftlichen Vorstufe von Eucharius Rösslins Hebammenlehrbuch *Der schwangeren Frauen und Hebammen Rosengarten* und des *Frauenbüchleins* Ps.-Ortolfs," *Sudhoffs Archiv* 78 (1994): 220–236.

131. I have used the German edition, *Der Swangern frawen und hebammen rossgarten* (Hagenau, 1529), bk. 2, chap. 11, fol. g iiiv, and the English edition, *The Byrth of Mankynd, Otherwise Named the Womans Boke* . . . (London, 1552), fols. 137–141.

132. Ibid.

133. See also discussion by Leibrock-Plehn, *Hexenkräuter*, pp. 136–141.

134. Walther Hermann Ryff, *Schwangerer Frauwen Rosengarten* (Frankfurt, 1569), fol. 109.

135. Ibid., fols. 108v–109.

136. Ibid., 120–121v.

137. For example, under colocynth, squirting cucumber, and tamarask, I found no mention of birth control uses, disguised or open. See Walther Hermann Ryff, *Confecbuch unnd Haus Apoteck* . . . (Frankfurt, 1610), fols. 156v–158, 164.

138. Girolamo Mercurio (Scipione), *La commare o riccoglitrice dell'eccmo* . . . (Venice, 1601), pp. 160–169, esp. pp. 161, 168.

139. Luius Mercado, *De secretis naturae*, in *Tractatus Henrici de Saxonia, Alberti Magni discipuli, De secretis mulierum* . . . (Frankfurt, 1602), pp. 58–61.

140. Ibid., p. 59.

141. Ibid., pp. 301–364; see also James V. Ricci, *The Genealogy of Gynaecology: History of the Development of Gynaecology throughout the Ages, 2000 B.C.–1800 A.D.* (Philadelphia, 1950), p. 262.

142. Jacobus Primerose (alias James Primerosius), *De mulierum morbus et symptomatis libri quinque* (Rotterdam, 1655), 1.2, pp. 5–15.

143. Ibid., p. 17.

144. Ibid., pp. 23 ff.

145. Ibid., 4.1, p. 235.

146. Ibid., 4.3, p. 269.

147. Ibid., 4.6, p. 289.

148. Vern L. Bullough, "An Early American Sex Manual, or, Aristotle Who?" *Early American Literature* 7 (1973): 236–246.

149. Pseudo-Aristotle, *Secretum secretorum*, in *The Works of Aristotle, the Fa-*

mous Philosopher in Four Parts (New England, 1813; rpt., New York, 1974), p. 16.

150. On its influence, see Otho T. Beall, "Aristotle's *Master Piece* in America: A Landmark in the Folklore of Medicine," *William and Mary Quarterly*, 20/3 (1963): 207–222; and Bullough, "Early American Sex Manual."

151. Pseudo-Aristotle, *Masterpiece*, in *Works of Aristotle*, p. 29.

152. *Experienced Midwife*, in *Works of Aristotle*, p. 141.

153. Ibid., p. 144.

154. Ibid., p. 145.

155. Ibid., p. 159.

156. Francis Mauriceau, *De praegnantium et parturientium et puerperarum morbis tractabus* (Paris, 1681), p. 54; *The Diseases of Women with Child*, Hugh Chamberlen, trans. (London, 1718), p. 25 (quotation cited from 1718 trans.).

157. Ibid., 1681 ed., p. 37; 1718 ed., p. 6.

158. Jane Sharp, *The Compleat Midwife's Companion: or, the Art of Midwifry Improv'd* . . . (London, 1725), fol. a1.

159. Jane Sharp, *Midwives' Book on the Whole Art of Midwifery* . . . (London, 1671; facsimile ed., New York, 1985), pp. 180–181; the plant *eringo* is also identified in the Middle Ages with *Senecio vulgaris* L., frequently found in medicines for women in the nineteenth century.

160. Norman R. Farnsworth, Audrey S. Bingel, Geoffrey A. Cordell, Frank A. Crane, and Harry H. S. Fong, "Potential Value of Plants as Sources of New Antifertility Agents," *Journal of Pharmaceutical Sciences* 64 (1975): 576; J. Jiu, "A Survey of Some Medicinal Plants of Mexico for Selected Biological Activities," *Lloydia*, 29 (1966): 256–257.

161. Sharp, *Compleat Midwife's Companion*, pp. 180–181.

162. Ibid., p. 182.

163. Ibid.

164. Roger Thompson, *Sex in Middlesex: Popular Mores in a Massachusetts County, 1649–1699* (Amherst, 1986), pp. 182–183.

165. Olva Thulesius, *Nicholas Culpeper: English Physician and Astrologer* (New York, 1992), p. 78.

166. Nicholas Culpeper, *Directory for Midwives: or, A Guide for Women, in their Conception, Bearing, and Suckling their Children.* . . (London, 1651), pp. 96, 202.

167. Ibid., p. 96.

168. Ibid., p. 142.

169. Thulesius, *Culpeper*, p. 88.

170. Daniel Defoe, *Conjugal Lewdness; or, Matrimonial Whoredom* (1727; repr. Menston, 1970), pp. 138–140.

171. Eve Levin, *Sex and Society in the World of the Orthodox Slavs, 900–1700* (Ithaca, 1989), p. 176.

172. James Reed ("Doctors, Birth Control, and Social Values: 1830–1970" in *The Therapeutic Revolution: Essays in the Social History of American Medicine*, Morris J. Vogel and Charles E. Rosenberg, eds. [Philadelphia, 1979], pp. 109–134) believes that physicians in the nineteenth century harbored fears that contraception was detrimental to the moral order, but whether this same emotion can be applied to the sixteenth and seventeenth centuries is conjectural.

173. Susan Cotts Watkins, "If All We Knew About Women Was What We Read in *Demography*, What Would We Know?" *Demography* 30 (1993): 551–577 at 554.

174. Nonnan, *Contraception*, p. 362.

175. Ibid., p. 363n.

176. Ibid., p. 363.

177. Quoted by John T. Noonan, Jr., "Abortion and the Catholic Church: A Summary History," *Natural Law Forum* 12 (1967): 111.

178. Noonan, *Contraception*, p. 373.

179. Joseph Needham, *A History of Embryology* (New York, 1959), p. 111.

180. Aristotle, *History of Animals*, 7.3.588b.

181. Jerome Bylebyl, "Harvey, William," in *Dictionary of Scientific Biography*, 6 (1972): 150–162 at 159–161.

182. Luigi Belloni, "Malpighi," in *Dictionary of Scientific Biography*, 9 (1974): 62–66 at 65–66.

183. Shirely Roe, *Matter, Life and Generation: Eighteenth-Century Embryology and the Haller-Wolff Debate* (Cambridge, 1981), p. 6.

184. L. W. B. Brockliss, "The Embryological Revolution in the France of Louis XIV: The Dominance of Ideology," in Dunstan, *Human Embryo*, 156–186 at 170.

185. Roe, *Matter, Life and Generation*, p. 4.

186. Brockliss, "Embryological Revolution," p. 170.

187. Roe, *Matter, Life and Generation*, p. 364.

188. Ibid., p. 370.

189. Ibid.

190. J. Hajnal, "European Marriage Patterns in Perspective," in *Population in History: Essays in Historical Demography*, ed. D. V. Glass and D. E. C. Eversley (Chicago, 1965), 101–143 at 101; Etienne van de Walle, "Marriage and Marital Fertility," *Daedalus*, 97 (1968): 486–501.

191. Midelfort, *Witch-Hunting*, p. 184; Hajnal, "European Marriage," p. 101 et passim, esp. p. 132; van de Walle, "Marriage"; on medieval marriage ages, see Frances Gies and Joseph Gies, *Marriage and the Faimly in the Middle Ages* (New York, 1987), pp. 33, 183–184, 207–208, 233, 283; Barbara Hanawalt, *The Ties That Bound: Peasant Families in Medieval England* (New York, 1986), pp. 95–100.

192. Hajnal, "European Marriage"; Michael W. Flinn, *The European Demographic System, 1500–1820* (Baltimore, 1981), p. 27.

193. Flinn, *European Demographic System*, p. 19.

194. Midelfort, *Witch-Hunting*, pp. 184–185.

195. H. J. Habakkuk, "The Economic History of Modern Britain," in Glass and Eversley, *Population in History*, pp. 147–158 at 151; Flinn, *European Demographic System*, p. 20.

196. Heinsohn and Steiger, *Vernichtung der weisen Frauen*, pp. 184–187, stresses the connection between pro-natalism and mercantile philosophy; see also Gunnar Heinsohn, Rolf Knieper, and Otto Steiger, *Menschenproduckton: Allgemeine Bevölkerungstheorie der Neuzeit* (Frankfurt am Main, 1979).

197. Charles Emil Stangeland, *Pre-Malthusian Doctrines of Population: A Study in the History of Economic Theory* (New York, 1966), pp. 118–137.

198. Heinsohn and Steiger, *Vernichtung der weisen Frauen*, 3d ed., pp. 264–271; and personal letter to author (19 April 1996).

199. Monter, *Witchcraft in France and Switzerland*, p. 198n.

200. The law cited is 21 Jac. 1, c. 27. See Hoffer and Hull, *Murdering Mothers*, p. 20; David Harley, "Provincial Midwives in England: Lancashire and Cheshire, 1660–1760," in Marland, *Art of Midwifery*, pp. 27–48.

201. Monter, *Witchcraft in France and Switzerland*, p. 198n; on rising infanticide cases in England, see Hoffer and Hull, *Murdering Mothers*.

202. Scot, *Discoverie of Witchcraft*, 2.5, p. 25.

203. Hoffer and Hull, *Murdering Mothers*, p. 27.

204. Leonard Arthur Parry, *Criminal Abortion* (London, 1932), p. 96.

205. Monter, *Witchcraft in France and Switzerland*, p. 198n.

206. Monter, "Protestant Wives," p. 216.

207. Richard C. Trexler, *The Women of Renaissance Florence*, 2 vols. (Binghamton, N.Y., 1993), 1: 31–65.

208. Lindsay Wilson, *Women and Medicine in the French Enlightenment: The Debate over Maladies des Femmes* (Baltimore, 1993), p. 118.

209. David Harley, "The Scope of Legal Medicine in Lancashire and Cheshire, 1660–1760," in *Legal Medicine in History*, ed. Michael Clark and Catherine Crawford (Cambridge, 1994), p. 56.

6.   The Broken Chain of Knowledge

1. Christina Larner, *Enemies of God: The Witch-hunt in Scotland* (Baltimore, 1981), p. 100. For a review of recent historiography, see Elsepeth Whitney, "International Trends: The Witch 'She' / the Historian 'He,' " *Journal of Women's History* 7 (1995): 77–101.

2. Gunnar Heinsohn and Otto Steiger, *Die Vernichtung der weisen Frauen: Beiträge zur Theorie und Geschichte von Bevölkerung und Kindheit* (Herbstein,

1985), pp. 13–17, 21–211; Gunnar Heinsohn and Otto Steiger, "The Elimination of Medieval Birth Control and the Witch Trials of Modern Times," *International Journal of Women's Studies* 5 (1982): 193–214.

3. Heinsohn and Steiger, "Elimination of Medieval Birth Control," p. 208.

4. Heinsohn and Steiger, *Vernichtung der weisen Frauen,* pp. 184–187; more detailed by Heinsohn and Steiger with Rolf Knieper, *Menschenproduktion: Allgemeine Bevölkerungstheorie der Neuzeit* (Frankfurt am Main, 1979), pp. 61–83 (not seen).

5. Claudia Honegger, *Die Hexen der Neuzeit: Studien zur Sozialgeschichte eines kulturellen Deutungsmusters* (Frankfurt, 1978), pp. 45–56, 116–126.

6. Selma R. Williams, *"Riding the Nightmare": Women and Witchcraft from the Old World to Colonial Salem* (New York, 1978), p. 111.

7. Karen Oppenheim Mason, "The Impact of Women's Position on Demographic Change during the Course of Development," in *Women's Position and Demographic Change,* ed. Nora Federici, Karen O. Mason, and Sølvi Sogner (Oxford, 1993), p. 31.

8. Heinsohn and Steiger, "Elimination of Medieval Birth Control," esp. pp. 202–207; Heinsohn and Steiger, *Vernichtung der weisen Frauen,* pp. 21–211, esp. 64–113; cf. also Heinsohn's examination (in the same book) of the connection between witch suppression, children, and education (pp. 213–309, esp. 235–244). For an appreciative review of the book, by Juergen Backhaus, see *The Wall Street Review of Books* 15 (1987): 101–104.

9. Wolfgang Behringer, "Die Vernunft der Magie: Hexenverfolgung als Thema der europäischen Geschichte," in *Frankfurter Allgemeine Zeitung,* no. 190, August 8, 1987, pp. 25–26.

10. For other critics, see Gerd Schwerhoff, "Erwiderung aud die Antikritik von G. Heinsohn/O. Steiger," in *Geschichtsdidaktik* 11 (1986): 422; Robert Jütte, "Die Persistenz des Verhütungswissens in der Volkskultur," *Medizinhistorisches Journal* 24 (1989): 214–231; Ritta Jo Horsley and Richard A. Horsley, "On the Trail of the 'Witches': Wise Women, Midwives and the European Witch Hunts," in *Women in German Yearbook 3: Feminist Studies and German Culture,* ed. Marianne Burkhard and Edith Waldstein (Lanham, 1986), 1–28 at 26–27.

11. See discussion, with references, by Ansley J. Coale, "The Decline of Fertility in Europe since the Eighteenth Century as a Chapter in Demographic History," in *The Decline of Fertility in Europe,* ed. Ansley J. Coale and Susan Cotts Watkins (Princeton, 1986), pp. 1–30.

12. John E. Knodel and Etienne van de Walle, "Lessons from the Past: Policy Implications of Historical Fertility Studies," *Population and Development Review,* 5 (1979): 217–245 at 226–227.

13. Roger Mols, "Population in Europe, 1500–1700: Two Centuries of

Demographic Evolution," in *The Fontana Economic History of Europe*, ed. Carlo M. Cipolla (Sussex, 1974), 2: 15–82 at 78.

14. Massimo Livi-Bacci, *Population and Nutrition: An Essay on European Demographic History*, trans. [from Italian ed., 1987] Tania Croft-Murray and Carl Ipsen (Cambridge, 1991), p. 8; Emmanuel Le Roy Ladurie, "Demographie et 'funestes secrets' le Lanquedoc (fin XVIIIe–début XIXe siècle)," in *Le territoire de l'historien*, 2 vols. (Paris, 1973), 1:328; Philippe Ariès, *Histoire des populations françaises et de leurs attitudes devant la vie dupuis le XVIIIe siècle* (Paris, 1948), pp. 496–497; Michael W. Flinn, *The European Demographic System, 1500–1820* (Baltimore, 1981), p. 43 et passim; on land use, see Colin Clark, *Population Growth and Land Use* (London, 1967).

15. E. A. Wrigley and R. S. Schofield, *The Population History of England, 1541–1871* (Cambridge, Mass., 1981), p. 417 (naming timing and incidence only); Mols, "Population in Europe," pp. 72–74.

16. Massimo Livi-Bacci, *A History of Italian Fertility* (Princeton, 1977), p. 16.

17. Flinn, *European Demographic System*, p. 46; Knodel and van de Walle, "Lessons from the Past," p. 232, suggest that neglectful and abusive child care may have been important factors in family limitation in premodern times.

18. Colin McEvedy and Richard Jones, *Atlas of World Population History* (New York, 1978), p. 22; cf. John D. Durand, "Historical Estimates of World Population: An Evaluation," *Population and Development Review*, 3 (1977): 253–296 at 256, for slightly different figures: 38 million for year 1000 and 68 million for 1500. Emmanuel Le Roy Ladurie (*The Peasants of Languedoc*, trans. John Day [Chicago, 1974], pp. 11, 52) reports the population in southern France as ebbing in the fifteenth century with a "truly considerable" increase in the sixteenth century.

19. Jean-Noël Biraben, "Essai sur l'evolution dur nombre des hommes," pp. 16–17; Livi-Bacci, *Population and Nutrition*, p. 5; McEvedy and Jones, *World Population*, pp. 24–26; Karl F. Helleiner, "The Population of Europe from the Black Death to the Eve of the Vital Revolution," in *Cambridge Economic History of Europe*, ed. E. E. Rich (Cambridge, 1967), pp. 1–95; Le Roy Ladurie, *Peasants of Languedoc*, p. 55.

20. H. J. Habakkuk, "The Economic History of Modern Britain," in *Population in History: Essays in Historical Demography*, ed. D. V. Glass and D. E. C. Eversley (Chicago, 1965), p. 147.

21. For example, Biraben ("Essai sur l'évolution," p. 16) estimates Europe's population in 1300 and 1500 as 70 million and 52 million, respectivly, compared with Heinsohn and Steiger's table with 73 and 45 million, but Biraben's table excludes the territory of Russia. Paul Mombert ("Die Entwicklung der Bevölkerung Europas seit der Mitte des 17. Jahrhunderts," *Zeitschrift für Nationalökonomie* 7 [1936]: 533–545 at 533) has slightly different figures but still they are approximate.

22. Durand, "Historical Estimates," p. 271.

23. Data for world estimates since 1750 with varying assumptions are presented by Jean Bourgeois-Pichat, "The Demographic Distress of the World," *Population Growth and Development: Research and Publication*, January 1966, no. 556.

24. J. Hajnal, "European Marriage Patterns in Perspective," in Glass and Eversley, *Population in History*, 101–143 at 130; cf. Mols, "Population in Europe," pp. 75–78; Clark, *Population Growth*, esp. pp. 180–181; Pierre Chaunu, *La civilisation de l'Europe classique* (Paris, 1966), pp. 204–205.

25. Wrigley and Schofield, *Population History of England*, p. 311.

26. Chaunu, *La civilisation*, p. 204.

27. Etienne Gautier and Louis Henry, *La population de Crulai Pariosse Normande* ([Paris], 1958), p. 232.

28. Knodel and van de Walle, "Lessons from the Past," p. 233.

29. E. A. Wrigley, *Population and History* (New York, 1969), p. 121.

30. Alfred Perrenoud, "Malthusianisme et protestantisme: un modèle démographique weberien," *Annales economies, sociétes, civilisations* 29 (1974): 975–988 at 980, calculated by averaging table for each period of time from 1625 to 1772; for other data on intervals between birth, see Pierre Goubert, "Legitimate Fecundity and Infant Mortality in France during the Eighteenth Century: A Comparison," *Daedalus* 97 (1968): 593–603 at 594–595; Louis Henry, *Anciennes familles Genevoises: Etude démographique, XVIe–XXe siècle*, Travaux et Documents, Cahier, no. 26 (Paris, 1956), pp. 85 ff.; Jütte, "Persistenz," p. 217.

31. Heinsohn and Steiger, *Vernichtung der weisen Frauen*, pp. 167–171.

32. David Herlihy and Christiane Klapisch-Ziber, *Tuscans and Their Families* (New Haven, 1985), p. 250, said that women of middle and low levels of wealth in the fifteenth century had "distinctly fewer babies than did their rich neighbors."

33. From Maine State Manuscripts Library, quoted in Brief 281, American Historians as Amici Curiae, Supporting Appellees, in *Webster v. Reproductive Health Service*, No. 88–605, Supreme Court of the United States, October Term, 1988, p. 6n (brief separately paged as pp. 1–31; pp. 339–369 in volume); see also Laurel Thatcher Ulrich, *A Midwife's Tale: The Life of Martha Ballard Based on Her Diary, 1735–1812* (New York 1991), p. 56.

34. Herlihy and Klapisch-Zuber, *Tuscans*, p. 251.

35. For a summary, see Flinn, *European Demographic System*; Jean-Louis Flandrin, "Contraception, mariage et relations amoureuses dans l'occident chrétien," *Annales economies, sociétés, civilisations* 24 (1969): 1370–1390; T. H. Hollingsworth, *Historical Demography* (Ithaca, 1969).

36. Geoffrey Robert Quaife, *Wanton Wenches and Wayward Wives: Peasants and Illicit Sex in Early Seventeenth Century England* (New Brunswick, 1979), p. 118.

37. McEvedy and Jones, *World Population*, pp. 42–43; Heinsohn and Steiger, *Vernichtung der weisen Frauen*, p. 104, has different estimates; Wrigley and Schofield's figures (*Population History of England*, pp. 208–209) do not begin until the year 1541.

38. K. H. Connell, "Land and Population in Ireland, 1780–1845," in Glass and Eversley, *Population in History*, 423–433 at 423.

39. Ibid., pp. 429–433.

40. E. A. Wrigley, "The Growth of Population in Eighteenth-Century England: A Conundrum Resolved," *Past and Present* 93 (1983): 121–150 at 122; Wrigley and Schofield, *Population History of England*, pp. 208–209.

41. Wrigley and Schofield, *Population History of England*, pp. 208–209, 213.

42. Wrigley, "Growth of Population," p. 129.

43. Ibid., p. 131.

44. Thomas McKeown and R. G. Brown, "Medical Evidence Related to English Population Changes in the Eighteenth Century," in Glass and Eversley, *Population in History*, 285–307 at 303–307.

45. Wrigley, "Growth of Population," p. 146.

46. Thomas Robert Malthus, *An Essay on the Principle of Population* (1st ed., 1789), in vol. 1 of *The Works of Thomas Robert Malthus*, 6 vols. (London, 1789; 1986), pp. 103–109 (pp. 40–41 in 1986 ed.).

47. Janet Farrell Brodie, "Family Limitation in American Culture, 1830–1900," Ph.D. diss. University of Chicago, 1982, p. 1; McEvedy and Jones, *World Population*, p. 288; for a slightly contrasting view, see J. Potter, "The Growth of Population in America, 1700–1860," in Glass and Eversley, *Population in History*, pp. 631–685.

48. Yasukichi Yasuba, *Birth Rates of the White Population in the United States, 1800–1860: An Economic Study* (Baltimore, 1962), p. 32.

49. Livi-Bacci, *Italian Fertility*, pp. 28–29, 53.

50. McEvedy and Jones, *World Population*, pp. 179–181; Hollingsworth, *Historical Demography*, pp. 76, 100; Clark, *Population Growth*, pp. 77–78; see contrasting figures in Durand, "Historical Estimates," p. 256.

51. Massimo Livi-Bacci, *Popolazione e forze di lavoro delle regioni italiane al 1981* (Rome, 1968), p. 524; slightly different figures using different dates as guideposts are in Wrigley, "Growth of Population," p. 122, and Mols, "Population in Europe," p. 38.

52. Louis Henry, "The Population of France in the Eighteenth Century," trans. Peter Jimack, in Glass and Eversley, *Population in History*, 434–456 at 442; Pierre Goubert, "Recent Theories and Research in French Population between 1500 and 1700," trans. Hargaret Hilton, in Glass and Eversley, *Population in History*, 457–473 at 469.

53. Jean Bourgeois-Pichat, "The Demographic Distress of the World," *Population Growth and Development: Research and Publication* 556 (January 1965): 489.

54. Gustaf Utterström, "Two Essays on Population in Eighteenth-Century Scandinavia," in Glass and Eversley, *Population in History*, p. 538; Sweden's actual census data begin in 1749, China about 1750, Austria 1754, Norway and Denmark 1769, Hungary 1777, the United States 1790, Great Britain 1801.

55. McKeown and Brown, "Medical Evidence," p. 298; Flandrin, "Contraception, mariage," pp. 1375, 1386–1388.

56. Etienne van de Walle, *The Female Population of France in the Nineteenth Century: A Reconstruction of 82 Départements* (Princeton, 1974), pp. 61–83, 259.

57. Charles Pouthas, *La population français pendant le première moitié du XIXe siècle*, Travaux et Documents, Cahier 25 (Paris, 1956), pp. 21–28; McEvedy and Jones, *World Population*, p. 56.

58. For political ramifications and recognition during the period, see Laure Chantrel, "Dépopulation et réforme de la fiscalité en France aux XVIe et XVIIe siècles," *Population* 49 (1994): 457–479.

59. Ralph A. Houlbrook, *The English Family, 1450–1700* (London, 1984), pp. 82–83, 116–117; Flinn, *European Demographic System*, p. 19.

60. Le Roy Ladurie, "Demographie et 'funestes secrets,'" p. 328; Ariès, *Histoire des populations*, pp. 496–497.

61. Henry, "Population of France," p. 452.

62. Alan Macfarlane, *Marriage and Love in England: Modes of Reproduction, 1300–1840* (Oxford, 1986), p. 62.

63. Peter Fryer, *The Birth Controllers* (New York, 1966), p. 36.

64. Ludwig Knapp, *Theologie und Geburtshilfe nach F. E. Cangiamila's Sacra Embryologia (Editio Latin, MDCCLXIV mit aktuellen Bemerkungen)* (Prague, 1908), pp. 60–61.

65. McKeown and Brown, "Medical Evidence," pp. 285–306, raise the question whether mortality rates changed significantly in the eighteenth century despite claims that living conditions improved in the second half.

66. On mortality rates, 1500–1820, see Flinn, *European, Demographic System*, pp. 47–64.

67. Massimo Livi-Bacci, "Social-Group Forerunners of Fertility Control in Europe," in Coale and Watkins, *Decline of Fertility in Europe*, pp. 182–200; restricted by Coale, "Decline of Fertility," p. 14.

68. Le Roy Ladurie, "Demographie et 'funestes secrets,'" p. 328; Ariès, *Histoire des populations*, pp. 496–497.

69. Ansley Coale, "The Demographic Transition Reconsidered," in *International Population Conference, Liège* 1 (1973): 53–72 at 65; discussion by Bruce W. Frier, "Natural Fertility and Family Limitation in Roman Marriage," *Classical Philology* 89 (1994): 318–333 at 327–328; George Alter, "Theories of Fertility Decline: A Nonspecialist's Guide to the Current Debate," in *The European Experience of Declining Fertility, 1850–1970*, ed. Jon R. Gillis, Louise A. Tilly, and David Levine (Cambridge, Mass., 1992), 13–27 at 21–23.

70. Theories revolving around the question of parents' motivation to limit size are discussed by Alter, "Theories of Fertility Decline."

71. Ibid., pp. 22–23; Frier, "Natural Fertility," p. 327; and, to some degree, Angus McLaren, *Reproductive Rituals: The Perception of Fertility in England from the Sixteenth to the Nineteenth Century* (New York, 1984).

72. Patricia Crawford, "Attitudes to Menstruation in Seventeenth-Century England," *Past and Present* 91 (1981): 47–73 at 70.

73. Heinsohn and Steiger, *Vernichtung der weisen Frauen*, p. 175, and personal letter from Otto Steiger (April 12, 1996).

74. Mark Jackson, "Suspicious Infant Deaths: The Statute of 1624 and Medical Evidence at Coroners' Inquests," in *Legal Medicine in History*, ed. Michael Clark and Catherine Crawford (Cambridge, 1994), 65–86 at 69.

75. R. S. Schofield, "Perinatal Mortality in Hawkshead, Lancashire, 1581–1710," *Local Population Studies* (1970): 11–16 at 12–14.

76. Ibid., p. 13; Angus McLaren, *A History Contraception from Antiquity to the Present Day* (Cambridge, 1990), p. 159, for comments.

77. John E. Knodel, *Demographic Behavior in the Past: A Study of Fourteen German Village Populations in the Eighteenth and Nineteenth Centuries* (Cambridge, 1988), p. 48.

78. Angus McLaren, "Policing Pregnancies: Changes in Nineteenth-Century Criminal and Canon Law," in *The Human Embryo*, ed. G. R. Dunstan (Exeter, 1990), 187–207 at 189.

79. L. Lewin, *Die Fruchtabtreibung durch Gifte und andere Mittel: ein Handbuch für Ärzte und Juristen* (Berlin, 1922), p. 138.

80. Jütte, "Persistenz," p. 227.

81. Ibid., pp. 224–225.

82. Ibid., p. 223.

83. Barbara Duden, *The Woman Beneath the Skin: A Doctor's Patients in Eighteenth-Century Germany* (Cambridge, Mass., 1991), pp. 77, 162–170.

84. Quaife, *Wanton Wenches*, p. 118.

85. Ibid.

86. Ibid., p. 120.

87. Roger Thompson, *Sex in Middlesex: Popular Mores in a Massachusetts County, 1649–1699* (Amherst, 1986), p. 26.

88. Quaife, *Wanton Wenches*, p. 119.

89. Ibid., pp. 119–120.

90. Duden, *Woman Beneath the Skin*, p. 77.

91. T. Brugis, *Vade mecum*, quoted by Audrey Eccles, *Obstetrics and Gynaecology in Tudor and Stuart England* (Kent, Ohio, 1982), p. 70.

92. McLaren, "Policing Pregnancies," p. 198; see full discussion by Knapp, *Theologie und Geburtshilfe*, pp. 56–60 (who gives 1764 as the date of Cangialmila's edition).

93. Roy Porter, *Health for Sale: Quackery in England, 1660–1850* (Manchester, 1989), pp. 146–86.

94. John Gerard, *The Herball or Generall Historie of Plantes* ... (London, 1597), bk. 2, chap. 386, p. 862; 2, 382, p. 864; 2, 399, p. 883; 2, 427, p. 926; 2, 221, p. 564; 2, 444, p. 962; 2, 465, p. 996; 3, 41, p. 1,184; 3, 47, p. 1,195; 3, 61, p. 1,219; 3, 64, p. 1,223; 3, 87, p. 1,257; 3, 141, p. 1,349.

95. Ibid., bk. 2, chap. 437, p. 946; 1, 22, p. 30; 1, 29, p. 40; 1, 35, p. 50; 1, 63, p. 87; 1, 90, p. 145; 2, 9, p. 190; 2, 71, p. 306; 2, 268, p. 668.

96. Ibid., bk. 2, chap. 221, p. 564; 2, 437, p. 946; 2, 243, p. 603.

97. Ibid., bk. 2, chap. 371, pp. 846–847.

98. Norman R. Farnsworth, Audrey S. Bingel, Geoffrey A. Cordell, Frank A. Crane, and Harry H. S. Fong, "Potential Value of Plants as Sources of New Antifertility Agents," *Journal of Pharmaceutical Sciences*, 64 (1975): 576.

99. Gerard, *Herball*, bk, 2, chap. 325, p. 762.

100. Ibid., bk. 3, chap. 50, p. 1,202; 2, 211, p. 546.

101. Ibid., bk. 3, chap. 46, p. 1,194.

102. Ibid., bk. 1, chap. 37, p. 54.

103. Ibid., bk. 2, chap. 411, pp. 898–899.

104. Ibid., bk. 2, chap. 511, p. 1,076.

105. Larissa Leibrock-Plehn, *Hexenkräuter oder Arznei: Die Abtreibungsmittel im 16. und 17. Jahrhundert* (Stuttgart, 1992), p. 128.

106. Jacobus Theodorus, *New vollkommen Kräuter Buch*, 2 vols. (Basel, 1664), bk. 2, sec. 4, chap. 32, pp. 389–390.

107. Ibid., 3.2.6, 2.2.41 (pp. 1,353, 1,142 respectively).

108. 1588 ed., p. 40, cited by Leibrock-Plehn, *Hexenkräuter*, p. 128.

109. References in Leibrock-Plehn, *Hexenkräuter*, p. 129.

110. John Peachey, *The Compleat Herbal of Physical Plants*, 2d ed. (London, 1707), pp. 42, 103, 117, 121, 130–131, 178, 188, 205, 207, 199, 326; in the edition I saw the pagination was confused with a reversion and repeated sequence.

111. Ibid., pp. 27, 45, 168–169, 228, 224.

112. Ibid., 90–91, 16–17, 143.

113. Ibid., p. 209.

114. Ibid., pp. 22–23, 84, 86.

115. Ibid., p. 89.

116. Ibid., p. 66.

117. Ibid., p. 203.

118. Ibid., p. 167.

119. Ibid., pp. 162–163.

120. Ibid, pp. 167–168.

121. Olva Thulesius, *Nicholas Culpeper: English Physician and Astrologer* (New York, 1992), p. 67.

122. Nicholas Culpeper, *A Physical Directory; or, A Translation of the Dispensatory Made by the College of Physicians of London* (London, 1650), pp. 7–9.

123. Ibid., pp. 9, 37, 15, 20, 35, 43, 45, 34 (in order of reference above).

124. Ibid., p. 35.

125. Ibid., pp. 45, 18 ("Abrotanum").

126. Ibid., p. 37.

127. Ibid., p. 63.

128. Ibid., p. 83.

129. Ibid., p. 171.

130. Ibid., pp. 171–172.

131. Ibid., pp. 93–94.

132. Nicholas Culpeper, *The English Physitian Enlarged . . .* (London, 1653), pp. 3, 12, 31.

133. Ibid., p. 42.

134. Ibid., p. 114; Nicholas Culpeper, *Culpeper's Complete Herbal, and the English Physician . . .* (Manchester, 1826), p. 68; similar remarks, p. 67.

135. Culpeper, *English Physitian*, pp. 299–300.

136. Ibid., pp. 24–25; in 1826 ed., p. 15.

137. Ibid. (1653), p. 97; (1826), p. 60.

138. Ibid. (1653), pp. 52–53.

139. Ibid. (1653), pp. 294–295; (1826), pp. 116–117.

140. Ibid. (1653), p. 325; (1826), p. 140.

141. Ibid. (1653), p. 352; (1826), pp. 177–178.

142. Ibid. (1653), pp. 374–379 (wormwood); (1826), pp. 48, 122, 202–203.

143. Ibid. (1653), p. 335.

144. Jean Prevost, *De remediorum cum simplicium, tum compositione materia . . .* (Venice, 1640), pp. 407–410.

145. Ibid., pp. 418–428.

146. Jean Prevost, *Medicina pauperum ac ejusdem De venenis ac eorundem alexipharmacis opusculum* (Frankfurt, 1641), pp. 123–124.

147. Jean Prevost, *Medicaments for the Poor: or, Physick for the Common People; Containing Excellent Recipes for Most Common Diseases*, trans. Nicholas Culpeper, 2d ed. (London, 1662), pp. 119–120.

148. Thulesius, *Culpeper*, p. 154.

149. Prevost, *Medicina pauperum*, pp. 124–128; cf. *De remediorum*, pp. 419–428; *Medicaments for the Poor* (trans. Culpeper), pp. 121–122.

150. Prevost, *Medicina pauperum*, pp. 127–128; *Medicaments for the Poor* (trans. Culpeper), pp. 122–123.

151. Prevost, *Medicina pauperum*, pp. 231–236.

152. Joseph Pitton de Tournefort, *The Compleat Herbal . . .* , 2 vols. (London, 1719), 1: 313. I have used the anonymously translated English edition, which includes texts of other writers, but the passages by Tournefort are clearly marked.

153. Ibid., p. 385.

154. Ibid., p. 433.

155. Ibid., p. 438.

156. Cf. Galen, *De simplicium medicamentorum temperamentis ac facultatibus*, 7.11.11 (Kühn ed., 12: 58–59).

157. Tournefort, *Compleat Herbal*, 1: 568.

158. Ibid., 1: 243; cf. Cicero, *De divinatione*, 1.16.10.

159. Ibid., 1: 244.

160. Ibid., 2: 284.

161. Ibid., 1: 522–524 (willow); 2: 4 (black hellebore).

162. Ibid., 2: 630.

163. Alfred Swaine Taylor, *The Principles and Practice of Medical Jurisprudence*, 2 vols., 5th ed. (London, 1865), 2: 782.

164. Tournefort, *Compleat Herbal*, 2: 84.

165. Ibid., 2: 52.

166. Ibid., 1: 336.

167. Ibid., 2: 142–147.

168. Ibid., 2: 149.

169. Pliny, *Natural History*, 27.93.139–140.

170. Vanni Beltrami, "Il silfio cirenaico dall' antichità classica all' ordierna farmacopea sahariana," *Sahara* 2 (1989): 87–94.

171. Ibid., p. 92.

172. John Freind, *Emmenologia: in qua fluxus muliebris menstrui phaenomena, periodi, vitia, cum mendendi methodo ad rationes mechanicas exiguntur* (London, n.d.), fol. A2; Freind, *Emmenologia: Written, In Latin, By the Late Learned Dr. John Friend*, trans. Thomas Dale (London, 1729), p. (A5).

173. Freind, *Emmenologia* (Latin ed.), p. 9.

174. Ibid., pp. 79–80.

175. Ibid., p. 123.

176. Ibid., p. 140.

177. Ibid., pp. 180–181.

178. Ibid., pp. 201–205.

179. Ibid., pp. 206–207.

180. Ibid., pp. 207–240.

181. On midwives in the seventeenth and eighteenth centuries in general, see Jacques Gélis, *History of Childbirth, Fertility, Pregnancy and Birth in Early Modern Europe* (Boston, 1991), pp. 104–111.

182. William Smellie, *A Treatise on the Theory and Practice of Midwifery* (London, 1752), p. 124.

183. Ibid., p. 109.

184. Henry Manning, *A Treatise on Female Diseases* (London, 1771), p. 75.

185. Ibid., p. 75.

186. See above, Chapter 3.

187. *Oxford English Dictionary* (1989 ed.), s.v.

188. Dioscorides, *De materia medica*, 5.80.

189. Manning, *Female Diseases*, pp. 75, 78, 80.

190. Ibid., pp. 78–79.

191. Ibid., p. 377.

192. Jean Astruc, *Traité des maladies des femmes, Où l'on a tâché de joindre à une Théorie solide la Pratique la plus sûre et la mieux éprouvée*, 6 vols. (Paris, 1761–1765), 1: 7, pp. 165–166.

193. Ibid., 1: 206.

194. Ibid., 1: 217.

195. *Inula* sp., known to Dioscorides (*De materia medica*, 3.121) as an emmenagogue and abortifacient, has been noted for the same in various modern folklore reports (L. Palma, *Le piante medicinale d'Italia: botanica, chimica, farmacodinamica, terapia* [Rome, 1964], p. 563), and in one science report it has been found to have antiovulatory activity (R. Chaudhury, "Plants with Possible Antifertility Activity," *Indian Council for Medical Research: Special Reports Series*, 55 [1966]: 11).

196. Astruc, *Traité des maladies des femmes*, 1: 223.

197. Ibid., 5: 326–344.

198. Thomas Forbes, *The Midwife and the Witch* (New Haven, 1966), p. 120, citing Francis Bacon (1676).

199. Jose Luis Valverde and Jose A. Perez Romero, *Drogas americanas en fuentes de escritores franciscanos y dominicos* (Granada, 1988).

200. Ibid.

201. Nicolas Monardes, *Herbolaria de Indias*, ed. and with commentary by Xavier Lozoya (Sevilla, 1574; rpt. [Mexico?], ca. 1990), p. 105; Nicolas Monardes, *Joyfull newes out of the new-found worlde* . . . , trans. John Frampton (London, 1596), fol. 27v.

202. Monardes, *Herbolaria*, p. 111; Frampton trans., fol. 30v.

203. Monardes, *Herbolaria*, pp. 128–129; Frampton trans., p. 35v.

204. Monardes, *Herbolaria*, p. 163; Frampton trans., fols. 53v–54.

205. Monardes, *Herbolaria*, p. 173; Frampton trans., fol. 58.

206. Monardes, *Herborlaria*, p. 180.

207. Cited by Walter H. Lewis and Memory P. F. Elvin-Lewis, *Medical Botany: Plants Affecting Man's Health* (New York, 1977), p. 324.

208. George B. Wood and Franklin Bache, *The Dispensatory of the United States of America*, 7th ed. (Philadelphia, 1847), p. 357; John K. Crellin and Jane Philpott, *Herbal Medicine Past and Present*, 2 vols. (Durham, 1989), 2: 176–178; Wolfgang Schneider, *Lexikon zur Arnzeimittelgeschichte*, 7 vols. (Frankfurt, 1974), 5/2: 141–144.

209. R. L. Badhwar, I. C. Chopra, and S. L. Nayar, "Reputed Abortifacient Plants of India," *Indian Journal of Agricultural Science* 16 (1946): 342–355 at 350.

210. Mary Kilbourne Matossian, *Poisons of the Past: Molds, Epidemics, and History* (New Haven, 1989), p. 67.

211. Edward Shorter, *A History of Women's Bodies* (New York, 1982), p. 184.

212. Friedrich Flückiger and Daniel Hanbury, *Pharmacographia: A History of the Principal Drugs of Vegetable Origin met with in Great Britain and British India*, 2d ed. (London, 1879), p. 740.

213. Leonard Arthur Parry, *Criminal Abortion* (London, 1932), p. 40; Paul Berman, "The Practice of Obstetrics in Rural America, 1800–1860," *Journal of the History of Medicine and Allied Sciences* 50 (1995): 175–193 at 189.

214. Amalie M. Kass, " 'Called to Her at Three O'clock AM': Obstetrical Practice in Physician Case Notes," *Journal of the History of Medicine and Allied Sciences* 50 (1995): 194–229 at 217.

215. Linda R. Caporael, "Ergotism: The Satan Loosed in Salem?" *Science*, 192 (1976): 21–26.

216. Ibid.; on the use and control of the drug ergot, see Oliver Prescott, *A Dissertation on the Natural History and Medicinal Effects of Secale cornutum, or Ergot* n.p., 1813).

217. I am grateful to Mrs. Yvonne Holland of New York City for calling my attention to this song and for the English translation.

218. Charles Knowlton, in *A Dirty, Filthy Book: The Writings of Charles Knowlton and Annie Besant on Reproductive Physiology and Birth Control and an Account of the Bradlaugh-Besant Trial*, ed. and with commentary by S. Chandrasekhar (Berkeley, 1981, on 1834 ed.), p. 138.

219. Lindsay Wilson, *Women and Medicine in the French Enlightenment: The Debate over Maladies des Femmes* (Baltimore, 1993), p. 118.

220. Tony Hunt, *Plant Names of Medieval England* (Cambridge, 1989), pp. 34–35.

221. Quaife, *Wanton Wenches*, p. 118.

222. But according to Marty Newman Williams and Anne Echols (*Between Pit and Pedestal: Women in the Middle Ages* [Princeton, 1994], p. 41), Spain was the only region where abortion was tried as a crime.

223. D. Feldman, *Birth Control in Jewish Law: Marital Relations, Contraception, and Abortion as Set Forth in the Classic Texts of Jewish Law* (New York, 1968), p. 237.

224. Wilson, *Women and Medicine*, pp. 118–119, from archival source.

225. Quoted by Shorter, *History of Women's Bodies*, p. 186.

226. Ibid., pp. 186–187.

227. Duden, *Woman Beneath the Skin*, p. 162.

228. Ibid., pp. 157–170.

229. John Tennent, *Every Man His Own Doctor, or, The Poor Planter's Physician* ... (Philadelphia, 1736), p. 40; for plant identification, see Hunt, *Plant Names*, p. 145.

230. John Lawson, *Lawson's History of North Carolina* (London, 1714), p. 198.

231. *Edinburgh New Dispensatory*, ed. William Lewis (Philadelphia, 1791), pp. 115, 137, 136, 145–146; rpt. (Philadelphia, 1796), pp. 88, 103, 104–105, 139–144, 153–154, 159–160, 176, 181, 190–191, 201–202, 211, 216–217, 222, 233.

232. Ibid. (1791), p. 268; (1796), pp. 228–229 (text the same in both editions).

233. Ibid. (1791), p. 136; (1796), p. 82; "The London College [of Pharmacy] has rejected it from their pharmacopoeia" (1791 ed., p. 103).

234. Ibid. (1791), p. 137.

235. Ibid. (1791), pp. 114–115.

236. Ibid. (1791), p. 448.

237. Ibid. (1791), p. 522.

238. Ibid. (1791), p. 526.

239. Philip M. Teigen, "This Sea of Simples—The Materia Medica in Three English Recipe Books," *Pharmacy in History*, 22 (1980): 104–108 at 107.

240. John K. Crellin, *Medical Ceramics: A Catalogue of the English and Dutch Collections in the Museum of the Wellcome Institute of the History of Medicine* (London, 1969), no. 80, p. 27.

241. Rudolf E. A. Drey, *Apothecary Jars: Pharmaceutical Pottery and Porcelain in Europe and the East, 1150–1850* (London, 1978), no. 35a, p. 78.

242. André Allard, *La boutique de l'apothicaire au XVIIe siècle* (Cahor, 1952), esp. pp. 99–110, for one detailed inventory.

243. M. Olivier, "Observation," *Journal de médecine, chirurgie, pharmacie*, 12 (1760): 129–131.

244. [Dr.?] Aigremont, *Volkserotik und Pflanzenwelt*, 2 vols. (Halle, 1908), 2: 19–20.

245. Wolfgang Behringer, "Die Drohung des Schadenzaubers: Von den Regeln wissenschaftlicher Arbeit—Eine Antwort auf Heinsohn und Steiger," in *Frankfurter Allgemeine Zeitung*, no. 232, October 7, 1987, p. 37; as reported by Heinsohn and Steiger, *Vernichtung der weisen Frauen*, 3d ed., p. 394.

246. Jütte, "Persistenz"; in the 3d edition of *Vernichtung der weisen Frauen* (Munich, 1989, pp. 385–398), Heinsohn and Steiger address this issue.

247. Cornelia Hughes Dayton, "Taking the Trade: Abortion and Gender Relations in an Eighteenth-Century New England Village," *William and Mary Quarterly*, 48 (1991): 19–49, esp. p. 23.

248. Jütte, "Persistenz," p. 216.

7. The Womb as Public Territory

1. 43 Geo. 3, c. 58 (*Statutes of the Realm*, pp. 203–204).

2. For a statement about English common law on abortion, see William

Hawkins, *A Treatise on the Pleas of the Crown* (London, 1762), 1.31.16, p. 80, reproduced in Eva R. Rubin, *The Abortion Controversy: A Documentary History* (Westport, Conn., 1994), p. 6.

3. Ibid.

4. *Times*, March 29, 1803, p. 2.

5. Angus McLaren, "Policing Pregnancies: Changes in Nineteenth-Century Criminal and Canon Law," in *The Human Embryo: Aristotle and the Arabic and European Traditions*, ed. G. R. Dunstan and Mary J. Seller (Exeter, 1990), 187–207 at 188.

6. Leonard Arthur Parry, *Criminal Abortion* (London, 1932), pp. 44–46.

7. Ibid.

8. Angus McLaren, *A History of Contraception from Antiquity to the Present* (Oxford, 1990), p. 162.

9. L. Lewin, *Die Fruchtabtreibung durch Gifte und andere Mittel: Ein Handbuch für Ärtze und Juristen* (Berlin, 1922), p. 139.

10. Ibid.

11. Ibid., p. 140.

12. Phillip A. Rafferty, *Roe v. Wade: The Birth of a Constitutional Right*, 2 vols. (Ann Arbor, 1992), 2: 483–490, esp. p. 486.

13. Helen Brock and Catherine Crawford, "Forensic Medicine in Early Colonial Maryland, 1633–83," in *Legal Medicine in History*, ed. Michael Clark and Catherine Crawford (Cambridge, 1994), 24–44 at 37.

14. Ibid.

15. *Public Statute Laws of the State of Connecticut, 1821, 152–3*, cited by James C. Mohr, *Abortion in America: The Origins and Evolution of National Policy, 1800–1900* (Oxford, 1978), p. 21.

16. Mohr, *Abortion in America*, p. 22.

17. Ibid., p. 27; see also article by a Professor of Midwifery, Charles Coventry, "History of Medical Legislation in the State of New York," *New York Journal of Medicine* 4 (1845): 151–161.

18. Mohr, *Abortion in America*, p. 27.

19. Ibid., p. 140.

20. 9 Geo. 4, c. 31 (1828); text in Parry, *Criminal Abortion*, p. 103.

21. 1 Vict., c. 85, in Parry, *Criminal Abortion*, pp. 103–104.

22. *Dispensatory of the Royal College of Physicians* (London, 1805), pp. 130–144.

23. Ibid., p. 311.

24. Ibid., p. 172.

25. *London Dispensatory*, 2d ed. (London, 1818), p. 256.

26. Ibid., p. 214.

27. Ibid., p. 397.

28. *Edinburgh New Dispensatory* (New York, 1818), pp. 159, 194, 190.

29. Ibid., pp. 259, 292, 298, 352–353.

30. Ibid., p. 293.

31. Ibid., pp. 326, 349.

32. Ibid., p. 397.

33. *Dispensatory of the United States of America* (Philadelphia, 1836), pp. 112–113, 115–117, 121, 169–170, 242, 282–284, 304–306, 326–328, 557.

34. Ibid., pp. 554–555.

35. Ibid., pp. 586–587.

36. Ibid., p. 334.

37. Ibid., pp. 437, 639, 553.

38. Ibid., pp. 667–668; the same statement is repeated in the fourth edition (1839), p. 66.

39. Ibid., pp. 282–284.

40. Roger Thompson, *Unfit for Modest Ears; A Study of Pornographic, Obscene, and Bawdy Works Written or Published in England in the Second Half of the Seventeenth Century* (Totowa, N.J., 1979), pp. 12–13, 33ff.

41. Lawrence Stone, *Uncertain Unions: Marriage in England, 1660–1753* (Oxford, 1992), p. 66.

42. P. E. H. Hair, "Bridal Pregnancy in Rural England Further Examined," *Population Studies* 24 (1970): 59–70 at 59; Hair, "Bridal Pregnancy in Rural England in Earlier Centuries," *Population Studies* 20 (1960): 233–243 at 235; accepted by E. A. Wrigley and R. S. Schofield, *The Population History of England, 1541–1871* (Cambridge, Mass., 1981), p. 304.

43. Andrew Blaikie, *Illegitimacy, Sex, and Society: Northeast Scotland, 1750–1900* (Oxford, 1993), pp. 100–101.

44. John T. Noonan, Jr., *Contraception: A History of Its Treatment by the Catholic Theologians and Canonists*, Enlarged ed. (Cambridge, Mass., 1986), pp. 306–311.

45. Ibid., p. 311.

46. Jean-Louis Flandrin, "Sex in Married Life in the Early Middle Ages: The Church's Teaching and Behavioural Reality," in *Western Sexuality: Practice and Precept in Past and Present Times*, ed. Philippe Ariès and André Béjin (Oxford, 1985), [114–129 at 115–116; Noonan, *Contraception*, pp. 323–326.

47. John T. Noonan, Jr., "Abortion and the Catholic Church: A Summary History," *Natural Law Forum* 12 (1967): 105–106.

48. Ibid., pp. 106–107.

49. Ibid., p. 107.

50. Ibid.

51. Noonan, *Contraception*, pp. 343–344.

52. Daniel Callahan, *Abortion: Law, Choice, and Morality* (New York, 1970), yp. 412, says that Sanchez argued that there was an absolute prohibition against contraception but not abortion.

53. Angus McLaren, *Reproductive Rituals: The Perception of Fertility in En-*

gland from the Sixteenth to the Nineteenth Century (New York, 1984); Thomas Laqueur, *Making Sex: Body and Gender from the Greeks to Freud* (Cambridge, Mass., 1992), p. 5.

54. Robert Martensen, "The Transformation of Eve: Women's Bodies, Medicine and Culture in Early Modern England," in *Sexual Knowledge, Sexual Science*, ed. Roy Porter and Mikulas Teich (Cambridge, 1994), 107–133 at 124, 128–129.

55. Laqueur, *Making Sex*, pp. 1, 8.

56. Hilda Smith, "Gynecology and Ideology in Seventeenth Century England," in *Liberating Women's History: Theoretical and Critical Essays* (Urbana, 1976), 97–114 at 107.

57. From unpublished notes of James King. I was unable to verify the reference in Morellet's works.

58. Laqueur, *Making Sex*, pp. 4–5.

59. Nemesius, *De natura hominis* (Tefler ed., p. 369).

60. Laqueur, *Making Sex*, p. 5.

61. On medieval gender differences, see Joan Cadden, *Meanings of Sex Difference in the Middle Ages* (Cambridge, 1993).

62. Patricia Crawford, "Sexual Knowledge in England, 1500–1750," in Porter and Teich, *Sexual Knowledge, Sexual Science*, 82–106 at 86. For a general picture of sexuality in the nineteenth century, see Alain Corbin, "Backstage," in *A History of Private Life* (Cambridge, Mass., 1990), pp. 577–613.

63. Peter Wagner, "The Pornographer in the Courtroom: Trial Reports about Cases of Sexual Crimes and Delinquencies as a Genre of Eighteenth-Century Erotica," in *Sexuality in Eighteenth-Century Britain*, ed. Paul-Gabriel Boucém (Manchester, 1982), 120–140 at 134.

64. Ivan Illich, *Gender* (London, 1982), p. 124.

65. "Accoucheuse," *Encyclopédie, ou Dictionnaire universel raissoné* (Paris, 1770), 1: 263.

66. McLaren, *History of Contraception*, p. 161.

67. H. H. Ploss, *Zur Geschichte, Verbreitung und Methode der Frucht-Abtreibung: Culturgeschichtelich-Medicinische Skizze* (Leipzig, 1883), p. 47.

68. Illich, *Gender*, p. 124.

69. Colin McEvedy and Richard Jones, *Atlas of World Population History* (New York, 1978), pp. 56–58; Charles H. Pouthas, *La population française pendant le première moitié du XIXe siècle*, Travaux et Documents, Cahier 25 (Paris, 1956), pp. 21–28 (who says there was a decline).

70. Pouthas, *Population française*, p. 21; the recognition of the decline and its political reactions are traced by Laure Chantrel, "Dépopulation et réforme de la fiscalité en France aux XVIe et XVIIe siècles," *Population* 49 (1994): 457–479. The invocation of fear of population decline through birth control, with France used as an example, is found in D. A. O'Donnell and W. L. Atlee,

"Report on the Committee on Criminal Abortion," *Transactions of the American Medical Association* 22 (1871): 239–258 at 243.

71. E. A. Wrigley, "The Growth of Population in Eighteenth-Century England: A Conundrum Resolved," *Past and Present* 93 (1983): 121–150 at 122.

72. Ibid., p. 122; McEvedy and Jones, *World Population*, p. 56.

73. Anonymous, "Why Not? A Book for Every Woman," *Boston Medical and Surgical Journal* 75 (1866): 273–276 at 274.

74. Malthus, *Essay* (1789 ed.), pp. 13–14; (1986 reprint), p. 9.

75. Charles Knowlton in *A Dirty, Filthy Book: The Writings of Charles Knowlton and Annie Besant on Reproductive Physiology and Birth Control and an Account of the Bradlaugh-Besant Trial*, ed. and with commentary by S. Chandrasekhar (Berkely, 1981; reprint of 1834 ed.), p. 12.

76. Illich, *Gender*, p. 124.

77. Michel Foucault, *Histoire de la sexualité*, 3 vols. (Paris, 1978), 1: 92ff.

78. Henry Wright, *The Unwelcome Child: or, The Crime of an Undesigned and Undesired Maternity* (Boston, 1858), pp. 38ff.

79. Malthus in 1840 edition of the *Encyclopaedia Britannica* and de Condorcet in *Esquisse d'un tableau historique du progrès de l'esprit humain*, both quoted by Gunnar Heinsohn and Otto Steiger, "The Rationale Underlying Malthus's Theory of Population," in *Malthus Past and Present* (London, 1983), 223–232 at 228–229.

80. Amos Dean, *Principles of Medical Jurisprudence* (Albany, 1854), pp. 56–57; for reading of the signs of pregnancy in early period, see Audrey Eccles, *Obstetrics and Gynaecology in Tudor and Stuart England* (Kent, Ohio, 1982), p. 61.

81. Henry Bracton, *De legibus et consuetudinibus angliae*, 4 vols., trans. Samuel E. Thorne (Cambridge, 1968), fol. 69b (2: 202).

82. Lucinda McCray Beier, *Sufferers and Healers: The Experience of Illness in Seventeenth-Century England* (London, 1987), p. 44 et passim.

83. Porter, "A Touch of Danger," p. 217; on English male midwives, see Ornella Moscucci, *The Science of Woman: Gynaecology and Gender in England, 1800–1929* (Cambridge, 1990), pp. 46–74.

84. Michael J. O'Dowd and Elliot E. Philipp, *The History of Obstetrics and Gynaecology* (New York and London, 1994), p. 97.

85. Roger Kervran, *Laennec: His Life and Times*, trans. D. C. Abrahams-Curiel (New York, 1960), pp. 139–141.

86. C. Keith Wilbur, *Antique Medical Instruments: Revised Price Guide* (Atglen, Pa., 1987), pp. 21–23; O'Dowd and Philipp, *History of Obstetrics*, p. 98.

87. Dean, *Principles of Medical Jurisprudence*, p. 60.

88. Diderot, *Encylopédie, ou dictionnaire raisonné* 7 (1757): 558, as cited by Bergues, *Prévention des naissances*, p. 104.

89. Shirely Roe, *Matter, Life and Generation: Eighteenth-Century Embryology and the Haller-Wolff Debate* (Cambridge, 1981), pp. 28–29.

90. Ibid., p. 41.

91. Joseph Needham, *A History of Embryology* (New York, 1959), pp. 221–223.

92. Roe, *Matter, Life and Generation*, p. 65.

93. Ibid., pp. 110–118; Needham, *History of Embryology*, p. 223.

94. McLaren, *History of Contraception*, p. 156; Noonan, *Contraception*, pp. 415ff; Laqueur, *Making Sex*, pp. 227–230; Théodore Tarczylo, "From Lascivious Erudition to the History of Mentalities," in *Sexual Underworlds of the Enlightenment*, ed. G. S. Rousseau and Roy Porter (Chapel Hill, 1988), 26–45 at 31–42.

95. Laqueur, *Making Sex*, pp. 172–174.

96. The difficulties of prosecution by the law was discussed in an article in *Lancet* (July 30, 1853, 2: 102).

97. "Report on Criminal Abortion," *Transactions of the American Medical Association* 12 (1859): 75–78.

98. I. T. Dana, "Report on Production of Abortion," *Transactions of the Maine Medical Association for the Years 1866, 1867, and 1868* (Portland, 1869), p. 37.

99. Ibid., p. 38.

100. O. Turner, "Criminal Abortion," *Boston Medical and Surgical Journal*, new ser. 5, no. 16 (1870): 299–301, but allowing a single exception: deformity of pelvis so severe that fetal death was certain.

101. J. B. W. Nowlin, M.D., "Criminal Abortion," *Southern Practitioner* 9 (1887): 177–182 at 179.

102. John P. Stoddard, "Foeticide: Suggestions Towards Its Suppression," *Detroit Review of Medicine and Pharmacy* 10 (1875): 653–658 at 658.

103. Hugh L. Hodge, *Foeticide or Criminal Abortion; Lecture Introductory to the Course of Obstetrics, and Diseases of Women and Children*, University of Pennsylvania, Session 1839–1840 (Philadelphia, 1869), p. 17.

104. E. Franke Howe, *Sermon on Ante-Natal Infanticide, Delivered by Rev. Frank Howe, at the Congregational Church in Terre Haute, on Sunday Morning, March 28th, 1869* (Terra Haute, 1869), p. 2.

105. Andrew Nebinger, *Criminal Abortion; Its Extent and Prevention, Read before the Philadelphia County Medical Society, February 9, 1870* (Philadelphia, 1870), p. 19.

106. "Report on Criminal Abortion," *New York Medical Journal* 15 (1872): 77–87 at 77.

107. Noonan, *Contraception*, p. 403.

108. McLaren, "Policing Pregnancies," p. 196.

109. *Codicis Iuris Canonici Fontes* (Vatican, 1933), 3: 28 (552.3).

110. Callahan, *Abortion*, p. 413.

111. McLaren, "Policing Pregnancies," pp. 201–203.

112. See Callahan, *Abortion*, p. 412 et passim.

113. Horatio Robinson Storer, *Criminal Abortion* (Boston, 1868), p. 72.

114. Edward H. Parker, "The Relation of the Medical and Legal Professions to Criminal Abortion," *Transactions of the American Medical Association* 31 (1880): 465–471 at 469.

115. Text of laws, usually in German translation, are reproduced by Lewin, *Fruchtabtreibung*, pp. 139–159.

116. D. Feldman, *Birth Control in Jewish Law: Marital Relations, Contraception, and Abortion as Set Forth in the Classic Texts of Jewish Law* (New York, 1968), p. 237.

117. Dana, "Report on Production of Abortion," p. 39: "when it is absolutely necessary to save the life of the mother . . . [is] the sole condition on which the physician is justified in inducing abortion."

118. Ibid., p. 139.

119. McLaren, "Policing Pregnancies," p. 189.

120. Alfred Swaine Taylor, *The Principles and Practice of Medical Jurisprudence* (London, 1865), pp. 786–787.

121. McLaren, *History of Contraception*, p. 189.

122. Gunnar Heinsohn and Otto Steiger, *Die Vernichtung der weisen Frauen: Beiträge zur Theorie und Geschichte von Bevölkerung und Kindheit* (Herbstein, 1985), pp. 12, 176.

123. Angus McLaren, *Birth Control in Nineteenth-Century England* (New York, 1978), p. 51.

124. Knowlton, *Dirty, Filthy Book*, p. 137.

125. Ibid., p. 138.

126. Ibid., p. 139.

127. Peter Fryer, *The Birth Controllers* (New York, 1966), pp. 141–172; Knowlton, *Dirty, Filty Book*, pp. 1ff; McLaren, *Birth Control in Nineteenth-Century England*, pp. 52–57, 82–85; Janet Farrell Brodie, *Contraception and Abortion in Nineteenth-Century America* (Ithaca, 1994), pp. 89–90.

8. Eve's Herbs in Modern America

1. Advertisement appearing in the *Indianapolis Daily State Sentinel*, January 1, 4, 1859; cited in James C. Mohr, *Abortion in America: The Origins and Evolution of National Policy, 1800–1900* (Oxford, 1978), p. 142.

2. H. Gibbons, "On Feticide," *Transactions of the Medical Society of the State of California During the Years 1877 and 1878*, vol. 7/8, 209–225 at 209.

3. Ibid., p. 32.

4. For testimony on physicians encountering the results of "irregulars and

persons outside of the profession of medicine proper," see S. K. Crawford, "Criminal Abortion," *Transactions of the Twenty-Second Anniversary Meeting of the Illinois State Medical Society* (Chicago, 1872), 74–81 at 74.

5. For an account of physicians and birth control, see John S. Haller, Jr., and Robin Haller, *The Physician and Sexuality in Victorian America* (Urbana, 1974), pp. 113–131.

6. John Burns, *Observations on Abortion Containing an Account of the Manner in which it takes Place* . . . (Troy, N.Y., 1808), pp. 74–75.

7. Ibid., p. 75.

8. John Brevitt, *The Female Medical Repository to which is Added a Treatise on the Primary Diseases of Infants; Adapted to the Use of the Female Practitioners and Intelligent Mothers* . . . (Baltimore, 1810), p. 117n.

9. Ibid., pp. 45–46.

10. Mohr, *Abortion in America*, n. 1 *et passim;* L. Lewin, *Die Fruchtabtreibung durch Gifte und andere Mittel: Ein Handbuch für Ärtze und Juristen* (Berlin, 1922), pp. 90 ff.

11. Samuel K. Jennings, *The Married Lady's Companion or Poor Man's Friend,* 2d ed. (New York, 1808), pp. 43–49.

12. William Buchan, *Domestic Medicine: or, A Treatise on the Prevention and Cure of Diseases by Regimen and Simple Medicines* (London, 1772).

13. Otho T. Beall, *"Aristotle's Master Piece* in America: A Landmark in the Folklore of Medicine," *William and Mary Quarterly* 20, no. 3 (1963): 207–222; Vern L. Bullough, "An Early American Sex Manual, or, Aristotle Who?" *Early American Literature* 7 (1973): 236–246.

14. Alfred G. Hall, *The Mother's Own Book and Practical Guide to Health: Being a Collection of Necessary and Useful Information. Designed for Females Only* . . . (Rochester, 1843), p. 51.

15. For medieval identifications, see Tony Hunt, *Plant Names of Medieval England* (Cambridge, 1989), p. 295 *et passim.*

16. James Duke, *Handbook of Medicinal Herbs* (Boca Raton, 1985), pp. 277–278.

17. Ibid., pp. 53–54.

18. Frederick Hollick, *Diseases of Woman, Their Causes and Cure Familiarly Explained* . . . (New York, 1847), p. 150.

19. Ibid., p. 151.

20. Ibid., p. 152.

21. Ibid., pp. 152–153.

22. Ibid., p. 156.

23. Ibid., pp. 156–157.

24. M. K. Hard, *Woman's Medical Guide; being a Complete Review of the Peculiarities of the Female Constitution* . . . (Mt. Vernon, 1848), p. 34.

25. Ibid., p. 302.

26. Ibid, p. 34.

27. Ibid., pp. 37ff.

28. Ibid., pp. 280–281, 294.

29. Ibid., pp. 288–289.

30. Buel Eastman, *Practical Treatise on Diseases Peculiar to Women and Girls: To Which is Added an Eclectic System of Midwifery* . . . (Cincinnati, 1848), p. 26.

31. John K. Crellin and Jane Philpott, *Herbal Medicine Past and Present*, 2 vols. (Durham, N.C. 1989), 2: 125; Henry De Laszlo and Paul S. Henshaw, "Plants Used by Primitive Peoples to Affect Fertility," *Science* 119 (1954): 626–631 at 627; V. J. Brondegaard, "Contraceptive Plant Drugs," *Planta Medica* 23 (1973): 167–172 at 168.

32. Crellin and Philpott, *Herbal Medicine*, 2: 426.

33. Ibid., 2: 27–28.

34. Ibid., 2: 186–187.

35. Mohr, *Abortion in America*, p. 48.

36. A. M. Mauriceau, *The Married Woman's Private Medical Companion* . . . (New York, 1847), p. 104.

37. Ibid., p. 105.

38. Ibid., pp. 127–142.

39. Ibid., p. 168.

40. Ibid., pp. 13–18.

41. Ibid., pp. 15–16.

42. Ibid., p. 18.

43. "Madame Restell, and Some of Her Dupes," Editorial in *New York Medical and Surgical Reporter* 1, no. 10 (1846): 158–165.

44. Ansley J. Coale and Melvin Zelnik, *New Estimates of Fertility and Population in the United States: A Study of Annual White Births from 1855 to 1960 and of Completeness of Enumeration in the Censuses from 1880 to 1960* (Princeton, 1963), p. 36; see also Wilson H. Grabill, Clyde V. Kiser, and Pascal K. Whelpton, *The Fertility of American Women*, Census Monograph Series (New York, 1958), p. 14.

45. Mary P. Ryan, "Reproduction in American History," *Journal of Interdisciplinary History* 10 (1979): 319–332, asserts that the basic change was not an increase in the practice of birth control but an adoption of new techniques.

46. Judith Walzer Leavitt, "Under the Shadow of Maternity: American Women's Responses to Death and Debility Fears in Nineteenth-Century Childbirth," *Feminist Studies* 12 (1986): 129–154 at 138.

47. Janet Farrell Brodie, *Contraception and Abortion in Nineteenth-Century America* (Ithaca, N.Y., 1994), pp. 67–79.

48. Vern L. Bullough, "A Brief Note on Rubber Technology and Contraception: The Diaphragm and the Condom," *Technology and Culture* 22 (1981): 104–111.

49. From *Low Life*, as cited by Angus McLaren, *Birth Control in Nineteenth-Century England* (New York, 1978), p. 31.

50. Editorial, "Criminal Abortions," *Buffalo Medical Journal and Monthly Review* 14 (1859): 248.

51. *Proceedings of the Tenth Annual Convention of the American Association of Spirtualists Held at Crow's Opera Hall, Chicago, on Tuesday, Sept. 16* [1873], p. 91.

52. McLaren, *Birth Control in Nineteenth-Century England*, p. 31; Mohr, *Abortion in America*, pp. 48–54; Brodie, *Contraception and Abortion*, p. 225; Cheri Kathleen Slocum, " 'Taking the Cold': Birth Limitation in North Carolina Nineteenth to Early Twentieth Centuries," unpublished M.A. thesis, North Carolina State University, Raleigh, 1992, pp. 58ff.; the formulas for some of these medicines are found in E. Woodruff, *The Female Medical Counselor, Being a Domestic Treatment on the Diseases of Females and Children* (San Francisco, 1885), pp. 263–365; Lawrence Stone, *The Family, Sex and Marriage in England, 1500–1800* (New York, 1977), p. 423.

53. James S. Whitwire, "Criminal Abortion," *Chicago Medical Journal* 31 (1874): 385–393 at 389.

54. "Quacks and Abortion: A Critical and Analytical Inquiry," *Lancet* 1 (June 24, 1899): 531.

55. Mohr, *Abortion in America*, pp. 52–57.

56. Slocum, " 'Taking the Cold,' " p. 61.

57. "Quacks and Abortion: A Critical and Analytical Inquiry," *Lancet* 1 (June 24, 1899): 1739.

58. Advertisement from the Boston *Daily Times*, January 23, 1845, reproduced in Mohr, *Abortion in America*, p. 57.

59. James Woycke, *Birth Control in Germany, 1871–1933* (London, 1988), p. 19.

60. Ibid., p. 55.

61. Wilson Yates, "Birth Control Literature and the Medical Profession in Nineteenth Century America," *Journal of the History of Medicine and Allied Sciences* 31 (1976): 42–54 at 50.

62. Ely Van de Warker, "Detection of Criminal Abortion," *Journal of the Gynecological Society of Boston* 4 (1871): 229–245 at 230.

63. Ibid., pp. 231–332.

64. Ibid., pp. 230–233.

65. Ely Van de Warker, *The Detection of Criminal Abortion and a Study of Foeticidal Drugs* (Boston, 1872), pp. 52–53.

66. Ibid., p. 71.

67. D. Feldman, *Birth Control in Jewish Law: Marital Relations, Contraception, and Abortion as Set Forth in the Classic Texts of Jewish Law* (New York, 1968), p. 237.

68. "Quacks and Abortion," pp. 182–183.

69. Joseph G. Pinkham, "The Very Frequency and Inexcusable Destruction of Foetal Life in Its Early Stages by Medical Men in Honorable Standing," *Journal of the Gynecological Society of Boston* 3 (1870): 374–377 at 374.

70. Patricia Crawford, "Sexual Knowledge in England, 1500–1750," in *Sexual Knowledge, Sexual Science*, ed. Roy Porter and Mikulas Teich (Cambridge, 1994), 82–106, reports that physicians were unwilling to advise women about menstruation in fear of providing information about an abortion (p. 86).

71. James Whitehead, *On the Causes and Treatment of Abortion and Sterility* (London, 1847), p. 254.

72. Ibid., p. 253.

73. Ibid., p. 253.

74. On the action of ergot (ergotamine) for abortions and hastening childbirth, see George B. Wood and Franklin Bache, *The Dispensatory of the United States of America*, 7th ed. (Phaladelphia, 1847), pp. 516–524; Walter H. Lewis and Memory P. F. Elvin-Lewis, *Medical Botany: Plants Affecting Man's Health* (New York, 1977), p. 321.

75. Whitehead, *Causes and Treatment*, p. 254.

76. Ibid., p. 143.

77. Ibid., p. 144.

78. "Quacks and Abortion: A Critical and Analytical Inquiry," *Lancet* 2 (1898): 1723–1725; discussed by Angus McLaren, *A History of Contraception from Antiquity to the Present* (Oxford, 1990), p. 189.

79. C. D. Meigs, *Females and Their Diseases* (Philadelphia, 1848), pp. 416–423, where he discusses emmenagogues, and p. 405, where he says that they cause abortions. See also discussion by Crellin and Philpott, *Herbal Medicine*, 1: 176–178.

80. I. T. Dana, "Report on Production of Abortion," *Transactions of the Maine Medical Association for the Years 1866, 1867, and 1868* (Portland, 1869), p. 1841.

81. Mohr, *Abortion in America*, p. 140.

82. "Abortion," *Bulletin of the International Medico-Legal Congress, Held June 4, 5, 6, and 7, 1889, at New York* (New York, 1891), 164–181 at 177.

83. Angus McLaren, *Reproductive Rituals: Perceptions of Fertility in England from the Sixteenth Century to the Nineteenth Century* (New York, 1984), pp. 104–105.

84. Brief 281, American Historians as Amici Curiae, Supporting Appellees, in *Webster v. Reproductive Health Service*, No. 88–605, Supreme Court of the United States, October Term, 1988, p. 10 (brief separately paged as 1–31; pp. 339–369 in volume). Their quotes are taken from Linda Gordon, *Woman's Body, Woman's Rights: A Social History of Birth Control in America* (New York, 1976), pp. 51–52.

85. W. A. Puckner and L. E. Warren, "Chichester's Diamond Brand Pills," *Journal of the American Medical Association* 56 (1911): 1591–1592.

86. Ibid.

87. Alfred Swaine Taylor, *The Principles and Practice of Medical Jurisprudence*, 5th ed. in 2 vols., ed. Frederick J. Smith (London, 1905), 2: 168–169.

88. Ibid.

89. *State of North Carolina v. Jacob F. Slagle* (1880), in *North Carolina Reports: Cases Argued and Determined in the Supreme Court of North Carolina* 83: 630–633 at 631.

90. Alfred Swaine Taylor, *The Principles and Practice of Medical Jurisprudence* (London, 1865), p. 786.

91. Taylor, *Principles and Practice of Medical Jurisprudence*, 2: 168.

92. For excellent, detailed studies of the politics of fertility and demography, see Richard Allen Soloway, *Birth Control and the Population Question in England, 1877–1930* (Chapel Hill, 1982), and *Demography and Degeneration: Eugenics and the Declining Birthrate in Twentieth-Century Britain* (Chapel Hill, 1990); David Levine, *Reproducing Families: The Political Economy of England Population History* (Cambridge, 1987).

93. *Laws of the State of Indiana* (1859), 59: 1–2; see also Eugene Quay, "Justifiable Abortion—Medical and Legal Foundations," *Georgetown Law Journal* 49 (1960, 1961): 173–256, 395–538 at 468.

94. Mohr, *Abortion in America*, p. 142.

95. *State v. Eliakim Cooper* (1848), *New Jersey Supreme Court* 22: 52–58 at 53–54; the importance of this case is discussed in *Keeler v. Superior Court of Amador County*, 2 Cal. 3d 619, in *West's California Reporter* 87 (1970): 7 Cal. App. 3d, p. 485.

96. *State v. Cooper*, p. 54.

97. *State v. Murphy*, *New Jersey Law Reports* 27 (1858): 112–116 at 114; discussion by Robert A. Destro, "Abortion and the Constitution: The Need for a Life-Protective Amendment," *California Law Review* 63 (1975): 1250–1351 at 1273–1275.

98. Texas Penal Code, Chap. 9, Title 15, Article 1192, in Eva R. Rubin, *The Abortion Controversy: A Documentary History* (Westport, Conn., 1994), p. 25.

99. N.C. Session Laws, Chap. 351, sections 1 and 2, cited in Quay, "Justifiable Abortion," p. 502.

100. *State vs. Slagle*, p. 632, citing a supreme court case in Pennsylvania (13 Penn. State Rep. 631).

101. Nebraska General Statutes, Chap. 58, sections 6 and 39 (1873), as cited in Quay, "Justifiable Abortion," p. 492.

102. Quay, "Justifiable Abortion," *passim*.

103. Quay, "Justifiable Abortion," p. 454.

104. Ibid., p. 454; Mohr, *Abortion in America*, p. 202.

105. James Harvey Young, *The Toadstool Millionaires: A Social History of Patent Medicines in America before Federal Regulation* (Princeton, 1961), pp. 40–41.

106. Brief 281, American Historians as Amici Curiae, pp. 13–16.

107. As reprinted by Rubin, *Abortion Controversy*, pp. 28–29.

108. William F. Howe and Abraham H. Hummel, *In Danger, or Live in New York: A True History of a Great City's Wiles and Temptations* (New York, 1888), p. 163.

109. Ibid., p. 167.

110. Mohr, *Abortion in America*, pp. 198–199.

111. Brief 281, American Historians as Amici Curiae, p. 348.

112. C. S. Bacon, "The Midwife Question in America," *Journal of the American Medical Association* 29 (27 November 1897): 1089–1093 at 1091.

113. Ibid.

114. Leslie J. Reagan, "Linking Midwives and Abortion in the Progressive Era," *Bulletin of the History of Medicine* 69 (1995): 569–598 at 569, 576–577.

115. "Quacks and Abortion: A Critical and Analytical Inquiry," *Lancet* 2 (December 24, 1898): 1723–1725 at 1723; reporting from "Owen v. Greenberg," [London] *Times*, March 10, 1898.

116. Justice Darling, [Report on] "Owen v. Greenberg," [London] *Times*, March 10, 1898, p. 13.

117. "Quacks and Abortion," 2: 1724; the story about the trial in [London] *Times* (March 10, 1898) reported that if a woman did not get satisfaction with the first bottle, she was to send for a stronger bottle for 10 shillings. If the second did not work, she was instructed to send for a still stronger bottle at 21 shillings. The contents of all three were found to be the same concentration.

118. Mohr, *Abortion in America*, pp. 224–225; the laws are reprinted by Quay, "Justifiable Abortion."

119. Quay, "Justifiable Abortion," p. 447 *et passim*.

120. Ibid., pp. 448, 509.

121. Ibid., pp. 466, 506; by 1845 the revised Statutes of Illinois specified a three-year prison penalty for anyone who gave, counseled another person to take, or took a poison to cause a "miscarriage," according to Crawford, "Criminal Abortion," p. 75.

122. Quay, "Justifiable Abortion," pp. 456, 488.

123. Wisconsin Statutes Annual, section 940.04, 6 (1958); Revised Statutes, Chap. 164, section 10.11 (1858), in Quay, "Justifiable Abortion," p. 518.

124. On the politics of the act, see James Harvey Young, *Pure Food: Securing the Federal Food and Drugs Act of 1906* (Princeton, 1989), pp. 146ff.

125. Arthur Cramp, *Nostrums and Quackery and Pseudo-Medicine*, 3 vols. (Chicago, 1936), 3: 62–66.

126. Ibid., 3: 66.

127. James Harvey Young, *The Medical Messiahs: A Social History of Health Quackery in Twentieth-Century America* (Princeton, 1967), pp. 67ff.

128. 25 Fed. Cas. 1140, 1141 (S.D.N.Y., 1876), in Brief 281, American Historians as Amici Curiae, p. 357.

129. Charles Wesley Dunn, *Dunn's Food and Drug Laws: Federal and States*, 3 vols. (New York, 1927), 2: 296; Quay, "Justifiable Abortion," p. 543, cites a statute as Colorado Laws, section 6687, without providing text.

130. Kansas Revised Statutes 1923, section 21–1101, cited in Dunn, *Dunn's Food and Drug Laws*, 2: 820.

131. Dunn, *Dunn's Food and Drug Laws*, 2: 755.

132. Iowa Code, sections 725.5, 725.6, 147.56, 205.1–3, cited in Quay, "Justifiable Abortion," p. 473.

133. Louisiana 1924, p. 385, Act 95 of 1920, cited in Dunn, *Dunn's Food and Drug Laws*, 2: 923–924.

134. Louisiana Revised Statutes Annual, sections 14:87–88, 37: 1285, cited in Quay, "Justifiable Abortion," pp. 476–477.

135. Sarah Stage, *Female Complaints: Lydia Pinkham and the Business of Women's Medicine* (New York, 1979), p. 32; Varro E. Tyler, "Was Lydia E. Pinkham's Vegetable Compound an Effective Remedy?" *Pharmacy in History* 37 (1995): 24–28 at 25.

136. Norman R. Farnsworth, Audrey S. Bingel, Geoffrey A. Cordell, Frank A. Crane, and Harry H. S. Fong, "Potential Value of Plants as Sources of New Antifertility Agents," *Journal of Pharmaceutical Sciences* 64 (1975): 535–598 at 560; Crellin and Philpott, *Herbal Medicine*, pp. 366–367. An earlier study concluded, however, that it had no effect on animals, but the study was based on anatomical dissections of uterine tissue and done at a time when plant antifertility drugs were discounted. See Edgar A. Kelly and E. V. Lynn, "The Value of Senecio in Medicine," *Journal of the American Pharmaceutical Association* 23 (1934): 113–118.

137. On estrogen activity in pleurisy root, see Christopher H. Costello and C. L. Butler, "The Estrogenic and Uterine-stimulating Activity of *Asclepias tuberosa*: A Preliminary Investigation," *Journal of the American Pharaceutical Association*, Scientific Edition 39 (1950): 233–237, who report the probable presence of estriol and a definite effect on uterine tissue *in vitro* and *in vivo*.

138. Tyler, "Pinkham's Vegetable Compound," p. 27.

139. Stage, *Female Complaints*, p. 127.

140. Young, *Medical Messiahs*, pp. 176–179 *et passim*.

141. Ibid., p. 178.

142. Tyler, "Pinkham's Vegetable Compound," p. 27. The formula sold in stores today has changed most ingredients except pleurisy root.

143. Cramp, *Nostrums and Quackery*, 3: 62; Anonymous, *Female Weakness Cures* (Chicago: American Medical Association, 1937), p. 46.

144. Frederick Joseph Taussig, *Abortion, Spontaneous and Induced; Medical and Social Aspects* (St. Louis, 1936), p. 352.

145. P. E. H. Hair, "Bridal Pregnancy in Rural England Further Examined," *Population Studies* 24 (1970): 59–70 at 65.

146. Margaret Sanger in *The Birth Control Review* 1 (1917): 4; 4 (1920): 1.

147. Ibid., 2 (1918): 3–4.

148. Ibid., 4 (1920): 3; Margaret Sanger, *My Fight for Birth Control* (New York, 1938), pp. 224–237.

149. *Birth Control Review* 5 (1921): 17.

150. James Reed, "Doctors, Birth Control, and Social Values: 1830–1970," in *The Therapeutic Revolution: Essays in the Social History of American Medicine*, ed. Morris J. Vogel and Charles E. Rosenberg (Philadelphia, 1979), 109–134 at 129.

151. Carole R. McCann, *Birth Control Politics in the United States, 1916–1945* (Ithaca, 1994), pp. 43–45; on Sanger see also Shirley Green, *The Curious History of Contraception* (New York, 1971), pp. 14ff.

152. Sanger, *My Fight*, pp. 48–49.

153. [Dr.?] Aigremont, *Volkserotik und Pflanzenwelt*, 2 vols. (Halle, 1908), 2: 27.

154. Paul, *Libri medicorum*, 2.222.5–6 (Heiberg ed.).

155. Aigremont, *Volkserotik*, A, 2: 29–30.

156. Ibid., A, 2: 18.

157. J. M. Watt and M. G. Breyer-Brandwijk, *The Medicinal and Poisonous Plants of Southern and Eastern Africa*, 2d ed. (Edinburgh, 1962), pp. 117–118; Duke, *Handbook of Medicinal Herbs*, p. 224.

158. Aigremont, *Volkserotik*, A, 1: 107.

159. Ibid., A, 1: 104.

160. Ibid., A, 1: 55–56.

161. Ibid., A, 1: 46.

162. Ibid. A, 1: 38.

163. James Woycke, *Birth Control in Germany, 1871–1933* (New York, 1988), p. 18.

164. Aigremont, *Volkserotik*, A, 2: 19–20.

165. Woycke, *Birth Control in Germany*, p. 17.

166. Retrogressive ejaculation induced by applying pressure to the base of the penis to force the stream of semen into the bladder.

167. Woycke, *Birth Control in Germany*, pp. 10ff.

168. James DeMeo, "The Use of Contraceptive Plant Materials by Native Peoples," *Journal of Orgonomy* 26 (1992): 152–176.

169. D. D. O. Oylebola, "Yorba Traditional Healers' Knowledge of Contraception," *East African Medical Journal* 58 (1981): 777–784.

170. Yun Cheung Kong, Jing-Xi Xie, and Paul Pui-Hay But, "Fertility Reg-

ulating Agents from Traditional Chinese Medicines," *Journal of Ethnopharmacology* 15 (1986): 1–44.

171. J. O. Kokwaro, "A Review of Research on Plants for Fertility Regulation," *Korean Journal of Pharmacology* 12 (1981): 1–44.

172. V. V. Kharkhov and M. N. Mats, "Pasteniaa kak potentsial'nye istochniki protivozachatochnhkh sredstv," *Rastite'nye Resursy* 17 (1981): 293–299.

173. B. Weniger, M. Haag-Berrurier, and R. Anton, "Plants of Haiti Used as Antifertility Agents," *Journal of Ethnopharmacology* 6 (1982): 67–84.

174. George A. Conway and John C. Slocumb, "Plants Used as Abortifacients and Emmenagogues by Spanish New Mexicans," *Journal of Ethnopharmacology* 1 (1979): 241–261.

175. P. Arenas and R. Moreno Azorero, "Plants Used as Means of Abortion, Contraception, Sterilization and Fecundation by Paraguayan Indigenous People," *Economic Botany* 31 (1977): 302–306.

176. K. C. Tiwari, R. Majumder, and S. Bhattacharjee, "Folklore Information from Assam for Family Planning and Birth Control," *International Journal of Crude Drug Research* 20 (1982): 133–137.

177. Carol Laderman, *Wives and Midwives: Childbirth and Nutrition in Rural Malaysia* (Berkeley, 1983).

178. C. D. Casey, "Alleged Anti-fertility Plants of India," *Indian Journal of Medical Sciences* 14 (1960): 590–600.

179. Told me in August 1994 by Betsy Williams (Andover, Mass.).

180. Mohr, *Abortion in America*, p. 276, n. 15.

181. Barbara Duden, *Disembodying Women: Perspectives on Pregnancy and the Unborn*, trans. Lee Hoinacke (Cambridge, Mass., 1993), p. 61.

182. Peter R. Braude and Martin H. Johnson, "The Embryo in Contemporary Medical Science," in *The Human Embryo*, ed. G. R. Dunstan (Exeter, 1990), 208–221 at 217–218.

183. Duden, *Disembodying Women*, p. 50.

Index

331